Youth Sports in America

Youth Sports in America

THE MOST IMPORTANT ISSUES IN YOUTH SPORTS TODAY

Skye G. Arthur-Banning, Editor
P. Brian Greenwood and Mary Sara Wells, Associate Editors

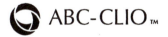
ABC-CLIO™

An Imprint of ABC-CLIO, LLC
Santa Barbara, California • Denver, Colorado

Library of Congress Cataloging-in-Publication Data

Names: Arthur-Banning, Skye G., editor.

Title: Youth sports in America : the most important issues in youth sports today / Skye G. Arthur-Banning, editor ; P. Brian Greenwood and Mary Sara Wells, associate editors.

Description: Santa Barbara, California : ABC-CLIO, 2018. | Includes bibliographical references and index.

Identifiers: LCCN 2017060192 (print) | LCCN 2017061466 (ebook) | ISBN 9781440843020 (e-book) | ISBN 9781440843013 (hard copy : alk. paper)

Subjects: LCSH: Sports for children—United States.

Classification: LCC GV709.2 (ebook) | LCC GV709.2 .Y677 2018 (print) | DDC 796.083—dc23

LC record available at https://lccn.loc.gov/2017060192

ISBN: 978-1-4408-4301-3 (print)
      978-1-4408-4302-0 (ebook)

22 21 20 19 18   1 2 3 4 5

This book is also available as an eBook.

ABC-CLIO

An Imprint of ABC-CLIO, LLC

ABC-CLIO, LLC
130 Cremona Drive, P.O. Box 1911
Santa Barbara, California 93116-1911
www.abc-clio.com

This book is printed on acid-free paper ∞

Manufactured in the United States of America

Contents

Preface

During America's colonial era and its first decades of existence, youngsters played sports in farm pastures or on frozen ponds, with no adult supervision and only a few loose rules that were enforced by the kids themselves. When it got dark, the children were forced to go inside and get cleaned up for bed, their thoughts already calculating the odds that they would be able to do it all over again the following day, after school or chores were completed. Flash forward to the early 1900s, when organized youth sport began to take shape in American communities. These competitions, which took place largely in the school setting, were seen as a way to enforce "American" values like respect, teamwork, and self-discipline. Organized youth sports quickly surged in popularity. Yet no one from a century ago could have predicted what youth sport would look like today: highly organized, ultra-competitive, and a significant economic force in many communities. Indeed, *Time* magazine estimated in 2017 that kids' sports in America has become a $15 billion industry. Not surprisingly, this environment has placed additional pressure on young athletes to perform and advance, and while the average high school athlete has only a 1–2 percent chance of ever getting an athletic scholarship for college, far too many parents and children believe that the football, volleyball, or soccer star in their household will someday be among that select company.

Some argue that this progression from backyard baseball games to Little League World Series on ESPN amounts to child exploitation, and that sport's capacity to deliver both fun and personal growth to young athletes has been somehow diminished. Others suggest that despite the excesses of modern youth sports, they remain a valuable vehicle for youth development, helping kids grow into responsible, hard-working adults. Which of these characterizations is true? Or are there elements of truth in both pictures? These questions are important ones for any parent, coach, administrator, or athlete looking to get involved in youth sports.

Youth Sports in America: The Most Important Issues in Youth Sports Today examines the most important topics and issues swirling around this cultural phenomenon. We have enlisted the help of many of the top experts in their respective fields to provide authoritative overviews about a broad range of topics. Although sport is the central theme for this book, it features essays written by distinguished psychologists, medical professionals, therapists, and professors in addition to practitioners and parents.

This book examines youth sport from a number of different angles, from the myriad potential benefits of youth sport to the injuries and harms that unfortunately also befall some participants. We sought to also approach youth sport from the perspective of many of the people involved in youth sport, from the athletes themselves to the parents, coaches, officials, and trainers who all play unique and pivotal roles in shaping the character and tenor of youth sports in America. We also have sought to address the many different young people who participate in youth sport, highlighting the unique experiences and challenges of boys, girls, LGBT athletes, and individuals with disabilities, for while we recognize sport is universal and provides an avenue for connection and challenge, it is often viewed and embraced differently by different populations.

In addition, we have provided a variety of entries that can serve as information resources for athletes, parents, and coaches on issues such as helping the youth sport athlete cope with failure, finding a competitive balance between what is needed and what is most enjoyable, or weigh the benefits and drawbacks of specializing in a single sport rather than participating in multiple sports. Finally, *Youth Sports in America* addresses many of the hot topics in modern youth sport, such as the influence of television and social media on youth sport, the escalating financial cost of youth sports, and problems such as concussions, hazing, bullying, and burnout that are all too common in the youth sport setting.

Packed with information and insights that will be of interest to everyone involved in the world of youth sports—athletes, parents, coaches, referees, and administrators—this book will thus be a valuable resource for anyone seeking a better understanding of youth sport in America.

Adaptive Sports

Sports involvement, ranging from recreational to competitive levels of play, has been promoted among children and adolescents because it has numerous benefits. For example, participation in sports—no matter the skill level—has been found to aid the development of important life skills including social skills, collaboration with others, commitment and follow-through to responsibilities, setting and achieving goals, character development, self-esteem, and improved academic performance. Although sports and recreational opportunities are readily available for youth without disabilities in school and community settings, fewer opportunities for participation exist among youth who have a disability or chronic health condition. Since the 1990s, civil rights legislation has been developed to ensure that persons who have a disability are provided with the same opportunities regarding education, employment, and sports and recreation involvement as their peers who do not have a disability. Therefore, the intent of this entry is to introduce readers to adaptive sports, more specifically Paralympic sports, and the positive impact participation in adaptive sports can have on youth who have a disability.

Who Participates in Adaptive Sport?

Individuals who have a physical and/or intellectual disability are eligible to participate in adaptive sports. It is estimated that approximately 5.2 percent of adolescents between the ages of 5 and 17 living in the United States have a physical and/or intellectual disability (U.S. Census Bureau, 2011). Physical disabilities may include sensory impairments and musculoskeletal, neuromuscular, or neurological health conditions. Sensory impairments are health conditions in which functional capacity is reduced in one or more of the five senses. For example, an individual may have a visual impairment or hearing impairment. Musculoskeletal, neuromuscular, and neurological health conditions are the result of injury to the central nervous system, peripheral nervous system, bones, muscles, and/or joints. Examples of these health conditions include amputation, spinal cord injury, traumatic brain injury, cerebral palsy, spina bifida, muscular dystrophy, multiple sclerosis, and cerebrovascular accident (stroke). An individual may be born with a physical health condition, or he or she may acquire it later in life as a result of an unanticipated circumstance (e.g., traumatic accident, bacterial infection).

In contrast to physical disabilities, intellectual disabilities refer to health conditions that result in altered cognitive functioning, potentially resulting in impaired communication skills, social skills, academic skills (e.g., reading/writing ability, mathematical processing), and/or skills associated with activities of daily living (e.g., self-care, organizational skills). Examples of intellectual disabilities include Down syndrome, autism, fetal alcohol syndrome, and fragile X syndrome. Intellectual disabilities may be present at the time of birth (i.e., congenital), or an individual may develop the intellectual disability during early childhood years before he or she reaches 18 years of age.

What Is Adaptive Sport?

Adaptive sport refers to "any modification of a given sport or recreation activity to accommodate the varying ability levels of an individual with a disability" (Lundberg, Taniguchi, McCormick, and Tibbs, 2011, 206). One common modification is to change the physical space or setting in which a sport is traditionally played to accommodate athletes with disabilities. For example, softball is traditionally played on dirt and grass surfaces, whereas wheelchair softball is played on a soft but firm rubberized surface. This modification in space allows for athletes who use assistive devices (e.g., wheelchair, walker, crutches) to more easily maneuver on the field of play.

A modification may also include altering the rules for a particular sport to increase accessibility. For example, volleyball is typically played from a standing position on a court that is 18×9 meters in size, with a net that is 7–8 feet off the ground. Sitting volleyball, an adaptive sport for athletes who have an injury and/or impaired functioning in their lower extremities (e.g., leg amputation), is played from a seated position on a court that is 10×6 meters in size, with a net that is located approximately 3 feet off the ground. These rule modifications allow for individuals with varied ability in their lower extremities to engage in the game of volleyball as any other athlete would with regard to court positions, serving, offensive and defensive skills (i.e., blocking, spiking, bump pass), and scoring.

Another modification may involve altering the equipment used for the sport. For example, the biathlon event combines cross-country skiing and target shooting. Individuals who have a visual impairment can participate in the shooting portion of biathlon events using an auditory rifle, in which headphones worn by the athletes signal via the frequency and tone of a beeping rhythm when the rifle is in line with the center of the target (indicating to the athlete when to pull the gun's trigger). This modification in equipment facilitates athletes with visual impairment to independently compete in the biathlon events in the same way any other athlete would, regardless of ability. Although many modifications to sport have been identified, the purpose of any modification is to (1) permit the athlete to independently participate in the sport, and (2) maintain the traditional rules and style of the game as much as possible.

Benefits of Participation in Adaptive Sport

Benefits of sports participation for youth who have a disability are similar to those experienced by youth who do not have a disability, and include improved physiological and psychosocial quality of life and well-being. Regardless of one's ability level, youth who participate in sport have an opportunity to (1) develop a sense of mastery in sports-specific skills, (2) increase competence in their abilities, (3) improve self-esteem, and (4) form their personal and/or athletic identity. These outcomes are significant for athletes progressing through childhood and adolescence. As Erickson's stages of psychosocial development (1959) propose: youth between the ages of 6 and 12 are seeking to learn and achieve, and youth between 13 and 18 are looking to become their own, autonomous person.

Through sports (be it at a recreational, intramural/club sports, or elite level), youth who have a disability demonstrate improved cardiorespiratory fitness, physical strength, and endurance. Youth who have a disability are at increased risk for developing secondary health conditions (e.g., diabetes, obesity, depression, pressures sores). Thus, active sports participation among youth with disabilities decreases sedentary behaviors, which then decreases the likelihood of their developing a secondary health condition. Furthermore, research indicates that youth who are physically active are more likely to remain physically active as adults, advancing the likelihood of the individuals maintaining positive health, while also preventing the onset of ill-health in the future. Having an opportunity to participate in sports is critical for youth who have a disability, as it introduces them to activities in which they can participate in the long term (e.g., high school, college, adulthood); it also creates an awareness of activities in which they can become elite level athletes and competitors, should they so choose.

Similar to their peers without disabilities, opportunities to engage in sports are meaningful for youth with disabilities in other ways as well. Sports provide an opportunity to socially interact with others, leading to improved social skills and an established network of friends. For youth with disabilities, social connections via sports participation can also develop due to their experiences feeling a sense of relatedness among their peers and teammates who (1) share the same sports/activity interests, and/or (2) have the same type of disability or health condition as they do. Also, as a result of participation in inclusive sports programs, preexisting assumptions and stereotypes regarding persons who have a disability are diminished when youth without disabilities recognize that their peers who have a disability have the same athletic desires, capabilities, and talents necessary for sports competition as they do. Consequently, social relations, increased advocacy, and respect among youth with and without disabilities naturally evolve due to the interactions and perspectives gained by participants of all abilities during inclusive sports programming.

Lastly, sports can be a positive outlet for youth who have a disability to learn to control and express their emotions in a positive way. Specific to sports, learning good sportsmanship associated with winning, losing, agreeing/disagreeing with coach's and/or referee's decisions is involved. Specific to their developing as an adolescent, and in their coping with their having a disability, sports can be an avenue through which youth who have a disability can learn to appropriately manage their stress, anger, and frustration in a healthy manner.

Adaptive Sports Programming

Typically, adaptive sports programs are presented as inclusive programs or specialized programs. Inclusive programs provide an opportunity for individuals with and without disabilities to participate in the same activities. Youth with disabilities enjoy participation in inclusive programs because it facilitates their engaging in sports alongside their peers and/or family members who have a similar interest and love for the recreational activity or sport. Inclusive programs tend to decrease marginalization that comes from separation from one's peers, establishes equality, and creates a sense of social relatedness among youth. Likewise, youth without disabilities who participate in inclusive programs report that they often evolve in their perspective regarding what it means to have a disability. By engaging in sport with peers who have a disability, youth who do not have a disability gain a greater awareness and understanding of what it means to have a disability, recognizing abilities and skills rather than limitations. Social acceptance occurs as peers with and without disabilities realize that they share the same interests, desires, and goals regarding skill progression and athletic development in their selected sport.

In contrast, specialized programs are sports programs provided solely for individuals who have a disability. For youth who have a disability, participation in specialized programs offers them social support that differs from the social support available to them in inclusive programs. In particular, specialized programs provide opportunities to develop relationships with peers who have experienced similar life circumstances as well as the shared understanding that comes in knowing the impact their having a disability has had on their physiological and psychosocial quality of life.

Although inclusive programs tend to occur at a recreational level for the purposes of enjoyment and social interaction, specialized programs tend to focus on athletic identity, sport-specific training, skill development, and competition. Thus, a second advantage to participation in specialized sports programs is the opportunity for youth to engage in higher levels of competition specific to adaptive sports where equipment, rules, sports classifications, and sport strategies specific to the sport being pursued are learned and repeatedly practiced often in preparation for an upcoming competition or event. In other words, youth who have a disability and are wanting to develop as an athlete and experience more significant competition in hopes of reaching an elite level (i.e., participation in varsity high school, collegiate programs, or community-based tournament teams) can do so by participation in specialized adaptive sports programs. Some well-known examples of competitive opportunities for individuals with disabilities include the Paralympics and the Special Olympics.

The Paralympics and Special Olympics

The Paralympics and Special Olympics serve as the main organizations that provide specialized programs associated with adaptive sports in school, community, and competition-based settings. The Paralympics is an international entity that is traditionally representative of community-based sports programming and elite-level sports competition for individuals with physical disabilities and/or visual and/or hearing impairments, although there are some Paralympic sports in which individuals with intellectual impairments are eligible to participate. The Special Olympics, also an international organization, offers community-based and competitive sports programming for individuals with developmental disabilities. In 1960 the first summer Paralympic Games were held in Italy with 400 athletes from 23 countries competing in eight sporting events. In 1976, the first winter Paralympic Games took place in Sweden with 53 athletes from 16 countries competing in two sporting events. During the most recent 2012 London summer Paralympic Games, 4,237 athletes representing 164 countries competed in 20 sporting events. In 2014, during the Sochi winter Paralympic Games, 547 athletes from 45 countries competed in five sporting events. At present, the summer and winter Paralympic Games are held

Table 1 Paralympic Sports

Summer Sports			Winter Sports
Archery	7-aside football	Swimming	Alpine skiing
Athletics	Goalball	Table tennis	Biathlon
Badminton	Judo	Taekwondo	Cross-country skiing
Boccia	Powerlifting	Triathlon	Ice sledge hockey
Canoe	Rowing	Wheelchair basketball	Wheelchair curling
Cycling	Sailing	Wheelchair dance	
Equestrian	Shooting	Wheelchair fencing	
5-aside football	Sitting volleyball	Wheelchair rugby	
		Wheelchair tennis	

every four years in the same geographic locations—and sports venues—as the Olympic Games (i.e., international competition for athletes who do not have a disability). The Paralympic Games typically take place two weeks following the Olympic Games. Paralympic athletes representing multiple nations from around the world have an opportunity to qualify and compete in both team-based and individual-based Paralympic sports (see Table 1).

The Paralympic Games represent the highest level of competition and achievement for athletes with disabilities. Many athletes spend years training to develop their sport-specific skills and abilities in order to work their way up to the elite-level status in which they become eligible to qualify for their national team.

Getting Involved in Adaptive Sports

For youth with disabilities, their first exposure to adaptive sports is often the result of participating in an introductory adaptive sports clinic, an adaptive physical education class within their school system, and/or a community-based recreational sports team. In addition, youth may become aware of adaptive sports through media coverage of adaptive sports events or a featured story about an athlete who has a disability. Information shared among other families with children who have a disability represents another way that youth become aware of adaptive sports opportunities. Finally, youth athletes may be encouraged to participate in adaptive sports from a variety of allied health professionals including, but not limited to, recreation therapists, physical therapists, and occupational therapists during the rehabilitation process postinjury.

After being introduced to adaptive sport, youth with disabilities who choose to pursue participation in adaptive sport should have an opportunity to do so within their elementary, middle, and/or high school physical education classes and athletic programs. Depending on the geographic location, youth with disabilities also have opportunities to engage in adaptive sports within local community-based organizations including Paralympic sport clubs, nonprofit adaptive sports organizations, county or city parks and recreation programs, or adaptive sports camps/clinics hosted by local rehabilitation hospitals. Youth with disabilities are able to hone their athletic skills, specific to their selected sport, in these targeted programs and can work their way into a more elite-level track. This includes competing in adaptive sports at the collegiate level and/or being recruited for national training camps, both of which can produce an opportunity to qualify for the national Paralympic team.

Civil Rights Legislation Related to Youth, Disability, and Adaptive Sports

In the last several decades, civil rights legislation specific to individuals who have a disability has been established within the United States to ensure that communities and educational, vocational, and recreation/sports programs housed within communities are accessible and inclusive of individuals who have a disability. This legislation also protects individuals who have a disability from discrimination and exclusion. In 1990, the Americans with Disability Act (ADA) was created. The purpose of the ADA is to ensure that public services, transportation, and employment opportunities for persons who have a disability are available to the same equivalent and quality as those provided to individuals who do not have a disability. In addition, the ADA developed the Standards for Accessible Design that outlines specific criteria that must be upheld within community structures to ensure that persons who have a disability can approach, enter, and use public facilities. More information regarding the ADA legislation can be found at http://www.ada.gov.

The Individuals with Disabilities Education Act (2004), first introduced as the Education for All Handicapped Children (1975), is legislation requiring that school systems provide education to children and youth who have a disability. This legislation encourages schools to develop individualized education plans, based on individual student abilities and needs, and to provide accommodations and supports in order to ensure that student education takes place in a "least restrictive environment." Access to participation in physical education is also included in this legislation, which addresses both mainstream (students with and without disabilities together) and special educational classroom settings. More information regarding the IDEA legislation can be found at http://idea.ed.gov.

In 2013, the U.S. Department of Education provided clarification regarding Section 504 of the Rehabilitation Act (1973). The reason for the clarification: to confirm that school systems understood their role and responsibility in offering students who have a disability the same opportunity for participation in school-based intramural and/or competitive sports programs as those provided to their peers without disability. More information explaining Section 504 legislation can be found at http://www2.ed.gov/about/offices/list/ocr/letters/colleague-201301-504.pdf.

These civil rights laws are important resources for youth who have a disability, their family members, and their school administrators to be aware of so that if need be, the student athletes and/or their support network can advocate for adaptive sports services on their behalf.

Barriers to Participation in Adaptive Sport

Unfortunately, there are a number of intrapersonal, interpersonal, environmental, and social barriers that can discourage and/or prevent youth who have a disability from pursuing participation in recreation and/or competitive sports programs. Intrapersonal factors that often inhibit youth who have a disability include lack of confidence in their abilities and hesitance to believe that they can engage in the sport to the extent that they would like to. Youth who have a disability may compare themselves to their peers who do not have a disability and erroneously self-impose negative perceptions of themselves, their abilities, and their potential for advancing in their selected sport. Also, depending on the nature of their disability (i.e., if they have an acquired injury vs. a congenital health condition), individuals may still be working through, adjusting to, coping with, and accepting that they have a disability and the life transitions that are subsequently involved for themselves and their extended family and friends.

Other personal factors that can impede participation in adaptive sports may include limited access to transportation or an inability to financially afford the costly adaptive equipment. Furthermore, program fees may be necessary for successful participation in the sport. Participation in inclusive programs may also be challenging for youth who have a disability because of protective parenting; their parents may be hesitant to allow them to participate in adaptive programs for fear that (1) their children will be at risk for further injury; (2) their children will be mistreated or lack acceptance among their peers who do not have a disability; or (3) that their children may not perform to the level that they personally expect of themselves, or to the level that others expect, resulting in disappointment and/or their feeling incompetent.

Interpersonal factors also play a significant role in either facilitating or hindering youth who have a disability and who wish to take part in adaptive sports. At times, the context (i.e., physical structures and/or social environment) in which community-based and/or school-based programs take place are not accessible to youth who have a disability. For example, facilities in which inclusive and/or specialized programs are offered may not be structurally accessible in that access to the facility may be limited due to accessible public transportation routes not providing services to the facility location; or the facility itself may not be accessible in accordance with the Americans with Disability Act Standards (1990; i.e., a building has stairs but no elevators or access ramps; restrooms do not have doors that are wide enough for persons who use a wheelchair to navigate).

Unfortunately, in some cases, communities and schools may lack sport programs or fail to provide adequate adaptive sports opportunities. Some programs that do offer inclusive or specialized programs are ineffective in marketing their program, resulting in poor enrollment due to youth who have a disability being unaware of opportunities in their hometown. Other community-based and/or school-based programs have a strong desire to provide adaptive sports to their constituents but lack the funding and/or administrative support to do so. In addition, often staff members and volunteers of programs that offer adaptive sports programming lack knowledge in how to best accommodate individuals who have a disability due to their having received minimal training specific to disability awareness/education, adaptive equipment, etc. As a result, youth who have a disability may feel unsupported when they attend these programs, and program staff do not feel qualified or prepared to deliver high-quality services, which can cause them to become hesitant in including youth who have a disability in future activities.

Similarly, attitudes within society can influence the success of inclusive sports programs. Too often, individuals assume that persons who have a disability are not capable of engaging in activities at the same level as individuals who do not have a disability. As a result, parents of athletes without a disability, or the athletes themselves, may be reluctant to enroll youth who have a disability into an athletic team. Subsequently, there may be concern that coaching and training necessary for qualifying and competing at advanced tournaments will be compromised due to the athletes who have a disability needing more time to obtain skills. Although this attitude is not held by all coaches, athletes without a disability, and/or parents of athletes without a disability, there are several misinformed stereotypes that exist regarding the presumed abilities (or lack of) of athletes who have disabilities. Thus, it is imperative that communities continue to provide education to citizens (e.g., community members, organizations/administrations, staff, coaches, parents, athletes) to dispel misunderstandings and falsehoods regarding the abilities of individuals who have a disability or health condition. Effective educational efforts can replace inaccurate assumptions and labels placed on youth who have a disability with an improved awareness of what it means to have a disability and a more accurate understanding that youth who have a disability often possess the same interests, goals, skills, and abilities as their nondisabled peers.

Conclusion

Youth with disabilities reap numerous benefits from participation in sport and recreational activities. Although all of the physical health benefits are important, such as obesity and diabetes prevention, sport participation also yields psychological benefits such as stress reduction. Moreover, sports provide a context for fostering positive social interactions and a sense of belonging. Adaptive sport opportunities in community and school settings are varied but may become more formalized and highly competitive.

Additional Resources

Parents of youth who have a disability should contact local allied health professionals (e.g., pediatrician, recreation therapist, physical therapist, occupational therapist), school officials, and/or parks and recreation sports leagues to learn about the inclusive and/or specialized sports programs being offered at their local community, state, and/or regional level. Parents can also visit Disabled Sports USA at http://www.disabledsportsusa.org/chapters for more information about the adaptive sports chapters (often in partnership with nonprofit adaptive sport organizations) offering adaptive sports events taking place in or near their local community. For information regarding the Paralympics, visit the International Paralympic Committee at http://www.paralympic.org or the United States Paralympic website at http://www.teamusa.org/us-paralympics. More specifically, U.S. Paralympics provides a detailed list of the Paralympic sports clubs within each state (http://www.teamusa.org/US-Paralympics/Community/Paralympic-Sport-Clubs); these programs offer entry to higher levels of competition for youth athletes interested in pursuing a more elite level of adaptive sports participation.

Brandi M. Crowe and Justine J. Reel

Further Reading

American Psychiatric Publishing. *Intellectual Disability.* Accessed August 1, 2015, at http://www.dsm5.org/documents/intellectual%20disability%20fact%20sheet.pdf.

American Psychological Association. *Individuals with Disabilities Education Act (IDEA).* Accessed August 1, 2015, at http://www.apa.org/about/gr/issues/disability/idea.aspx.

Anderson, Denise. 2009. "Adolescent Girls' Involvement in Disability Sport: Implications for Identity Development." *Journal of Sport and Social Issues, 33*(4): 427–449.

Anderson, Denise M., Angela Wozencroft, and Leandra A. Bedini. 2008. "Adolescent Girls' Involvement in Disability Sport: A Comparison of Social Support Mechanisms." *Journal of Leisure Research, 40*(2): 183–207.

Bedini, Leandra A., and Ashley Thomas. 2012. "Bridge II Sports: A Model of Meaningful Activity through Community-Based Adapted Sport." *Therapeutic Recreation Journal, 46*(4): 284–300.

Blauwet, Cheri, and Stuart E. Willick. 2012. "The Paralympic Movement: Using Sports to Promote Health, Disability Rights, and Social Integration of Athletes with Disabilities." *The American Academy of Physical Medicine and Rehabilitation, 4*: 851–856.

Crowe, Brandi, and Marieke Van Puymbroeck. 2015. "Physical Medicine and Rehabilitation Practice." In David R. Austin et al. (Eds.), *Recreation Therapy: An Introduction* (4th ed., pp. 235–251). Urbana, IL: Sagamore Publishing.

Eime, Rochelle M., Janet A. Young, Jack T. Harvey, Melanie J. Charity, and Warren R. Payne. 2013. "A Systematic Review of the Psychological and Social Benefits of Participation in Sport for Children and Adolescents: Informing Development of a Conceptual Model of Health through Sport." *International Journal of Behavioral Nutrition and Physical Activity, 10*: 98–118.

Erikson, E. H. (1959). *Identity and the life cycle: Selected papers.* With a historical introduction by David Rapaport. New York: International University Press.

Groff, Diane G., Neil R. Lundberg, and Ramon B. Zabriskie. 2009. "Influence of Adapted Sport on Quality of Life: Perceptions of Athletes with Cerebral Palsy." *Disability and Rehabilitation, 31*(4): 318–326.

Ketteridge, Asha, and Kobie Boshoff. 2008. "Exploring the Reasons Why Adolescents Participate in Physical Activity and Identifying Strategies That Facilitate Their Involvement in Such Activities." *Australian Occupational Therapy Journal, 55*: 273–282.

Law, Mary, Theresa Petrenchik, Gillian King, and Patricia Hurley. 2007. "Perceived Environmental Barriers to Recreational, Community, and School Participation for Children and Youth with Physical Disabilities." *Archives of Physical Medicine and Rehabilitation, 88*: 1636–1642.

Losinski, Mickey, Antonis Katsiyannis, and Mitchell L. Yell. 2014. "Athletics and Students with Disabilities: What Principals Should Know." *NASSP Bulletin, 98*(4): 310–323.

Lundberg, Neil R., Stacy Taniguchi, Bryan P. McCormick, and Catherine Tibbs. 2011. "Identity Negotiating: Redefining Stigmatized Identities through Adaptive Sports and Recreation Participation among Individuals with Disability." *Journal of Leisure Research, 43*(2): 205–225.

Mayer, Whitney E., and Lynn S. Anderson. 2014. "Perceptions of People with Disabilities and Their Families about Segregated and Inclusive Recreation Involvement." *Therapeutic Recreation Journal, 48*(2): 150–168.

Rimmer, James A., and Jennifer L. Rowland. 2008. "Physical Activity for Youth with Disabilities: A Critical Need in an Underserved Population." *Developmental Neurorehabilitation, 11*(2): 141–148.

Shapiro, Deborah R., and Jeffery J. Martin, J. J. 2014. "The Relationships among Sport Self-Perceptions and Social Well-Being in Athletes with Physical Disabilities." *Disability and Health Journal, 7*: 42–48.

Stumbo, Norma, and Carol A. Peterson. 2009. *Therapeutic Recreation Program Design: Principles and Procedures* (5th ed.). San Francisco: Pearson Benjamin Cummings.

United States Census Bureau. 2011. *School-Aged Children with Disabilities in U.S. Metropolitan Statistical Areas: 2010.* Accessed August 1, 2015, at https://www.census.gov /prod/2011pubs/acsbr10-12.pdf.

Verschuren, Olaf, Lesley Wiart, Dominique Hermans, and Marjolijn Ketelaar. 2012/ "Identification of Facilitators and Barriers to Physical Activity in Children and Adolescents with Cerebral Palsy." *The Journal of Pediatrics, 161*(3): 488–494.

Wilhite, Barbara, and John Shank. 2009. "In Praise of Sport: Promoting Sport Participation as a Mechanism of Health among Persons with a Disability." *Disability and Health Journal, 2*: 116–127.

Body Image and Eating Disorders

The importance of having proper nutrition as a competitive athlete has been emphasized for all sports and levels of competition. Food is used by active youth and adults alike to fuel the body's systems to aid in a successful sport performance. Although having adequate energy intake is critical to performing at a high level, athletes may be expected to eat more or less depending on the demands of their sport related to energy expenditure or the expected body type. Many sports associate a particular physique with an athlete's height or weight. For example, adolescent figure skaters in a 2014 study reported the need to be short and thin in order to execute spins and jumps effectively. Although youth participants may be diverse in terms of the height and weight percentiles for their age, athletes from certain sports may feel pressured to change their body weight, size, or shape to meet a perceived sport ideal.

In attempts to "fit in" with other athletes or to "look" the part, athletes may alter their eating patterns or exercise behaviors to change their bodies. Body image has been defined as one's perception about his or her appearance. Positive body image can contribute to overall self-confidence and having the right psychological mindset to perform well in sports and other activities. Unfortunately, negative body image is common among youth athletes. Negative body image is often referred to as body dissatisfaction. It is the result of a discrepancy between one's perceptions of his or her actual body compared to a perceived ideal body and has been associated with attempts to change one's body size, shape, or weight, which can have a negative effect on one's athletic performance. For example, adolescent dancers who expressed negative body image were more likely to experience difficulty with concentration before and during competitions and practice. Youth male athletes who reported body image dissatisfaction also scored lower on measures of perceived and actual physical ability than male athletes who were satisfied with their bodies. Young female athletes who reported being unhappy with their appearance or were teased about their bodies were less likely to continue participating in sport. Furthermore, negative body image was associated with a lack of confidence throughout one's performance. Finally, body dissatisfaction has consistently been shown to be the strongest predictor of eating disorders. Therefore, the body image and eating behaviors of our youth athletes—whether positive or negative—have powerful implications for both performance and health.

What Is an Eating Disorder?

Generally, in order to fuel the body for maximum performance, an athlete needs to eat the right kinds of food—and in sufficient quantities—to handle the demands of his or her sport. Eating patterns for youth athletes exist along a continuum from so-called healthy eating to clinical eating disorders diagnosed by a medical professional. Healthy eating refers to eating an adequate amount of nutrients (carbohydrates, protein, and fat) to maintain the body's systems, body weight, and provide enough energy for high-level athletic performance. According to the United States Department of Agriculture, Americans are encouraged to eat a well-balanced diet of grains, fruits, and vegetables. Having a healthy relationship with food consists of eating regular meals, eating when hungry, and stopping when full rather than participating in yo-yo dieting and emotional eating.

In contrast to healthy eating, disordered eating may involve restricting the intake of certain kinds of foods or overall intake. Disordered eating may also include binge eating or excessive food intake that is driven by one's emotions. Finally, disordered eating behaviors may include behaviors used to purge food such as vomiting, laxatives, or diuretics. Compensatory behavior may also include excessively exercising to reduce or eliminate food intake.

In order to qualify for a diagnosis of a clinical eating disorder, a list of criteria needs to be met. One requirement for an eating disorder is that a youth athlete must report a fear of gaining weight and exhibit intense body dissatisfaction. When an athlete is underweight and not eating enough to maintain a healthy weight for his or her height and bodily systems, he or she may be classified as suffering from a disorder known as anorexia nervosa. Anorexia nervosa includes extreme caloric restriction with the result of significantly low body weight. The fear of becoming fat and negative body image prevent the athlete with anorexia nervosa from achieving a healthy weight even though this low weight is associated with negative health consequences.

Another eating disorder is bulimia nervosa, which is characterized by binge eating and purging behaviors. For example, a youth athlete who regularly overeats to a point beyond fullness, and who then exercises out of guilt, may exhibit some signs of bulimia nervosa. Bulimia nervosa involves binge eating and compensatory behaviors on a weekly basis for at least three months. Like anorexia nervosa, negative body image is a key feature of bulimia nervosa.

Finally, some athletes will fit the criteria for a third type of eating disorder commonly known as binge eating. In this case, athletes engage in overeating but do not use a compensatory method to counteract the binge episode. Binge episodes involve eating rapidly, eating beyond the point of fullness, and experiencing the sense that one cannot stop eating (feeling out of control). Binge eating typically occurs at least weekly for three months or longer to meet the diagnosis of binge-eating disorder.

Prevalence of Eating Disorders among Youth Athletes

The onset of puberty, which may bring with it upwards of 50 percent of adult body weight, often results in struggles with body image dissatisfaction. This is worrisome given the relationship between body image dissatisfaction, disordered eating (irregular eating behaviors), and eating disorders (specifically diagnosed conditions such as anorexia nervosa or bulimia nervosa). For adolescents, in general, prevalence rates for anorexia and bulimia are approximately 1 percent and 4 percent, respectively. The percentage of adolescents, regardless of athletic standing, who exhibit nonclinical eating disorders, or disordered eating, is closer to 10 percent (Zachrisson, Vedul-Kjelsas, Götestam, and Mykletun, 2008). The age of onset for eating disorders was once thought to be in middle to high school. However, recent reports indicate that children as young as 5 years of age have been diagnosed with eating disorders.

Prevalence rates for eating disorders in athletes are rather wide-ranging, depending on the study sample and methods of data collection. Generally, rates of clinical eating disorders in athletes range from 5 percent to 33 percent. However, many athletes exhibit disordered eating behaviors that do not align with the standard criteria for an eating disorder diagnosis. In fact, as many as 60 percent of female adolescent athletes exhibited disordered eating behaviors on a nondiagnostic level in one study. This discrepancy between eating disorder rates in athletes versus nonathletes tends to relate to the types of athletes included in the study. For example, some studies tend to include athletes (e.g., gymnasts) who have much higher rates of disordered eating due to the nature of the sport. Interestingly, dieting, preoccupation with food, and bulimic symptoms were higher in female athletes than male athletes or nonathletes. Moreover, nonathlete adolescent males had higher rates of binge eating than their athlete counterparts. However, the challenge of mixed results in the larger body of research makes it difficult to determine whether sport is a protective or risk factor to disordered eating in adolescent athletes. Regardless of the methodological challenges, negative body image and disordered eating remain a challenge to adolescent athletes for a variety of reasons, leaving athletes identified as an at-risk group in school counseling research and other areas.

Types of Sport Categories and At-Risk Athletes

The popular debate about whether athletes are more or less likely to develop disordered eating or an eating disorder is unresolved, as findings have been mixed related to prevalence for athletes versus nonathletic populations. However, certain athletes have been considered more vulnerable for the potential development of negative body image and disordered eating behaviors. Specifically, athletes who fit a psychological profile characterized as being highly perfectionistic, and highly achievement-oriented along with being sensitive to criticism and having low self-esteem, may be more at risk for engaging in disturbed eating patterns. Additionally, athletes in individual sports had higher levels of social physique anxiety and disordered eating attitudes and behaviors than athletes in team sports. Furthermore, certain sports tend to be associated with more direct pressures to fit a particular physique to compete.

Sports have been commonly divided into the following categories when analyzing the prevalence of disordered eating among athletes: ball sports (or team sports), aesthetic sports, weight class sports, and endurance sports. Ball sports such as basketball and softball are believed to have less clearly identified pressures to lose or gain weight for youth athletes. Although no athlete is immune from developing negative body image or eating disturbances, it is believed that athletes who participate in ball sports, which are often team sports, tend to be at less risk than aesthetic and endurance athletes. In fact, research has shown that male team sport athletes have less body image dissatisfaction and greater perceived physical ability than individual sport athletes.

Aesthetic sports represent a category of sports that values a particular look or appearance that goes along with the competitive outcome. Popular aesthetic sports include figure skating, diving, synchronized swimming, and gymnastics, which all include being judged for how their bodies are positioned during their competitions. Although this way of scoring may seem subjective, the athletes are often encouraged to demonstrate "long lines" and to look lean in the air while performing moves. Athletes who believe that they should be leaner in order to improve sport performance are at greater risk for disordered eating and eating disorders than athletes who desire to be leaner for any other reason. A recent study on youth athletes confirmed this hypothesis, with athletes participating in aesthetic activities scoring higher on measures of drive for thinness, bulimic symptomology, and drive for muscularity than athletes who participated in any other nonaesthetic activity. As a result, aesthetic athletes registered higher levels of body image dissatisfaction and disordered eating behaviors than nonaesthetic athletes, regardless of gender.

Another category of sports that is important to consider are sports competitions that are arranged in strictly defined weight classes, such as wrestling and boxing. These athletes may face intense pressures to lose or gain weight to compete in another weight class or division that will help the team or an individual athlete's performance standing and may engage in a variety of disordered behaviors such as excessive exercise in rubber suits, spitting and dehydration strategies, and sitting in a sauna, to lose weight prior to a weigh-in. Because there is such large attention devoted to the number on the scale, these athletes are considered to be "at risk" for disordered eating and eating disorders. Consequently, national governing bodies have made changes to sport policies to minimize the health risks associated with rapid weight-cycling; however, many weight class athletes continue to engage in disordered eating behaviors.

Endurance athletes comprise the final category of sports. Endurance sports such as cross-country running may imply that performance will be affected by one's body weight. Coaches and other athletes may reinforce the perception that performance will improve if one loses weight and is thereby lighter. Cross-country runners, in particular, have been found to have increased risk for disordered eating and eating disorders.

Influences of Coach and Significant Others on Youth Athletes

Coaches and other significant others such as parents and teammates also can be sources of significant pressure to change one's weight, shape, or size. It is common for performance in sports to be associated with one's body weight in a positive or negative way. Comments from coaches about one's body and how it looks can affect children from a young age. Parents who have a lot invested in their son's or daughter's success in sport may begin to take on the role as food or weight police for youth athletes. Finally, teammates may reinforce strict weight policies and a negative body image culture by discussing weight loss "strategies" and their perceived bodily flaws.

Pressures to look a certain way, both in the sport and the nonsport contexts abound. Thus, youth athletes' body image and eating behaviors are influenced by family, peers, and media to coaches and teammates. Those pressures may take the form of comments directed to the athlete or other indirect comments or behaviors. The degree of influence of a particular source varies based on individual athlete characteristics and specific environmental differences; nonetheless, research consistently indicates that family, friends, media, and coaches affect athletes' perceptions about themselves, their bodies, and their abilities.

Research has shown that athletes who recalled negative comments from their coach related to athlete body shape or weight were more likely to engage in disordered eating and weight control behaviors and experience feelings of anxiety and shame. These negative comments might include those targeting athlete appearance or commenting on the connection between weight loss or gain and performance improvement. These types of comments are rarely mentioned with the intention of improving the athletes' health. Finally, it is unfortunate, but often these types of negative comments are given in public settings, which may contribute to the negative emotions associated with the specific comments.

Parents influence their children through direct comments or behaviors related to the child's body size, shape, or weight, or implicitly through indirect comments or behaviors related to the size, shape, or weight of other bodies. Teasing, encouragement to change body size, shape, or weight, and negative comments have all been related to negative body image and disordered eating or eating disorders. Unfortunately, teasing and other criticisms from parents have been identified as a common source of negative body image for women. Specific to aesthetic athletes, parents' weight-related comments are often couched within the thin sport subculture and are less related to overall body size, weight, or shape. Nevertheless, weight-related parental pressure has been cited as a greater contributor to negative body image and disordered eating in aesthetic athletes than in their nonathlete counterparts. Even when parents are not focused on their child's body, they may have a negative impact on their child's body image. For instance, mothers' self-criticism of their own bodies has been identified as a source for body image dissatisfaction in young women.

Similar to the influence of parents, peers may negatively impact body image and eating behaviors both through direct comments and through modeling poor body image and weight control habits. When friends directly comment about an athlete's body size, shape, or weight, or when they model negative body image or weight control habits, girls learn to engage in fat talk as a social expectation, which further negatively impacts their own body image and weight control habits. When nonfriend peers, male or female, tease athletes about their body size, shape, or weight, they also have a negative impact on body image, as well as self-esteem and continued sport participation. Peer relationships are also affected by athletes' perceived competence and body image.

Media, in the form of TV, magazines, video games, Internet, and other outlets, provide youth with idealized forms of how bodies should look. That is, media serve to promote the thin ideal, or the idea that thinner is better in terms of body size, shape, and/or weight. Unfortunately for some athletes, the thin ideal may compete with their sport ideal, further complicating their ideas about how their bodies should look and the methods they use to achieve a certain body size, shape, or weight. For instance, a thrower in track and field may receive media messages that thinner is better, but requires significant strength—and thus body mass—to be successful in her event. She may then feel conflicted over how her body is supposed to look and may feel forced to choose between athletic success and appearance-based social status. Combined with fat talk with friends and teasing or other criticism from peers, weight-related media pressure contributes to a culture of appearance that negatively affects adolescent body image, especially in girls.

Athletes may face weight-related pressures from their coaches, their uniforms, their teammates, or the nature of the sport, itself. Although uniforms and sport type have been discussed previously, a deeper examination of the influence of coaches and teammates on athlete body image and disordered eating behaviors is required. Similar to weight-related pressure from parents and peers, coach and teammate weight pressure may be either explicit, in the form of direct comments about body size, shape, or weight or recommendations to manage weight, or implicit, in the form of comments about other athletes' body size, shape, weight or self-criticisms. Because coaches are seen as authority figures who have a significant effect on athletes' performance successes, they tend to have a large impact on athlete behavior. Teammates, too, have an important impact on athletes' body image and eating behaviors for a variety of reasons. For one, interactions with teammates may contribute to a culture of appearance given the conversations athletes have with one another about their own bodies or the teasing some athletes may endure from their teammates. As a result, athletes' body image may be markedly shaped by their interactions with their teammates. For another, athletic teams may provide an environment where athletes can share weight loss secrets with one another, allowing weight control methods to spread through the team from one teammate to the next, placing athletes at particular risk for disordered eating and eating disorders. In the long run, body image dissatisfaction and teasing from others have been shown to negatively affect female adolescent athletes' sport participation, indicating that a positive body image and social support network are necessary to improving body image and long-term physical activity.

Body Image and Eating Disorders among Male Athletes

Although female athletes are the focal point of most discussions about eating disorders, male athletes are not immune from developing negative body image or disordered eating behaviors. In fact, some groups of males are particularly at risk for eating disorders. Male athletes like wrestlers and boxers who compete in weight class sports are highly focused on their weight and size. The consequences of those practices have even prompted governing bodies to revise weight-management regulations. Male jockeys have also been found to engage in restrictive weight practices to be lighter on their horse. Ski jumping, which historically was a male-only sport in the Olympics, had a reputation for dieting, disordered eating, and weight loss with the goal of traveling a greater distance in the air. Finally, male athletes in aesthetic sports such as bodybuilding have been found to be highly focused on appearance and their diet.

Although male athletes such as male jockeys may be pressured to lose weight to optimize performance, some male athletes may actually be encouraged to gain weight for their sport. Researchers have argued that male athletes may strive for a different body ideal than their female counterparts. In some cases, male athletes described their body ideal as large, lean, and muscular with low body fat. Specifically, male athletes wanted to lose weight while gaining muscle, which is difficult to achieve without performance-enhancing drugs like steroids. Therefore, it is important to recognize that both male and female youth athletes from a variety of sports may be at risk for developing disordered eating and eating disorders.

Potential Resources and Referral Strategies

Coaches and parents should be aware of available resources for addressing eating disorders in the event they arise within an athletic team. One place information on professionals who treat eating disorders can be found is on EDReferral.com. It is important that an athlete who is suspected to have disordered eating behaviors be confronted in a way that directly identifies the problem while offering support. A referral to the school counselor or the athlete's pediatrician can be a first step if an eating disorder resource in the community is not readily available. Finally, it is important for individuals to recognize that eating disorders represent a complex problem. It is unlikely that the athlete will be able to stop without some comprehensive treatment.

Justine J. Reel, Ashley M. Coker-Cranney, and Brandi M. Crowe

Further Reading

American Psychiatric Association. 2013. *Diagnostic and Statistical Manual of Mental Disorders* (5th ed.). Washington, D.C.: American Psychiatric Association.

Cook, Brian, Heather Hausenblas, Ross D. Crosby, Li Cao, and Stephen A. Wonderlich. 2015. "Exercise Dependence as a Mediator of the Exercise and Eating Disorders Relationship: A Pilot Study." *Eating Behaviors, 16*: 9–12. doi:10.1016/j.eatbeh.2014.10.012

Curtis, Cate, and Cushla Loomans. 2014. "Friends, Family, and Their Influence on Body Image Dissatisfaction." *Women's Studies Journal, 28*(2): 39–56.

Fransisco, Rita, Isabel Narciso, and Madalena Alarcao. 2013. "Parental Influences on Elite Aesthetic Athletes' Body Image Dissatisfaction and Disordered Eating." *Journal of Child and Family Studies, 22*: 1082–1091. doi:10.1007/s10826-012-9670-5

Khan, Saira, and Andrea Pretróczi. 2015. "Stimulus-Response Compatibility Tests of Implicit Preference for Food and Body Image to Identify People at Risk for Disordered Eating: A Validation Study." *Eating Behaviors, 16*: 54–63. doi:10.1016/j.eatbeh .2014.10.015

Krentz, E. M., and P. Warschburger. 2013. "A Longitudinal Investigation of Sports-Related Factors for Disordered Eating in Aesthetic Sports." *Scandinavian Journal of Medicine & Science in Sports, 23*: 303–301. doi:10.1111/j.1600-0838.2011.01380x

Petrie, Trent A., Nick Galli, Christy Greenleaf, Justine J. Reel, and Jennifer Carter. 2014. "Psychosocial Correlates of Bulimic Symptomatology among Male Athletes." *Journal of Psychology and Sport Excellence, 15*(6): 1–8. doi:10.1016/j.psychsport.2013.09.002

Selby, Christine, and Justine J. Reel. 2011. "A Coach's Guide to Identifying and Helping Athletes with Eating Disorders." *Journal of Sport Psychology in Action, 2*(2): 100–112. doi:10.1080/21520704.2011.585701

Theander, Sten S. 2004. "Trends in the Literature on Eating Disorders over 36 Years (1965–2000): Terminology, Interpretation, and Treatment." *European Eating Disorders Review, 12*: 4–17. doi:10.1002/erv.559

United States Department of Agriculture. *Teen Nutrition.* Last modified June 15, 2015, at http://fnic.nal.usda.gov/lifecycle-nutrition/teen-nutrition.

Voelker, Dana, Daniel Gould, and Justine J. Reel. 2014. "Weight Pressures and Disordered Eating among Sub-Elite Female Figure Skaters." *Journal of Psychology and Sport Excellence, 15*(6): 696–704. doi:10.1016/j.psychsport.2013.12.002

White, Hannah J., Emma Haycraft, Sloane Madden, Paul Rhodes, Jane Miskovic-Wheatley, Andrew Wallis, Michael Kohn, and Caroline Meyer. 2015. "How Do Parents of Adolescent Patients with Anorexia Nervosa Interact with Their Child at Mealtimes? A Study of Parental Strategies Used in the Family Meal Session of Family-Based Treatment." *International Journal of Eating Disorders, 48*: 72–80. doi:10.1002/eat.22328

White, Sabrina, Jocelyn B. Reynolds-Malear, and Elizabeth Cordero. 2011. "Disordered Eating and the Use of Unhealthy Weight Control Methods in College Students: 1995, 2002, and 2008." *Eating Disorders, 19*: 323–334. doi:10.1080/10640266.2011.584805

Zachrisson, Henrik D., Einar Vedul-Kjelsas, K. G. Götestam, and Arnstein Mykletun. 2008. "Time Trends in Obesity and Eating Disorders." *International Journal of Eating Disorders, 41*(8): 673–680. doi:10.1002/eat.20565

Boys in Sports

Boys enter youth sports as they begin to negotiate a life that is filled with gendered expectations. The traditional "boy code" equates masculinity with athletic competence and success, but experts within the field of youth development point out that this view is now outdated. Boys also need to be nurtured and taught to be more open with their emotions, which is a critical piece to their holistic growth into masculinity. In most cases, sport can serve as a valuable vehicle for both the emotional and physical health and development of boys. Some boys thrive in sports, learning how to deal openly with feelings of failure and accomplishment while also discovering their physical limitations. However, others may succumb to the stress and burnout of heightened sports workloads before they even reach adolescence. As youth sports have grown in popularity and intensity, so have criticisms that boys are being overscheduled and turned into performance-driven monsters. Fathers can play a key role in their sons' development in sports, as it is one aspect of parenting in which men sometimes feel more capable. Sports present unique environments that allow fathers to demonstrate their commitment and involvement in their son's development while maintaining their own masculinity. The need for involved fathers is critical, particularly in minority and low socioeconomic communities where boys can be hypnotized by the extremely remote possibility that participation in youth football and basketball will eventually lead to a glamorous career in professional sports.

Sports Participation Trends for Boys

Estimates reveal that almost 20 million 6- to 16-year-old children play organized sports in America (Coakley, 2009). When the Women's Sports Foundation (2008) surveyed more than 1,000 3rd- through 12th-grade boys on the recreational sports they participated in over the past year, basketball and football were the top answers (see Table 1). At the high school level, the 10 most popular

Table 1 Most Frequent Physical Activities (Boys)

Physical Activity	Participation, %
Basketball	71
Football	65
Soccer	51
Jogging/running	49
Swimming/diving	48
Baseball	48
Bowling	48
Weight training	42
Cycling/mountain biking	33
Skateboarding	29

Source: Women's Sports Foundation, 2008.

interscholastic sports for boys in terms of participation in 2014 were (in order): football, track and field, basketball, baseball, soccer, wrestling, cross country, tennis, golf, and swimming and diving (National Federation of State High School Association, 2014). In contrast to girls, boys are more likely to be involved in sport at an earlier age, play multiple sports, and stay in sports in later years. In 1995, eight was the average age that boys began playing sports. More recently, 8 is the age where boys are engaging in competitions for national championships (Farrey, 2008). Age 10 is the approximate age when a boy's true competitiveness begins to show—"It's only a game" is a hard thing for many 10-year-old boys to hear. Organized games also help to occupy boys' emerging testosterone, which otherwise might be channeled into more aggressive and/or mischievous pursuits.

At their best, youth sports can foster healthy and supportive relationships between boys and other family members, help them to maintain a healthy weight, instill qualities such as self-discipline that can foster success later in life, and help them develop a healthy sense of self-worth. It is widely accepted that childhood physical activity through sport contributes to the quality of life of boys when all of the associated benefits are emphasized, not just some of them. Furthermore, sports participation can build character, friendship, and a sense of achievement and belonging. Considering the potential pitfalls and dangers that boys face, these life skills are particularly important.

Steve Biddulph, a veteran psychologist with expertise in the development of boys and men, notes that the domain of sports is the main place where boys can practically work through learning how to:

- Be a good loser (and not cry, punch someone, or run away if you lose).
- Be a good winner (to be modest and avoid making others feel bad).

- Be part of a team (to play cooperatively, recognize your limitations, and support others' efforts).
- Give it your best effort (to train even when you are tired and continue to try your hardest).
- Work for a long-term goal or objective (and make sacrifices to achieve it).
- See that almost everything you do in life improves with practice (Biddulph, 2013, 186).

Parents and coaches often laud what they see their boys learning through sports—socialization, interpersonal skills, commitment, and discipline. Sports can be one of the most important activities in transforming boys, yet it is also important to understand that sports rarely have that transformational power alone. The key is for sport administrators and coaches to foster environments designed specifically to do so.

Sports have traditionally served as a training and proving ground for boys to establish their masculinity. In American culture, boys' sports have been valued for promoting and instilling "male" characteristics such as toughness and athleticism. Boys use physical performances and achievements that occur in sports to "size each other up" and develop their own masculine identity. There is a diversity of masculine identities that are formed through sport. Some boys place enormous emphasis on toughness and skill, some on building muscle mass, some on winning/competition, some on social relationships, and others on increased social status among peer groups (i.e., BMOC or Big Man on Campus). However, the most dominant form of masculinity seen in youth sports is hegemonic masculinity—the culturally idealized form of masculine character centered on toughness and competitiveness. Many boys place higher importance on playing aggressive and violent sports versus those characterized by technique and finesse. In the sporting context, good performance is most frequently associated with authority and power. In the lives of many boys, a home run or a touchdown can validate their manhood much more than receiving an "A" on a geometry test.

William Pollack's seminal book *Real Boys* (1998) pointed to a gender gap that existed in American public schools in terms of academic performance. From elementary to high school, boys received lower grades and were held back more frequently than girls, and boys also accounted for the majority of school suspensions and misbehavior. Two decades later, not much has changed; boys continue to lag behind academically in comparison to their female counterparts. In assessing this trend, some observers have identified sports as the perfectly designed tool to aid boys' achievement in the classroom. Pollack, for example, identified four major areas in which sports are transformational for boys: (1) freedom to express emotions, (2) freedom to share love and affection, (3) boosts in self-esteem, and (4) teaching them how to handle failure (Pollack, 1998, 275). For some boys, sports offer opportunities for emotional closeness too often lacking in other areas of their lives. They often feel more comfortable caring about one another in the context of playing sports than in almost any other area of life. Sports help boys handle the feelings of joy, despair, pride, anger, humility, and give them an outlet to show affection that they don't tend to feel comfortable expressing in other contexts. Consistent involvement also elevates boys' self-esteem as they begin to master something, particularly for those who struggle academically. Some boys may discover that sports give them a platform for learning and applying new skills, leading to positive feedback and attention as well as an increased feeling of self-worth. However, sports also allow boys to experience loss and disappointment. "If sports were only about glorious victory and humiliating one's opponents (or one's less capable teammates), they would not help a boy to confront his fears and vulnerabilities. But sports in fact do involve loss" (Pollack, 1998, 279). A healthy sports environment allows boys to learn that losing is a part of life.

The Role of Fathers

Some fathers have used sports to produce both male cultures and identities in their sons from generation to generation. At around 6 years of age (right about the time many enter organized youth sports for the first time), some boys experience a "switching on" of masculinity; they essentially want to study how to be "male." If a boy succeeds in football, baseball, basketball, or any other sport, he often receives praise and attention from male role models such as a father and/or male coach. No matter what one's skill level, however, there is almost always someone stronger, faster, or better coordinated. When boys encounter this reality, the approval a young boy once received from the men in his life may then fade, and his self-confidence in playing/performing in the sport may be damaged, if not shattered. Other boys may feel like they do not fit the stereotypical image of masculinity; they might not feel competitive or tough enough. Some boys may reject certain sports that they otherwise might enjoy (e.g., volleyball, cross country, tennis) because they feel that they are insufficiently masculine. Unfair or not, sports have become the quintessential "measure of maleness" (Biddulph, 2013, 184). In fact, some fathers use sports as a tool to teach their sons how to act tough and endure pain silently, persevere, and act "masculine." Sports that emphasize aggression and domination, however, can stunt emotional growth and place youth at increased risk of serious or chronic injuries.

Through the vehicle of youth sports, some fathers can be more prominently involved with their children in a way that feels traditionally "masculine." In other child-centric arenas of American society, some fathers might feel like they are on the outside looking in; the daily operation of schools, churches, and child care have traditionally been largely dependent on the labor of women. As noted youth sports expert Jay Coakley (2006) argues, "In each of these feminized contexts many fathers continue to feel out of place even though there has been an emerging cultural consensus that they should be there" (157). One environment that may be unique, in that it has traditionally been both organized and controlled by men, is sports. Through participating in their children's sports, fathers can both fulfill their responsibility to assume a more significant role in child care and at the same time make fathering seem manly, heroic, and appealing.

On the other hand, sports have often been viewed as an environment in which societal perspectives about masculinity are loosened, and boys are allowed to freely express a full range of emotions and feelings. Pollack argues that sports provide boys with an arena to express their feelings, be spirited, emotive, and passionate. Max, a 12-year-old boy interviewed by Pollack summed this up:

> During school we have to be quiet and raise our hands to talk. It's boring and sometimes I feel like there's nobody to talk to. I love doing sports after school because we can all be together. We get to run fast, shout things out, scream, whatever. It lets me be me. (Pollack, 1998, 272)

Similarly, sports provide fathers with an opportunity to demonstrate their domesticity while maintaining their sense of masculinity.

As with any aspect of raising boys, parental involvement in sports can be viewed from several perspectives. For instance, some fathers may use sports to teach their sons about what it means to be a man. Sports in this context are most often used to reinforce a gender ideology that men need to be physically tough and talented and emotionally competitive to succeed in the real world. There is even some evidence that while both parents may appear to be involved in their children's sport, mothers tend to assume more supportive child care tasks (i.e., providing transportation, ironing shirts, making lunches) while fathers assume more sport-specific tasks (i.e., teaching playing techniques and sporting behavior). Fathers may be using their children's sports to accommodate the demands of child care and other domestic responsibilities imposed by a new perspective on fatherhood. Coakley (2006) reports that some

> . . . fathers use youth sports and a wide range of away-from-the-home recreational activities as experiences that they can enjoy as they spend 'quality parenting time' with the children. This often occurs at the same time that these fathers expect their wives to take care of in-and-around-the-home aspects of childrearing. (158)

Without challenging the cultural expectations of this new notion of fatherhood, men can engage in activities that they both enjoy and feel competent with.

The connection to sport is easy for many fathers primarily because it is grounded in their own childhood experiences. Pollack exemplified this connection in an interview with the parent of an adolescent son. The parent, John, had fond memories of playing ice hockey and suggested that he introduced his son Sean to the sport in an effort to build his self-confidence. As John stated, "I could see that Sean was enjoying just getting out alone with me, there aren't as many chances for that in a large family. And I could have talked his ear off—I love talking sports" (Pollack, 1998, 278). Men and women may differ in the priority they give to life domains, and while some of today's fathers may have retained their function as the primary income earner in their families, they are also facing expectations to be more involved in other domains of their children's lives. Youth sports may be centrally positioned as a primary site through which fathers can meet these new parenting expectations but do so in a way that minimizes a perceived emasculation.

There is little dispute that healthy fatherly involvement is associated with significant social, emotional, and cognitive gains for their sons. Consequently, there is a need to discover more opportunities for facilitating and enhancing a father's parental involvement in his son's sport experiences. The following are some of the key contemporary issues surrounding boys playing sports.

Hyperperformance

When a young boy walks off the court after playing an organized basketball game, the first question often asked of him is something to the effect of "Did you win? How many points did you score?" These priorities reflect the importance that American society places on competition and performance over whether the boy in question had fun or improved in fundamental skill development. Coakley (2009) refers to this as the performance ethic—a set of beliefs emphasizing that the quality of the sport experience can be measured in terms of becoming a better athlete, becoming more competitive, and being promoted into more highly skilled training. Pollack refers to this phenomenon as the "cult of competition" (Pollack, 1998, 284). As spectators, we tend to categorize boys based on their skill levels and production. Jimmy scored 15 points, while Corey scored 3 points; so, logic says Jimmy must be the better athlete. Parents can use the performance ethic to justify their investment in youth sports, which can ultimately lead to more educational and occupational opportunities. The parents of Jimmy may feel they got a better return on their investment than Corey's parents based on their son's individual performance. Boys playing youth sports are driven by statistical measurements of skill as well.

Statistics serve as a symptom of their boyish competitive nature and a direct reflection of the larger social culture in America.

The pressures from parents, peers, and coaches have elevated the competitive attitude within the realm of boys playing youth sports. Youth sports are organized, facilitated, and coached by adults who can often, whether intentionally or not, project their own competitive agenda on to the kids playing the game. Boys can be overwhelmed with a feeling that they must do well at sports. It is important to understand the value of creating sport options for boys that are not "based exclusively on a power and performance model" (Coakley, 2009, 256).

Boys in American sports are in danger of being overprogrammed athletically and underdeveloped emotionally. That's why the American Academy of Pediatrics recommends that organized youth sports focus on enjoyment rather than competition through age 9 (Farrey, 2008). Pollack (1998) has recommended that coaches push for "personal bests" from boys rather than stressing fierce competition and winning. In this way, boys can begin to see sports as an opportunity for all-around development rather than as an outright test of masculinity. Although parents serve as the primary line of influence for shifting boy's mindset in sports, coaches have a central role to play too.

Coaches can be guilty of gender role stereotyping, in which they place heavier pressure on boys than girls to win and excel. Girls do experience this pressure, especially in highly competitive club and school environments. Generally speaking, however, girls are more likely to participate in a more relaxed atmosphere that places

Table 2 Survey of Boys Playing Youth Sports on the Reasons for Participating

Rank	1989*	2010**
1	To have fun	To have fun
2	To improve my skills	To improve my skills
3	For the excitement of competition	To stay in shape and get exercise
4	To do something I'm good at	For the excitement and challenge of competition
5	To stay in shape	To be part of a team and learn teamwork
6	For the challenge of competition	To make friends
7	To play as part of a team	To go to a higher level of competition
8	To win	To win
9	To go to a higher level of competition	To earn a college scholarship
10	To get exercise	To increase my self-confidence

* *Source:* Ewing and Seefeldt, 1990.
** *Source: Hyman, 2010.*

a higher emphasis on having fun and being with friends. The truth, however, is that both boys *and* girls usually have the same goals when playing sports: to be with friends and to have fun. Two similar surveys (1989 and 2010; see Table 2) asked elementary school-aged children to rank the reasons why they play sports. The results from the boys are seen in Table 2. The answers "to have fun" and "to improve my skills" remain at the top of the list, but the emergence of new reasons such as "to go to a higher level of competition" and "to earn a college scholarship" deserve attention. These results point toward an emerging motivation trend for boys playing sports where competing at the next level is becoming a more important factor when choosing to play a particular sport. Nevertheless, in the 2010 study, 95 percent of boys cited fun as the reason for playing, twice the number of boys who mentioned winning.

Upward Mobility

Sport plays a pivotal role in American society, and its influence trickles down to American youth. In today's culture, the explosion of technology, smartphones, and social media has allowed instant access and live streaming of games and highlight videos. Most of these sports media outlets disseminate dominant masculine norms among boys and young men through what Messner, Dunbar, and Hunt (2000) refer to as the "television sports manhood formula" built around the themes of militarism, aggression, and violence (380). Especially in male sports, impressionable boys may be receiving messages from men "who never really grew up" (Biddulph, 2013, 181).

A relevant issue with this massive exposure to the "wide world of sports" is that it can give a distorted view to boys about the viability of sports as a career path. Young boys in America have long identified strongly with their sport heroes, but the 24-hour sports news cycle in the Internet age makes it even easier now. Within some low-income African American communities, there exists a widely held belief that sport is one of the few paths to upward mobility, even when there is evidence that suggests otherwise. African American athletes dominate the most popular mainstream sports such as football and basketball, acquire endorsements, earn extraordinarily high salaries, and are largely viewed as beloved celebrities. The many stories of male athletes coming from impoverished situations in their youth and succeeding in pro sports as adults is one of the reasons why noted sociologist Stanley Eitzen (2016) found that two-thirds of African American adolescent males believe that they will be a professional athlete when they grow up. However, according to Eitzen, the odds of an African American boy making it to the NFL are 10,000 to 1, and the odds of playing in the NBA are 20,000 to 1. In addition, only

Table 3 Odds of High School Boy Varsity Athletes Playing College or Pro Sports

	Basketball	Baseball	Football	Soccer	Hockey
Playing in any division in college	17:1	9:1	12:1	11:1	9:1
Playing in NCAA Division I	99:1	47:1	41:1	73:1	30:1
Going pro	1,860:1	764:1	603:1	835:1	170:1

Source: Scholarship Stats. 2014. http://www.scholarshipstats.com/varsityodds.html

1 out of every 225 boys who play in the Little League World Series will ever make it to Major League Baseball (Farrey, 2008). The truth is, all but a handful of parents and children chasing the proverbial professional sports carrot will be sorely disappointed (see Table 3).

Some parents are less concerned with their boy's development in a wide range of cognitive, social, and emotional skills and worry more about whether their child will be the next LeBron James. Much of this is guided by hopes of gaining college scholarships, or the slight possibility of their child making it to the "big" leagues. Boys, in addition to their coaches and parents, can easily fall into the trap of hyperfocusing on sports performance, leaving other important developmental aspects of childhood, like education, by the wayside.

Parents and young athletes also view youth sports as a way to obtain college scholarships. This may be particularly true for boys who do not perform as well in the classroom as their peers. However, the percentage of all American children who will end up playing high school sports is under 50 percent; and of those high school athletes, only 2 percent go on to play at an NCAA Division I university. Additionally, out of that 2 percent, only 3 percent of college athletes make it to the professional ranks (Farrey, 2008). A poll by the Harvard T. H. Chan School of Public Health revealed that 26 percent of parents with high school athletes hope their child will one day become a professional athlete (Robert Wood Johnson Foundation, 2015). The numbers were even higher for parents with a high school education or less (44 percent) and those with a household income less than $50,000 a year (39 percent).

The belief that sport is the only—or at least the most likely—path to social and financial mobility for boys (especially from impoverished backgrounds) continues to be a difficult message to combat. Experts point out that upward mobility is much stronger in other reputable industry sectors like engineering, medicine, law, and education just to name a few, and these are career fields that are egregiously underrepresented by minority groups. Ultimately, the proper message is that boys should approach sports as a means, not an end.

Overuse Injuries and Burnout

Sports-related overuse injuries and burnout are also causes for concern for boys, particularly those who specialize early. Being overly competitive in boys' sports leads to risk-taking, aggression, and pushing physical limitations. Young boys too often see playing through injuries and concussions as acts that affirm their masculinity and value. Boys are seen as less masculine when displaying visible signs of pain from an injury, so they hide it as much as possible for fear of being labeled as "soft." Unfortunately, this machismo "jock culture" of high school boys athletics in particular has helped contribute to an increase in the rates of ACL (knee) and UCL (elbow) injuries. Physicians have gone on record opposing sports specialization before boys turn 12 years old. As noted youth sports expert, author, and former ESPN contributor Tom Farrey (2008) stated, "our doctors should be specialists, not our children" (18).

Too much of a single sport at early ages can also cause burnout among both boys and girls. Adolescents who have burned out often choose to reduce the stress of year-round play and high expectations by withdrawing from the sport altogether. Almost three out of four adolescents drop out of youth sport programs by high school (Woods, 2016). A variety of factors have been cited for this trend, but experts in the field have speculated that the overemphasis on winning, specialization at an early age, increased injury incidents, and the high costs of participating in private clubs have all contributed to dropout in some capacity.

The irony with having boys specialize in one sport in hopes of gaining college scholarships is that many of the most successful college football coaches in America openly recruit multisport athletes more heavily than single-sport athletes. An infographic shared by the Ohio State University athletic department went viral in 2015 after it portrayed that 42 out of the 47 recent football players recruited by head coach Urban Meyer played more than one sport in high school (O'Sullivan, 2015). In the 2016 NFL Draft, almost 90 percent of the 253 total drafted players played multiple sports in high school (Vannini, 2016). An American Medical Society for Sports Medicine survey in 2013 found that 88 percent of college athletes surveyed participated in more than one sport as a child (DiFiori et al., 2014). This certainly counters the argument that if parents want their son to play major Division I college football, they need to get him to focus on that single sport at an early age. In fact, Babe Ruth, Roger Federer, Michael Jordan, and most U.S. Olympic male athletes played multiple sports through their adolescent years. Regardless of the facts in support of multisport athletes, some practices in American youth sport programs are designed to not only funnel boys into specific sports, but also into narrow positions within that sport.

Stacking

Another youth sport phenomenon, one that is tinged with racial discrimination and is most prevalent in some boys' sports, is known as stacking. This practice is defined as the disproportionate allocation of athletes to central and noncentral positions as a function of their race or ethnicity (LaVoi and Kane, 2014). Stacking occurs in team sports where there are multiple positions to be filled. Essentially, minority or underrepresented groups are steered away from or into certain positions on the field. Although the phenomenon has waned in recent years due to breakthroughs by high-profile professional sport athletes who break racial and other stereotypes, traditional practices typically take a very long time to be completely phased out. The following scenarios still occur in boy-specific youth sports around the country:

- In football, the best-looking, tall, Caucasian boy from a well-to-do family is picked to play quarterback. The speed positions (e.g., wide receiver, running back, defensive backfield) are saved for the black players, since they are seen as having the most athletic prowess. For the boys who show little promise with hand-eye coordination, they are asked to rarely touch the football and just block for the better athletes. These are also traditionally the most heavyset boys, and they are not encouraged to get into better shape but instead "bulk up" in order to protect the quarterback and/or clog the running lanes on defense.
- In baseball, the biggest/strongest boys are automatically assigned to be the pitchers on their respective teams. After all, they can be viewed as intimidating figures to the opposing batters when standing on the mound. They can also throw the ball the fastest, getting more batters out. The more athletically gifted boys are usually delegated to the shortstop and centerfield positions—the spots that get the most action in the game. The larger/heavyset kids are given the positions that require the least amount of quickness and agility (catcher, first base, and third base). Lowest on the totem pole are the smaller boys who may not be as proficient in catching and throwing as some of their other teammates are at their age. These boys are typically relegated to the two corner outfield positions (right and left field) and second base (due to the short throw to first base). These spots receive the least amount of baseballs hit to them, which can help the team reduce its defensive liabilities and increase the team's chances of winning.

Although these examples are not as prevalent as they once were, they still exist in youth football and baseball around the country. The major problem with the stacking philosophy is that it prematurely funnels boys into very skill-specific positions for the purposes of winning a game or tournament. In the end, the offensive line-man will never get the chance to catch a touchdown pass, the left fielder will never experience the thrill of pitching a baseball, and so on. At such a fragile and critical age, stacking can seriously damage a boy's confidence and psyche for life.

When stacking occurs, it is possible that sports then become an area in life where boys are encouraged *not* to try new things or expand their horizons since many of the variables of sport such as a new coach or different teammates year after year remain the same. Stacking can also help explain why, despite signs of progress, minorities remain underrepresented in certain team sports (e.g., soccer, lacrosse, and baseball). In the *Best Practices for Coaching Soccer in the United States,* a document released by U.S. Soccer, the organization advised coaches not to assign players into specific positions until the teenage years. Such an approach minimizes the likelihood that a young player will come to feel left out, unworthy, or ashamed as a result of his or her role on the team. It also takes into consideration "late bloomers," adolescent boys who have their growth spurts after 15 years of age (Smoll and Smith, 2002, 263). Research is clear that many late bloomers may not grow into their full physiological potential until well into their high school years. Many such boys, however, drift away from sports before reaching this plateau due to coaches who focus their attention on players who mature earlier. As a result, there exists a deficit of late-maturing boys participating in sport around 12 to 15 years of age (Smoll and Smith, 2002).

What happens on the road from middle to high school? Boys who mature early are more commonly seen on the upper level elite teams by high school, and these boys also enjoy enhanced social status among their peers. Late bloomers are discriminated against, encouraged to drop out by high school before their growth spurt, or are cut because they are not yet good enough. The bottom line is: science tells us that the most athletic boy at age 8 may not be the most athletic boy at age 14 when the rest of the field has time to catch up. In fact, jumping ability in all boys continues to improve through 19 years old. All boys eventually reach physical maturity, but adults involved with youth sports too often do not show the patience to wait for them to reach it. This problem is not only exacerbated by the phenomenon of stacking but also by early specialization.

To overgeneralize the problems related to stacking by saying that all youth football and baseball teams in the United States are guilty of the practice would be inaccurate. Indeed, many coaches make it a priority to play every boy at each position that the sport offers so as not to unfairly limit any boy's experience. Some youth sports programs even make it mandatory for all coaches to allow players to experiment playing at every position on the field, both for maximum skill development and fun. Most of the time, this involves a boy playing a handful of positions within the same game. Some coaches and parents laud this strategy, saying it yields the benefits of challenging the player to be a well-rounded athlete, builds self-confidence, and creates a more even playing field among the team. Even so, the practice has not been widely adopted across all of youth sports.

Rise of Alternative Sports

Given some of these issues experienced by boys in youth sports, more and more boys are exploring other participatory sport options to satisfy their competitive needs while also allowing for more freedom and creativity. The current generation of boys are the first to be raised in a world where parents dictate or direct more of their free time than ever before, a dynamic that leaves only fleeting moments of unstructured/unsupervised play for many. Seeking a refuge from the increased structure placed on them in the adult-centric youth sports environment, some boys have chosen to play and compete in the less-traditional realm of so-called alternative sports and eSports. This shift toward alternative or "action sports" is siphoning off boys who might have once played traditional team sports. For example, skateboarding has exploded as an alternative sport since the late 1990s, with many communities nationwide investing in skate parks that have become centers of teen recreational activity. Other alternative sports such as disc golf appeal to boys seeking a sport that costs almost nothing to play and comes free of coaches, schedules, referees, and unrealistic expectations. Many boys thrive in these nontraditional settings, as Coakley (2009) noted: "When I observe children in action sports, I'm regularly amazed by the physical skills that they develop without adult coaches and scheduled practices and contests" (133).

The cultural norm of today's youth sports in America is performance-based, particularly with young boys. Understandably, alternative sports also attract boys who value facing one's fears, taking risks, and earning respect for acts of bravery. Popular examples include skateboarding, snowboarding, surfing, BMX bicycling, mountain biking, climbing, and paintball. Action sports were once viewed as pursuits for outsiders and rebels but are now considered more mainstream than ever before. Action sports are thriving among boys predominantly because they are youth-controlled and not adult-controlled and have little emphasis on ultra-competitiveness.

Sports are beloved American institutions that are widely valued for their potential in helping mold boys into healthy and responsible young men. As boys continue to struggle to keep up with girls in school in some topics, sport is seen as a potential mechanism for boosting educational achievement and fostering masculine development in a respectful manner. When used correctly, advocates say that sports can drastically enhance the development of boys across a wide range of wellness dimensions, while still catering to their prototypical boyish wants and needs.

Troy Carlton, Michael Kanters, and Jeff James

Further Reading

Biddulph, Steve. 2013. *Raising Boys: Why Boys Are Different—and How to Help Them Become Happy and Well-Balanced Men.* New York: Ten Speed Press.

Buller, Leonard T., Matthew J. Best, Michael G. Baraga, and Lee D. Kaplan. 2015. "Trends in Anterior Cruciate Ligament Reconstruction in the United States." *The Orthopaedic Journal of Sports Medicine, 3*(1): 1–8.

Coakley, Jay. 2006. "The Good Father: Parental Expectations and Youth Sports." *Leisure Studies, 25*(2): 153–163.

Coakley, Jay. 2009. *Sports in Society: Issues and Controversies* (10th ed.). New York: McGraw-Hill Higher Education.

DiFiori, John P., Holly J. Benjamin, Joel Brenner, Andrew Gregory, Neeru Jayanthi, Greg L. Landry, and Anthony Luke. 2014. "Overuse Injuries and Burnout in Youth Sports: A Position Statement from the American Medical Society for Sports Medicine." *Clinical Journal Sports Medicine, 24*(1): 3–20.

Drummond, Murray J. N. 2016. "The Voices of Boys on Sport, Health, and Physical Activity: The Beginning of Life through a Gendered Lens." In Michael A. Messner and Michela Musto (Eds.), *Child's Play: Sport in Kids' Worlds* (pp. 144–164). New Brunswick, NJ: Rutgers University Press.

Eitzen, D. Stanley. 2016. *Fair and Foul: Beyond the Myths and Paradoxes of Sport* (6th ed.). Lanham, MD: Rowman & Littlefield.

Ewing, Martha, and Vern Seefeldt. 1990. *American Youth and Sports Participation.* Lansing, MI: Youth Sports Institute at Michigan State University.

Farrey, Tom. 2008. *Game On: The All-American Race to Make Champions of Our Children.* New York: ESPN Publishing.

Fleisig, Glenn S., and James R. Andrews. 2012. "Prevention of Elbow Injuries in Youth Baseball Pitchers." *Sports Health, 4*(5): 419–424.

Hyman, Mark. 2010. *A Survey of Youth Sports Finds Winning Isn't the Only Thing.* Accessed July 27, 2016, at http://www.nytimes.com/2010/01/31/sports/31youth.html?_r=0.

LaVoi, Nicole M., and Mary J. Kane. 2014. "Interscholastic Athletics." In Paul M. Pedersen and Lucie Thibault (Eds.), *Contemporary Sport Management* (5th ed., pp. 427–449). Champaign, IL: Human Kinetics.

Leff, Stephen S., and Rick Hoyle. 1995. "Young Athletes' Perceptions of Parental Support and Pressure." *Journal of Youth and Adolescence, 24*(2): 187–203.

Messner, Michael A., Michele Dunbar, and Darnell Hunt. 2000. "The Televised Sports Manhood Formula." *Journal of Sport and Social Issues, 24*(4): 380–394.

National Federation of State High School Association. 2014. *Athletics Participation Summary.* Accessed December 1, 2014, at www.nfhs.org/ParticipationStatics/PDF/2013 -2014_Participation_Survey_PDF.pdf.

O'Sullivan, John. 2015. *The Perils of Single-Sport Participation.* Accessed on July 27, 2016, at http://changingthegameproject.com/the-perils-of-single-sport-participation.

Pollack, William. 1998. *Real Boys: Rescuing Our Sons from the Myths of Boyhood.* New York: Owl Books.

Robert Morris University. 2014. *RMU Becomes First University to Offer Gaming Scholarships with the Addition of eSports to Varsity Lineup.* Accessed July 27, 2016, at http://www.rmueagles.com/article/907.php.

Robert Wood Johnson Foundation. 2015. *Sports and Health in America.* Accessed July 18, 2016, at http://media.npr.org/documents/2015/june/sportsandhealthpoll.pdf.

Scholarship Stats. 2014. *Odds of a High School Athlete Playing College Sports.* Accessed July 18, 2016, at http://www.scholarshipstats.com/varsityodds.html.

Smoll, Frank L., and Ronald E. Smith. 2002. *Children and Youth in Sport: A Biopsychosocial Perspective* (2nd ed.). Dubuque, IA: Kendall Hunt Publishing.

Vannini, Chris. 2016. *Nearly 90 Percent of 2016 NFL Draft Picks Played Multiple Sports in High School.* Accessed September 2, 2016, at http://coachingsearch.com/article?a =Nearly-90-percent-of-2016-NFL-Draft-picks-played-multiple-sports-in-high-school.

Women's Sports Foundation. 2008. *Go Out and Play: Youth Sports in America.* Accessed June 24, 2016, at www.womenssportsfoundation.org/Content/Research-Reports/Go-Out -and-Play.aspx.

Woods, Ronald B. 2016. *Social Issues in Sport.* Champaign, IL: Human Kinetics.

Bullying

Bullying is a regrettable but not uncommon problem in youth sports. In the past, coaches and even parents sometimes dismissed bullying as "kids just being kids." But things have changed, and there is now total agreement that bullying has no place in sports. There are many desirable physical, psychological, and social effects that can be gained from participation in youth sports. If children get bullied in sports, though, all of the potentially valuable outcomes get canceled out. In addressing the issue of bullying, youth sport coaches have a particularly prominent role to play. By utilizing antibullying resources like StopBullying, a special website maintained by the U.S. Department of Health and Human Services, coaches (and parents and administrators) can take steps to mitigate bullying.

Definition, Types, and Effects of Bullying

Bullying is defined as "unwanted, aggressive behavior among school aged children that involves a real or perceived power imbalance. The behavior is repeated, or has the potential to be repeated, over time" (StopBullying, 2016). This definition includes three key elements. First, bullying is a form of *aggression*. Its purpose is to deliver physical or psychological harm to another person. Bullying is an intentional behavior; it is not an accident. Second, there is an *imbalance of power*. Bullies use their power to control or harm others. Power can include such things as physical strength, popularity, cognitive ability, or access to embarrassing information. It is important to note that those who bully do not need to be stronger or bigger than those they bully. Rather, the power imbalance can come from a number of sources. Third, bullying behavior involves *repetition*. It happens more than once or has the potential to happen more than once.

There are three main types of bullying. In youth sports, the most common forms of *verbal bullying* are name calling, nasty and cruel nicknames, taunting, rudeness, and threats of violence and/or harm to another athlete. *Social* (or relational) bullying involves hurting someone's reputation or relationships. It includes excluding another athlete on purpose, gossiping, hurtful trash talk, and embarrassment of an athlete in front of others. *Physical* bullying involves hurting a person's body or possessions. It includes hitting, slapping, tripping, head butting, towel snapping, spitting, stealing, and making rude hand gestures.

Bullying is a serious problem that has harmful effects on both the victim and the bully. Boys typically bully using physical threats and actions, while girls are more likely to engage in social bullying. Yet, it is also important to note that the label *typically* is used here purposefully, and coaches and administrators should not fall into the all too easy gender stereotype trap and ignore signs of physical bullying from girls or social bullying from boys. Bullying can occur in virtually any setting, including the sport environment. Social media have magnified the problem, with the Internet enabling an epidemic of *cyberbullying* that can follow children into their home, once a safe haven from bullying for most children.

Regardless of the form it takes, bullying takes a terrible emotional and physical toll on children. Victims of bullying feel hurt, angry, afraid, helpless, hopeless, isolated, and ashamed. They may even feel guilty that the bullying is somehow their fault. Victims of bullying are at greater risk of developing mental health problems, such as depression, anxiety, and low self-esteem. In some cases, child and adolescent suicide is linked to bullying. When it occurs in sport settings, victims are more likely to skip practices and games to avoid being bullied. Not surprisingly, bullying is one of the reasons youngsters cite for quitting sports. Moreover, the scars inflicted by bullying can persist long into the future and can predispose a young person to develop psychological problems in adulthood.

Roles Children Play in Bullying

There are many roles that children can play. Being a *perpetrator* is one of the direct roles played in bullying. No single factor puts a child at risk of engaging in bullying. But some athletes who are more likely to bully others are well connected to their teammates, have social power, are overly concerned about their popularity, and like to dominate or be in charge of others. Others are more isolated from their teammates, have low self-esteem, and do not identify with the emotions or feelings of others. They tend to be aggressive or easily frustrated, have issues at home or school, have difficulty following rules, view violence in a positive way, and have friends who bully others.

Another direct role played by children is to be the *victim* of bullying behavior. Some factors put children at greater risk, but not all children with these characteristics will be bullied. Generally, young athletes who are bullied are perceived as "different" from their teammates (e.g., overweight or underweight, wear glasses, lesbian/gay/bisexual/transgender/questioning [LGBTQ] in sexual orientation or identification), and they are perceived as weak or unable to defend themselves. Some bullied children suffer from low self-esteem, are less popular than others and have few friends, do not get along well with others, or are perceived to be annoying or antagonizing to others.

Even if a child is not directly involved in bullying, he or she may be contributing to the behavior by performing several roles as a *witness*. *Assistants* in bullying may not start the action, but they may encourage the bullying behavior. *Reinforcers* are children who give an audience to bullying. They will often laugh or provide support for those who are engaging in bullying and may encourage it to continue. *Bystanders* are children who remain separate from the bullying situation. They neither reinforce the bullying behavior nor defend the child being bullied. But by providing an audience for the bully, bystanders may in fact encourage the bullying behavior. Finally, *defenders* are children who actively come to the aid of victims of bullying.

Children often play more than one role in bullying over time. In some cases, they may be directly involved as a perpetrator; they may be the victim; or they may witness bullying and play the role of assistant, reinforcer, bystander, or defender. Every situation is different. Some children are both perpetrators and victims of bullying. There are two reasons why it is important to recognize the multiple roles children play. First, those who are both bullied and bully others may be at more risk for negative outcomes. Second, it highlights the need to engage all children in prevention efforts, not just those who are known to be directly involved.

Guidelines for Preventing Bullying

As part of their sport safety responsibilities, coaches should take a proactive role in reducing the likelihood that bullying will occur on the teams for which they are responsible. This can be accomplished by devoting the necessary time and effort to implementing the following guidelines:

1. Establish a zero-tolerance policy. At the beginning of the season, coaches must clearly communicate that bullying in any form will not be tolerated. It is impossible to specify every potential behavior that constitutes bullying, but athletes have to understand they must conform with acceptable standards of behavior, both on and off the field/court.

It is well known that people acquire a greater sense of personal accountability if they are given a share of the responsibility for determining their own governance.

In view of this, an effective approach to setting a zero-tolerance policy is for coaches to incorporate it into a system of team rules that are developed with cooperative input from their athletes. Step-by-step procedures for forming team rules are presented elsewhere (Smith and Smoll, 2012, 38–40; Smoll and Smith, 2009).

With the support of parents and administrators, creating a bully-free environment is the responsibility of every youth sport coach. Consequently, team rules (including a zero-tolerance policy) should be shared, in writing, with everyone involved in the program.

2. *Educate young athletes about bullying.* Promoting athletes' understanding of bullying can help sustain prevention efforts over time. Coaches can contribute to this by talking with athletes about what bullying is and what to do if they are the target of bullying or a witness to its occurrence. In team meetings, which are typically short and held on a fairly regular basis, coaches can do the following:

- Provide an opportunity for athletes to express themselves. This can be accomplished by setting aside part of meetings to talk about bullying. Coaches can start conversations with open-ended questions like these: (a) "What does 'bullying' mean to you? What does it feel like to be bullied?" (b) "Have you ever felt scared to come to a practice or game because you were afraid of bullying? What have you done to try to change things?" (c) "Have you or your teammates left other kids out on purpose? Do you think that was bullying? Why or why not?" (d) "Do you ever see kids on our team being bullied? How does it make you feel?" (e) "What do you usually do when you see bullying going on?" and (f) "Have you ever tried to help someone who is being bullied? What happened? What would you do if it happens again?" In leading the discussions, coaches should assure athletes that they are not alone in addressing any problems that arise.
- Encourage athletes to speak to the coach if they are bullied or see others being bullied. The coach can give comfort, support, and advice, even if they might not be able to immediately solve the problem.
- Talk about how to stand up to bullies. Give tips, such as (a) look at the bully and say "stop" in a calm, clear voice, or (b) try to use humor and laugh it off, which could catch the bully off guard. If speaking up seems too hard or not safe, the victim should not fight back. Rather, they should walk away and go directly to the coach.
- Talk about strategies for staying safe. The strategies can include (a) telling coaches about the problem, so they can help athletes make a plan to stop the bullying, (b) avoiding situations in which bullying occurs, and (c) staying near coaches, as most bullying happens when adults are not around.

- Urge athletes to help others who are bullied. The assistance can involve (a) letting the bully know that such behavior is a violation of the zero-tolerance policy, (b) creating a distraction or focusing attention on something else, (c) helping the athlete being bullied escape the scene, (d) finding the coach, or asking a teammate to find the coach as soon as possible, and (e) simply being nice to the bullied athletes, which goes a long way toward letting them know they are not alone.

3. Put an emphasis on team building and creating a "family" atmosphere. One of the keys to preventing bullying is to create a safe and socially supportive sport environment. This involves establishing a culture of inclusion and respect that welcomes all athletes. The basic approach is encompassed in what is known as a *mastery climate*. In such a climate, the goal is to foster positive growth as an athlete and as a person. The emphasis is on effort, learning, and personal improvement—doing what it takes to be *your* best. To be sure, winning is valued, but in a mastery climate, the adults realize that winning takes care of itself if athletes are having fun, improving their skills, giving maximum effort, and are not shackled with fear of failure. Mastery climates foster an atmosphere of mutual support and encouragement, and everyone, regardless of ability, is made to feel an important part of the team. Detailed instructions for creating mastery climates appear elsewhere (Smith and Smoll, 2012, 29–51; Smoll and Smith, 2009).

Within the context of a caring environment, coaches can work to increase athletes' empathy based on the golden rule: "Do unto others as you would have them do unto you." Athletes should be instructed to never treat others in a manner they would find hurtful if it were done to them. They should be encouraged to regularly place themselves in the shoes of others. It is well known that lack of empathy lies behind bullying, and that empathy inhibits bullying. Moreover, empathy learned in sports creates better people outside of sports as well.

4. Be aware that coaching behaviors impact athletes. Children learn from adults' actions. By treating others with kindness and respect, coaches demonstrate the opposite of bullying. All coaching actions, including tone of voice and body language, set the standards of behavior for their team. For example, if coaches tease or yell at an athlete, they are giving subtle permission for youngsters to do the same thing. The point is that coaches have to consistently model how to treat others appropriately.

5. Keep the lines of communication open. Athletes need to know they should come to their coach if they see bullying or are the victim of it. Athletes should understand that they can play an important role in helping to prevent bullying, that coaches welcome their input, and that coaches will take action to stop bullying.

6. Look for warning signs of bullying. There are many "red flags" that may indicate someone is either being bullied or bullying others. Recognizing the warning signs is an important first step in combating bullying.

With respect to signs that an athlete is a victim of bullying, coaches should look for changes in the youngster. However, they should be aware that not all athletes who are bullied exhibit warning signs. Some signs that may point to a bullying problem are (a) unexplainable injuries; (b) lost or destroyed uniforms or equipment; (c) frequent headaches or stomach aches, feeling sick or faking illness; (d) loss of interest in the sport, or not wanting to go to practices and games; (e) expressed feelings of helplessness or decreased self-esteem; and (f) decreased or inconsistent performance.

Coaches also have a responsibility to look for signs that an athlete is a perpetrator of bullying. Athletes may be bullying others if they (a) frequently get into physical or verbal fights, (b) have unexplained new belongings, (c) have disciplinary problems in school, (d) blame others for their shortcomings, (e) don't accept responsibility for their actions, and (f) are overly competitive and worry about their reputation or popularity.

If any of the danger signals listed above appear, coaches should not ignore the problem. Rather, they should take immediate corrective or remedial actions.

Remedial Actions to Take in Response to Bullying

Despite the best efforts of coaches, the reality is that bullying is a frequent occurrence in organized sports. In view of this, the recommendations in this section, adapted from the StopBullying website to fit youth sports, are intended to correct the problem behavior, prevent another occurrence of bullying, and protect and support the children involved in the incident.

1. Recognize that coaches have the right and the responsibility to intervene. As adult supervisors, coaches are responsible for the behavior of their athletes, and combating bullying is part of their job. If coaches see bullying, they should not assume the athletes will work it out themselves. Rather, coaches have the authority and the obligation to step in and put a stop to bullying.

2. Get involved immediately. When coaches respond quickly and consistently to bullying, they send a message that the behavior is unacceptable. There are simple procedures that can be used to stop bullying on the spot and keep athletes safe. The actions include the "dos" and "don'ts" presented as follows:

Do:

- Intervene immediately. If necessary, get another adult to help.
- Separate the athletes involved.
- Make sure everyone is safe.
- Meet any immediate medical or psychological needs.
- Stay calm. Reassure the athletes involved, including bystanders.
- Model respectful behavior when intervening.

Avoid these common mistakes:

- Don't ignore it. Don't think athletes can work it out without adult help.
- Don't immediately try to sort out the facts.
- Don't force other athletes to say publicly what they saw.
- Don't question the children involved in front of others.
- Don't talk to the athletes involved together, only separately.
- Don't make the youngsters involved apologize or "patch things up" on the spot.

3. Find out what happened. Whether the coach just stopped bullying or an athlete reached out to the coach for help, the best way to proceed is to get the facts. This involves (a) keeping all the involved athletes separate; (b) getting the story from several sources, both athletes and adults; (c) listening without blaming; and (d) not calling the act "bullying" while trying to understand what happened. It may be difficult to get the whole story, especially if multiple athletes are involved, but coaches should collect all available information.

After getting the facts, coaches can then determine whether the situation is bullying or something else. This can be done by reviewing the definition of bullying and considering whether there is a power imbalance and/or history of bullying between the athletes involved. Also, if any of the athletes are in a gang, coaches should get police help, as gang violence has different ramifications and interventions.

4. Address bullying behavior with the perpetrator. The following guidelines are intended to assist coaches in working with athletes who have engaged in bullying behavior:

- Show athletes that bullying is taken seriously. Remind them of the zero-tolerance policy, and calmly tell the youngster that bullying is unacceptable. Model respectful behavior when addressing the problem.

- Make sure the athlete knows what the problem behavior is and how hurtful such behavior can be. Athletes who bully must learn their behavior is wrong and harms others. In admonishing bullying behavior, coaches should explain why the behavior is wrong. The explanation is intended to promote under-standing and (hopefully) "shaping-up."
- Foster empathy by encouraging the athletes who bullied to look at their actions from the victim's perspective. Ask them how they would feel if they were treated in that way. The goal is to help them understand how their actions affect others.
- Work with the athletes to understand some of the reasons they bullied. For example, sometimes athletes bully to fit in. These athletes can benefit from taking leadership roles, such as assistant team captain (coaches would not, however, want to reward an athlete who engaged in bullying with such a lead-ership position). Other times athletes act out because something else is going on in their lives—issues at home, abuse, stress. They also may have been bullied themselves. These children will likely need to be referred to mental health services for professional counseling.
- Involve the athlete who bullied in making amends, or repairing the situa-tion. For example, the athlete can write a letter apologizing to the teammate who was bullied, or do a good deed for the child who was bullied.
- Use consequences to teach. An effective behavior change procedure is to withdraw privileges from the offending athlete. In response cost (also called negative punishment or punishment by removal), an unwanted behavior is decreased by removal of something that an individual finds satisfying (i.e., "that'll cost you"). In sports, coaches can deprive athletes of things they value. For example, participation can be temporarily suspended by having the athlete who bullied sit off to the side, preferably in isolation ("time out" or "penalty box"). Taking away playing time or a starting position are also effective penalties. Temporary removal of the athlete from the team (i.e., withdrawing the privilege of sport participation) is an advanced form of response cost that may be necessary.
- Follow-up. After the bullying issue is resolved, coaches should continue to help the athletes who bullied to understand how their behavior affects other people. Along with this, coaches should liberally praise acts of thoughtful-ness or other evidences of positive behavior toward teammates.
- Permanently expel the athlete from the team. Elimination from a program is a last resort that should occur only after diligent efforts have been made to correct the problem. The situation is complicated by the fact that sports may be the only avenue for reaching the child, and a coach's relationship with the youngster may turn out to be a curative one.

5. Support athletes who are bullied. The following guidelines are intended to assist coaches in working with athletes who are the victims of bullying:

- Listen and focus on the athlete. Coaches should never tell athletes to ignore bullying. They should learn what has happened, show they want to help, and let victims of bullying know they are going to intervene and stop the bullying.
- Assure the athletes that bullying is not their fault. Coaches should not blame the athletes for being bullied. Even if they provoked the bullying, no one deserves that kind of treatment. The bullied athlete may be doing things that evoke negative responses and dislike from others. For example, some children may be seen as annoying or aggravating. If the athlete has been irritating others, counsel them on how to change the offending behaviors and become more socially successful. However, it is critically important not to do this in the moment directly after the bullying has occurred, as it will assuredly serve as unintended support for the notion that the bullying was their fault.
- Know that youngsters who are bullied may struggle with talking about it. In such cases, coaches should consider referring them to a school counselor or a psychologist.
- Give advice about what to do. Coaches should not tell the athlete to physically fight back against the youngster who is bullying, as it could spur violence. Rather, they can talk about the recommendations presented in the earlier section on how to "Educate young athletes about bullying." More exactly, coaches should (a) encourage bullied athletes to speak to them, (b) talk about how to stand up to bullies, and (c) discuss strategies for staying safe.
- Work together to resolve the situation and protect the bullied athlete. It may help to ask the child being bullied what can be done to make him or her feel safe. It is also beneficial to develop an action plan that includes steps to be taken to stop bullying and to maintain open communication with the athlete.
- Be persistent and follow up. Bullying will not likely end overnight. Coaches must commit to making it stop and consistently support the bullied athlete. Because bullying behavior repeats or has the potential to be repeated, it takes consistent effort to ensure that it stops.

6. Support athletes who witness bullying. Even if athletes are not perpetrators or victims of bullying, they can be affected by it. Many times, when athletes see bullying, they may not know what to do to stop it. They may not feel safe stepping in at the moment, but there are many other steps they can take. In regard to this, coaches can give advice about (a) reporting incidents of bullying to them, (b) how to stand up to bullies, and (c) strategies for staying safe. For details, see the earlier section on how to "Educate young athletes about bullying."

7. Report the incident to the sport program administrator. It is unfair to subject athletes to intolerable situations, and it is not the coach's responsibility to shoulder the burden of dealing with bullying alone. Coaches have plenty of things to do, so they shouldn't hesitate to seek assistance from program administrators.

8. Report the incident to the athletes' parents. As mentioned earlier, consideration of the responsibilities of parents is beyond the scope of this entry. However, when incidents of bullying occur, coaches should have a conference with parents to determine whether they can help. In regard to this, parents should be instructed to resist the urge to contact the other parents involved, as it may make matters worse. Instead, coaches or program administrators can act as mediators between parents.

Finally, some coaches find it helpful for parents to form a team safety committee—a small group of people focused on sport safety concerns. In addition to monitoring factors involved in preventing sport injuries, the committee could assist coaches in planning bullying prevention and intervention programs, and in educating athletes and parents about bullying.

Frank L. Smoll and Ronald E. Smith

Further Reading

Smith, Ronald E., and Frank L. Smoll. 2012. *Sport Psychology for Youth Coaches: Developing Champions in Sports and Life.* Lanham, MD: Rowman & Littlefield.

Smoll, Frank L., and Ronald E. Smith. 2009. *Mastery Approach to Coaching: A Self-Instruction Program for Youth Sport Coaches* [Video]. Accessed at http://www.y-e-sports.org.

Smoll, Frank L., and Ronald E. Smith. *Coaching and Parenting Young Athletes* [Blog]. Accessed at https://www.psychologytoday.com/blog/coaching-and-parenting-young-athletes.

StopBullying. 2016. U.S. Department of Health & Human Services. Accessed September 19, 2016, at http://www.stopbullying.gov.

Burnout among Child and Adolescent Athletes

Youth team sport is an enormous industry in the United States, serving an estimated 29.4 million participants ages 6 to 17 in 2016 (Sports and Fitness Industry Association, 2017), with the total industry estimated at over $9.0 billion in team sports equipment. Despite recent declines in overall youth sports participation, sports remain popular with an estimated 57 percent of children ages 6 to 17 participating in at least one of the 24 sports examined by the Sports and Fitness Industry Association in 2016. Sports media coverage also continues to grow for all levels, most notably youth, with increasing television coverage for state, regional, national, and international competitions.

Most parents, children, and coaches indicate that the most important aspects of sport participation for youth are social, psychological, and physical development. Specifically, some of the commonly perceived benefits of youth sport participation include moral and character development, increased opportunities for socialization with other children, learning about hard work and discipline, learning about winning and losing in a mature fashion, learning to deal with pressure, and physical health and well-being. Although these altruistic motives are often stated by adults as the primary goals for children participating in sport, the participants themselves often perceive a much stronger focus on winning than they do on these other benefits. With the increased popularity of youth sports also comes a stronger focus on winning and success at all levels. This focus on winning comes from many sources, including the players themselves, their parents, coaches, schools, and communities. It can take the form of pressure-filled exhortations from parents, the behavior of fans on the sidelines at competitions, playing-time decisions made by coaches, the practice strategies and techniques used by coaches, and the rules enacted by youth sport organizations.

One of the youth sport trends that has been increasingly linked to the prioritization of winning has been sport specialization among youth sport athletes. Sport specialization is the process of youth sport athletes training intensely, year-round, for one sport, to the exclusion of other activities and sports. With the increasing media attention and money associated with sports, parents may perceive that early sport specialization will increase the chances of their children receiving college scholarships or playing sports professionally, despite the fact that research has not supported this claim. Although literature on the topic of youth sport specialization is becoming more common and more cases are being written about athletes who specialize at a young age, little data exists to suggest the percentage of youth sport athletes who specialize in one sport. However, evidence does suggest that youth athletes who *do* specialize in one sport may be at a higher risk for experiencing burnout.

Children discontinue their sport participation for many different reasons. Among these reasons are a loss of interest, not having fun, feeling as if too much pressure is put on them to perform, and dissatisfaction with coaching. However, the impact of burnout on youth sport athletes should not be overlooked as one of the reasons why children discontinue participation. There are many factors associated with the current structure of youth sport programs that could lead athletes to experience burnout. As such, the following sections will examine the relevant definitions of burnout for youth athletes, in addition to the characteristics and correlates of youth athlete burnout. Finally, practical suggestions and recommendations are forwarded for youth sport stakeholders to consider in order to minimize the likelihood of burnout occurring.

Defining Athlete Burnout

Several terms are often used interchangeably in youth sport when referencing burnout, when in fact the phenomenon is something quite specific in terms of its root cause and the symptoms a young athlete would experience. For example, those unfamiliar with burnout may use this term to describe a young athlete's experience, when what is actually occurring would be what the literature refers to as *overtraining, staleness,* or *dropout.* Although some may consider each of these as being associated with burnout, they all likely represent a different set of characteristics that differentiate them from athlete burnout.

Truth be told, a uniform definition of burnout has been difficult to formulate because of its complexity; in fact, across the sport burnout research it has yet to be consistently, operationally defined. However, there appears to be some consensus among professionals that the various definitions of burnout typically consider the phenomenon as a multidimensional experience; thus, there are likely several components that distinguish athlete burnout from other negative sport outcomes such as overtraining and staleness.

One of the earlier and nonsport definitions of burnout was forwarded by Christina Maslach and Susan Jackson (1981). They suggested that burnout was a syndrome consisting of emotional exhaustion, depersonalization, and a reduced sense of personal accomplishment. This conceptualization has since been adapted within sport-specific contexts and led to definitions more applicable to athletic populations. For example, Ronald Smith (1986) asserted that burnout be considered a multidimensional experience that includes emotional, psychological, and occasionally physical withdrawal (e.g., dropout) from a previously enjoyable activity due to extreme and persistent stress. Although it is likely that stress is involved in the experience of burnout, researchers have also presented conceptualizations of burnout that are more inclusive of additional characteristics of this phenomenon. This is particularly true as one critique of Smith's widely used definition has been that it fails to differentiate athletes who withdraw from sport due to burnout versus dropping out for other reasons.

Extending the definitions from Smith (1986) and Maslach and Jackson (1981), Thomas Raedeke (1997) created one of the most widely used perspectives of athlete burnout. Basing his work on a series of previously published sport burnout studies, Raedeke conceptualized burnout as a process consisting of (1) emotional and physical exhaustion, (2) a reduced sense of sport accomplishment, and (3) a devaluation of one's sport that all occur over time. This definition also represents the components included in the Athlete Burnout Questionnaire (Raedeke and Smith, 2001) that sport and exercise psychology professionals use to measure burnout among athletes.

In contrast to some of the stress-based definitions and perspectives of burnout, noted youth sports expert and sociologist Jay Coakley (1992) suggested that burnout might best be viewed as a sociological phenomenon; this appears to be particularly important as it pertains to the experience of burnout among youth athletes. Although he acknowledged stress as an important component in understanding burnout, Coakley suggested burnout is best explained as a social phenomenon and proposed that burnout may be associated with the social development of young athletes, the social relationships involved with participating in sport, and the social structure of sport itself. More specifically, youth athletes may experience burnout and withdraw from sport due to dissatisfaction with a sense that they are leading a restricted set of life experiences centered exclusively around athletics; for these youth this may result in what he referred to as a unidimensional identity based solely on their role as an athlete. Furthermore, Coakley suggested that burnout occurred from an athlete's perceived lack of autonomy and control over his or her involvement in sport, particularly in relation to the influence of other youth sport stakeholders (e.g., coaches and parents).

As the definitions and frameworks used to conceptualize burnout vary, so may the signs and symptoms of the phenomenon among youth athletes according to the theoretical framework used. Yet, there are several common characteristics considered by most researchers to be representative of athlete burnout among youth athletes, which shall be summarized in the following section. However, as a note of caution, it is important to be aware that burnout is not experienced in the same way by all athletes and could therefore occur with different symptoms or warning signs among youth.

Potential Signs and Symptoms of Burnout

There is a general belief that chronic stress plays some role in the symptoms, signs, and consequences of burnout among athletes, although the degree of its influence may vary. In one of the earlier published findings about burnout within sport environments, David Feigley (1984) suggested that burnout among athletes be considered a progressive experience that occurs in stages. More specifically, those experiencing burnout in its beginning stages may experience an increasing state of fatigue and irritability as well as a loss of enthusiasm for their sport. Physically, athletes may notice minor body aches as well as changes in their eating habits. Feigley also suggested that some athletes may feel less successful in their sport, in addition to increased frustration and anger associated with their athlete role. During the intermediate stage, athletes may show signs of being more withdrawn or apathetic toward their sport. Physical symptoms at this stage include more excessive disordered eating behaviors and severe fatigue. Finally, at its advanced stage, athletes might experience cynicism and avoidant behavior toward their sport.

Other researchers have identified similar symptoms and signs of athlete burnout. For example, a wide array of physical characteristics has been identified such as fatigue, injury, sleeplessness, headaches, shortness of breath, and weight fluctuations. Behaviorally, athletes may become more easily angered or frustrated, experience performance inconsistencies or decrements, and possibly drop out or withdraw from the sport altogether. Emotionally, those experiencing burnout may feel helpless, depressed, irritable, and experience negativity and less enjoyment toward their sport.

In summary, the sport psychology literature has seen several theoretical frameworks emerge over the past three decades, each attempting to define and explain the burnout experiences among athletes. Many of these frameworks have utilized a stress-based perspective to explain the burnout experience. However, given the sociological and motivational influences that appear to be relevant for youth sport participants, Coakley's (1992) unidimensional identity model will be used as a mechanism to examine the correlates and realities of burnout unique to youth athlete populations.

Correlates and Realities of Burnout

When considering the main tenets associated with Coakley's model for burnout among youth athletes, specific variables appear to be particularly relevant to examine. These include the strength and exclusivity of one's athletic identity and early sport specialization, the role of other sport stakeholders in the youth athlete experience, and the perceived control and autonomy youth athletes have regarding their sport involvement.

Athletic Identity and Early Sport Specialization

Relatively few studies have addressed the influence of a unidimensional identity centered on the development of athlete burnout; further, these findings have yielded mixed results. However, there is some evidence to support assertions that unidimensional identity (i.e., defining one's self in an exclusive manner, like through a single sport) contributes to the occurrence of burnout among youth. This is particularly true considering the fact that this identity is based solely on that of an athletic role rather than a more diversified series of roles or experiences outside of sport. This can also be compounded by the process of early sport specialization, in which athletes restrict their participation in athletics to one single sport at a young age, often using a regimented protocol for their training with the hopes of gaining expertise and attaining status as an elite athlete. Although not uncommon to youth sport environments, this process becomes particularly problematic when young athletes make this commitment to specialize prematurely in their development. Developmental psychologists and researchers have found sport sampling to be more appropriate for younger athletes. In fact, it has been suggested that one of the many potential negative consequences of early sport specialization among youth athletes is burnout.

The Role of Sport Stakeholders

The influence of other sport-related stakeholders (e.g., parents and coaches) may also contribute to burnout among youth athletes. For example, one study found that 90 percent of the burned-out adolescent athletes they interviewed described their parental influences as being negative, stressful, inhibiting of autonomy, and delivering harmful feedback with respect to their self-esteem as an athlete (Udry et al., 1997). Another qualitative study of burned-out elite junior tennis players described the experiences of an athlete who reported negative pressure and overinvolvement by the mother and the coach as contributing factors (Gould et al., 1997). Thus, it seems feasible that one negative outcome of what has been termed the "helicopter parent" in youth sport may be the inhibition of the autonomy of young athletes. This could undermine athletes' perception of control, thereby contributing to the potential of experiencing burnout.

In addition to the potential impact of parents, coaches may also play an important role in burnout among youth athletes. For example, one study examined the impact that coaching behaviors have on both anxiety and burnout among female varsity soccer players. Coaches perceived as using more autocratic decision-making styles and giving less training and instruction, less social support, and less positive feedback were all associated with increased levels of burnout and anxiety for these athletes (Price and Weiss, 2000). Thus, given the important role coaches play as a key stakeholder in the experiences of youth athletes, it appears that in addition to parental influences, coaches have the potential to also play a role in the development of burnout.

Perceived Control and Autonomy

The degree to which athletes have control over their sport involvement and the ability to make decisions pertaining to their sport participation also appears to be important when it comes to the experience of burnout. In 1996, for example, researchers examined burnout among elite junior tennis players. They found that athletes reporting higher levels of burnout also noted having less input into their own training (Gould, Tuffey, Udry, & Loehr, 1996). This perceived lack of control over their sport participation might contribute to the presence of burnout as explained by self-determination theory (SDT). In fact, previous research using SDT to study athlete burnout has revealed important findings. For example, research has consistently found a positive association between athlete burnout and less self-determined forms of motivation, in addition to a negative relationship between burnout and more autonomous forms of motivation. Thus, it appears that athletes who have more control over the nature and extent of their sport participation are less likely to experience burnout.

Practical Recommendations for Youth Sport Stakeholders

For sport advocates who believe in the value of sport in the lives of youth, the associated negative by-products of burnout through sport have the potential to impact other aspects of an individual's life. Therefore, it is essential that steps be taken to decrease the likelihood of burnout in youth sport athletes. This section provides information and suggestions from previous research studies (see Further Reading) and extrapolates information from burnout theory to create suggestions for helping important youth sport stakeholders decrease the likelihood of youth sport athletes burning out. The major stakeholders involved in youth sport who may have the ability to decrease the likelihood of youth sport athletes experiencing burnout include the athletes, their parents and coaches, and youth sport administrators.

Athletes

Several suggestions have been provided by researchers to help athletes decrease the likelihood of experiencing burnout. The primary suggestions for youth athletes would include the following:

- Remember that sport is just a game and not a job.
- Ensure that you are playing for your own reasons.
- Focus on additional areas/topics outside of your sport.
- Try to make sport fun, and if it is not fun, don't play.
- Remember that year-round participation is not necessarily better; consider taking some time off from your sport periodically.
- Learn how to relax and enjoy sport.
- Focus more on the development of skills and the effort to be successful rather than the outcome of competitions.
- Make time for other commitments (e.g., school).
- Spend time with friends away from sport.
- Eat healthy and remember to get an appropriate amount of sleep.

Parents

Parents play an important role in the growth and development of their children in all areas of their lives. As such, parents spend a great deal of time around their children in both sport and nonsport environments and can provide a great deal of influence on how children and adolescents experience sport. With this in mind, it is essential that parents understand the role that they play in the development and identification of burnout in their children. Some of the suggestions for parents to help decrease the likelihood of their children experiencing burnout include:

- Provide the optimal amount of push to give their children with regard to sport.

- Be willing to reduce their involvement in sport.
- Encourage children to see themselves as much more than only an athlete.
- Talk with their children to find out what they want rather than telling them what to do.
- Either avoid coaching or separate the roles of coach and parent.
- Don't emphasize the outcome of competition but rather the development of skills and the effort exerted to be successful.
- Be supportive and empathize with their children.
- Promote their child's engagement in other activities.
- Provide opportunities for their children to "act" like kids and enjoy typical developmentally appropriate activities.
- Encourage their children to express themselves and their feelings about their sport.
- Ensure they are receiving proper nutrition and sleep.
- Provide structure to allow them time to complete other work (e.g., school).
- Take steps to keep them with coaches whom they respect and respect them.
- Allow their children to compete in sport at a level that is appropriate and enjoyable to them.

Coaches

Coaches often spend more time with youth athletes in the sporting environment than any other adults. As such, they have a strong influence over the sport setting and the way athletes view sport. With this in mind, several suggestions for coaches to help them decrease the likelihood of burnout include:

- Develop a personal involvement with the athlete that involves discussions about topics outside of sport.
- Encourage athletes to take time off to help refresh themselves.
- Develop two-way communication with the athlete that allows the athlete to make some decisions.
- Work to understand their players' feelings.
- Coach the athletes at the right level.
- Promote a positive atmosphere.
- Vary training methods and time requirements to avoid overtraining and boredom.
- Ensure that athletes are competing at the proper level.

- Find ways to reward athletes for effort and the development of new skills rather than the outcome of competitions.
- Promote the development of resilience and perceived competence in athletes.

Administrators

Many youth sport programs are run through leagues directed and managed by league administrators. Given the control that league administrators have over the structure and function of the league, they can indirectly have a strong impact on the overall competitive and training experiences of young athletes. Some suggestions for administrators to help decrease burnout among their athletes include:

- Write and publicize a mission and vision for the league that promotes a focus on youth development.
- Make all rules and decisions based on this mission and vision.
- Develop rules that allow athletes to compete in a safe environment with athletes of a similar maturity and ability level.
- Seek out qualified coaches to coach each team.
- Provide training for coaches to help them understand and abide by the mission and vision for the league.
- Provide training to parents to help promote a positive sport environment for the children.
- Enforce an environment that allows children to participate in a positive and supportive environment.

Conclusion

In sum, the physical, psychosocial, and developmental benefits associated with youth sport involvement have been well documented over the years. It is unfortunate that staleness and burnout can be realistic, yet unintended consequences for youth athletes. However, remaining aware of the aforementioned risk factors, symptoms, and suggestions for prevention and treatment of burnout can help many youth sport stakeholders ensure that youth sport experience remains a positive one for youth athletes across the developmental life span.

Brandonn S. Harris and Jack C. Watson II

Further Reading

Black, Jennifer M., and Alan L. Smith. 2007. "An Examination of Coakley's Perspective on Identity, Control, and Burnout among Adolescent Athletes." *International Journal of Sport Psychology, 38*: 417–436.

Coakley, Jay. 1992. "Burnout among Adolescent Athletes: A Personal Failure or Social Problem?" *Sociology of Sport Journal, 9*: 271–285.

Côté, Jean. 2004, January. *Education through Sport Participation: A Developmental Perspective.* European Lunch of the European Year of Education through Sport (EYES), Dublin, Ireland.

Cresswell, Scott L., and Robert C. Eklund. 2005a. "Motivation and Burnout among Top Amateur Rugby Players." *Medicine & Science in Sports & Exercise, 37*: 469–477.

Cresswell, Scott L., and Robert C. Eklund. 2005b. "Changes in Athlete Burnout and Motivation over a 12-Week League Tournament." *Medicine & Science in Sports & Exercise, 37*: 1957–1966.

Cresswell, Scott L., and Robert C. Eklund. 2006. "Athlete Burnout: Conceptual Confusion, Current Research, and Future Research Directions." In Sheldon Hanton and Stephen D. Mellalieu (Eds.), *Literature Reviews in Sport Psychology* (pp. 91–126). New York: Nova Science Publishers.

Deci, Edward, and Richard M. Ryan. 1985. *Intrinsic Motivation and Self-Determination in Human Behavior.* New York: Plenum.

DiFiori, John P., Holly J. Benjamin, Joel S. Brenner, Andrew Gregory, Neeru Jayanthi, Greg L. Landrey, and Anthony Luke. 2014. "Overuse Injuries and Burnout in Youth Sports: A Position Statement from the American Medical Society for Sports Medicine." *British Journal of Sports Medicine, 48*: 287–288.

Dubuc, Nicole G., Robert J. Schinke, Mark A. Eys, Randy Battochio, and Leonard Zaichowski. 2010. "Experiences of Burnout among Adolescent Female Gymnasts: Three Case Studies." *Journal of Clinical Sport Psychology, 4*: 1–18.

Feigley, David A. 1984. "Psychological Burnout in High-Level Athletes." *The Physician and Sportsmedicine, 12*: 109–119.

Fraser-Thomas, Jessica L., Jean Côté, and Janice Deakin. 2005. "Youth Sport Programs: An Avenue to Foster Positive Youth Development." *Physical Education and Sport Pedagogy, 10*: 19–40.

Gould, Daniel. 1996. "Personal Motivation Gone Awry: Burnout in Competitive Athletes." *Quest, 48*: 275–289.

Gould, Daniel, Suzanne Tuffey, Eileen Udry, and James Loehr. 1996. "Burnout in Competitive Junior Tennis Players: II. A Qualitative Analysis." *The Sport Psychologist, 10*: 341–366.

Gould, Daniel, Suzanne Tuffey, Eileen Udry, and James Loehr. 1997. "Burnout in Competitive Junior Tennis Players: III. Individual Differences in the Burnout Experience." *The Sport Psychologist, 11*: 257–275.

Gould, Daniel, Eileen Udry, Suzanne Tuffey, and James Loehr. 1996. "Burnout in Competitive Junior Tennis Players: I. A Quantitative Psychological Assessment." The Sport Psychologist, *10*: 322–340.

Harris, Brandonn S., and Andrew C. Ostrow. 2007. "Coach and Athlete Burnout: The Role of Coaches' Decision-Making Style." *Journal of Contemporary Athletics, 2*: 393–412.

Harris, Brandonn S., and Jack C. Watson II. 2011. "Self-Determination Theory and Coakley's Unidimensional Identity Model: An Evaluation of Relevant Measures for the Assessment of Youth Sport Burnout." *Journal of Clinical Sport Psychology, 5*: 117–133.

Harris, Brandonn S., and Jack C. Watson II. 2014. "Developmental Considerations in Youth Athlete Burnout: A Model for Youth Sport Participants." *Journal of Clinical Sport Psychology, 8*: 1–18.

Malina, Robert M. 2010. "Early Sport Specialization: Roots, Effectiveness, Risks." *Current Sports Medicine Reports, 9*: 364–371.

Maslach, Christina, and Susan E. Jackson. 1981. "The Measurement of Experienced Burnout." *Journal of Occupational Behaviour, 2*: 99–113.

National Council of Youth Sports. 2008. *Report on Trends and Participation in Organized Youth Sports.* Accessed June 30, 2015, at http://www.ncys.org/publications/2008-sports-participation-study.php.

NCYS Report on Trends and Participation in Organized Youth Sports. 2008. Accessed June 30, 2015, at http://www.ncys.org/pdfs/2008/2008-ncys-market-research-report.pdf.

Organized Youth Sports. Market Research Report. NCYS Membership Survey—2008 Edition. Accessed at http://www.ncys.org/pdfs/2008/2008-ncys-market-research-report.pdf.

Price, Melissa, and Maureen Weiss. 2000. "Relationships among Coach Burnout, Coach Behaviors, and Athletes' Psychological Responses." *The Sport Psychologist, 14*: 391–409.

Raedeke, Thomas. 1997. "Is Athlete Burnout More Than Just Stress? A Sport Commitment Perspective." *Journal of Sport & Exercise Psychology, 19*: 396–417.

Raedeke, Thomas, and Alan Smith. 2001. "Development and Preliminary Validation of an Athlete Burnout Measure." *Journal of Sport & Exercise Psychology, 23*: 281–306.

Sabo, Don, and Phil Veliz. 2008. *Go Out and Play: Youth Sports in America.* Women's Sports Foundation. Accessed June 30, 2015, at http://www.womenssportsfoundation.org/en/home/research/articles-and-reports/mental-and-physical-health/go-out-and-play.

Sage, George H., and Stanley D. Eitzen. 2013. *Sociology of North American Sport.* New York: Oxford University Press.

Smith, Ronald. 1986. "Toward a Cognitive-Affective Model of Athletic Burnout." *Journal of Sport Psychology, 8*: 36–50.

Sports and Fitness Industry Association (SFIA). 2017. *2017 Sports, Fitness, and Leisure Activities Topline Participation Report.* Data provided on August 24, 2017, by SFIA.

Udry, Eileen, Daniel Gould, Dana Bridges, and Suzanne Tuffey. 1997. "People Helping People? Examining the Social Ties of Athletes Coping with Burnout and Injury Stress." *Journal of Sport & Exercise Psychology, 19*: 368–395.

Vealey, Robin, Comar L. Armstrong, and Christy Greenleaf. 1998. "Influence of Perceived Coaching Behaviors on Burnout and Competitive Anxiety in Female College Athletes." *Journal of Applied Sport Psychology, 10*: 297–318.

Vitali, Francesca, Laura Bortoli, Luciano Bertinato, Claudio Robazza, and Federico Schena. 2015. "Motivational Climate, Resilience, and Burnout in Youth Sport." *Sport Sciences for Health, 11*: 103–108.

Wiersma, Leonard D. 2000. "Risks and Benefits of Youth Sport Specialization: Perspectives and Recommendations." *Pediatric Exercise Science, 12*: 13–22.

Character Development

A common misperception in society is that youth sports inevitably build character. Although one of the benefits of youth sport participation is the opportunity to build desirable qualities and characteristics, this does not always happen; the process of character development does not occur automatically. Young people who engage in sport have a wide range of experiences that are influenced by a number of factors—age, coaching style, level of competition, parents, peers, etc. The youth sport experience is often determined by the combined interaction of these factors and does not always yield benefits to character. In fact, some studies indicate that the longer youth participate in sport, the lower their moral maturity. Thus, although a number of social and psychological benefits are *possible*, there is a need to understand how to structure youth sport programs to ensure that these benefits are fully realized. Additionally, an overemphasis on winning and an unclear understanding of the term *character* make it difficult to take advantage of personal growth opportunities through sport experiences. Many of the psychosocial benefits of youth sport participation are predicated on fostering an administrative culture that is supportive of character education in sport. Further, it is clear that the optimization of character building in youth sport is a function of personal interactions and not simply by virtue of participation.

The association between character and sport did not originate in the 21st century. This concept has been recognized as early as Plato in his book *The Republic,* written in 380 CE. More recently, as Pierre de Coubertin (1863–1937) promoted the modern Olympics in 1890, he did so by asserting that through sport participation, important values would be cultivated and people would be beneficiaries of moral growth. This idea was embraced by many cultures around the world and has been embedded in modern society, where it continues to be a common adage to promote sport participation. Given current events, however, in which high-profile athletes or coaches have behaved in ways that would suggest poor character and moral development (e.g., Tiger Woods's extramarital affairs, Ray Rice's assault of his fiancé, Hope Solo's arrest for beating up her sister and nephew, New Orleans Saints' bounty scandal), many observers are calling on Americans to reexamine their assumptions that sport participation is a foolproof means of developing good character traits. Despite the negative media attention given to athletes who misbehave, however, there is also evidence for the potential good that can come from sport participation. What is it that determines either the development of positive character traits or the demonstration of poor character? How can positive character be fostered in sports?

Dimensions and Definitions of Character

It may be important to first elucidate a clear understanding of what is meant by *character*. Research has suffered from the ambiguous meaning of the term *character development*. Undefined or unclear meanings lead to vague and imprecise findings. The etymology of the word *character* from Greek suggests a marking tool. This has evolved over the years into a description of people's traits that set them apart from others. Often character is formed around the core values of an individual. Principles that are most important to us create a set of behavioral rules that guide our living. Formal ways of delineating character and its dimensions vary as well. In order to focus this discussion of character, four dimensions of character will be described: intellectual character, moral character, civic character, and performance character.

Briefly, *intellectual character* focuses on the degree to which individuals are driven to consider intellectual issues. Athletes with highly developed intellectual character may carefully consider the rationale behind the game strategies provided by the coach. They may also ponder the larger social issues surrounding involvement in sport. *Moral character* is what many people think of when they say character. Issues of moral behaviors and choices are at the forefront of this dimension. Athletes with highly developed moral character are more likely to value fair play over cheating to win. *Civic character* refers to a mindset of active engagement in the community or groups to which they belong. Athletes who want to serve in leadership positions in order to be helpful (rather than gain status for themselves) may have a high sense of civic character. *Performance character* is a combination of psychological traits that motivate individuals to achieve. These psychological traits include common skills that are associated with sport participation such as perseverance, resilience, and courage. Athletes with developed performance character are more likely to achieve their goals based on their use of these psychological traits. When character building is associated with sport, it is likely that they are referring to performance character. The present entry will consider character as a multidimensional construct, wherein the development of character may encompass all these factors or just one.

The study of moral development in a more general context was pioneered by Jean Piaget (1896–1980) and Lawrence Kohlberg (1927–1987). Their central focus on age-related moral developmental stages has been important in catapulting morality research to its current state. Kohlberg's six stages of moral development can be divided into three levels (preconventional, conventional, and postconventional), each with two stages. He theorized that as individuals progress through these stages they are able to handle increasingly complex moral dilemmas.

Within sport, Brenda Bredemeier and David Shields are prominent researchers who have examined aspects of morality in a sports context. They postulate that moral reasoning within sports contexts may be different than that done in every other aspect of our lives. Sport is often considered separate from other domains of life and allows participants to "bracket" their moral decisions within this context, arguing that within the confines of sport competition participants can temporarily suspend usual moral obligations. For example, many sport participants consider "trash talking" a part of the game. Long-time NBA coach, Lionel Hollins, said, "I've heard Larry Bird talk trash, Charles Barkley, Michael Jordan. All those guys. It's just part of sports, part of competition." Yet we do not often hear of business women and men exchanging words to gain an advantage over competitors using "psychological warfare." This *bracketed morality*, where moral brackets are created based on lines drawn around certain sports situations, is a part of what Bredemeier and Shields (1986) call *game reasoning*. Essentially, game reasoning is a set of thought processes focused around morality within the game itself, which often assumes an egocentric line of thinking, but often includes some reflection after competition ends.

Using Competition as a Vehicle for Teaching Character

Sports participation can facilitate the development of important positive character traits. The primary reason for this is the striving for achievement that is so central to sports. Competition facilitates opportunities to develop character because of the frequent encounters with adversity and continual striving for perfection. Within the context of sport, athletes learn valuable life skills. Gould and colleagues (2007) and Gould and Carson (2008) have examined the proposition that athletes learn life skills through sport experience. They suggest that athletes learn skills such as dealing with increased pressures (time and stress management), communication skills, leadership skills, and decision-making skills. Hansen and colleagues (2003) have also developed a list of skills that sport participation might develop, which includes goal setting, emotional regulation, social skills, and a sense of responsibility. Shields and Bredemeier, perhaps the most prominent researchers on sport and character

development issues, have suggested that sport and physical activity may offer opportunities to develop the skill of perspective-taking. Although not inherent in the
domination-laden ethos of sport, it may be possible to facilitate the development of
perspective-taking (a cognitive skill) and even empathy (Shields and Bredemeier,
1995).

Character development is closely intertwined with the notion of positive youth
development (PYD), an approach to adolescent development suggesting that youth
have potential for positive growth (Lerner, Brown, and Kier, 2005). Rather than
viewing young people as problems, a PYD perspective suggests that by participating
in organized activities, youth can develop a range of desirable qualities. The aim of
developing character is a core concept of PYD. Thus, character development may
be seen as an important outcome or goal of PYD. The Search Institute, a nonprofit organization dedicated to promoting positive change for young people, has
identified a set of developmental assets that describe the building blocks of
healthy development. The research of Peter Benson, Peter Scales, Dale Blyth, and
Nancy Leffert—among others such as Daniel Gould, David Shields, and Brenda
Bredemeier—has contributed immensely to moving our knowledge of PYD forward. Forty developmental assets are identified as significant predictors of thriving behaviors among youth (Benson, 1997). This body of research suggests that as
youth develop more of these essential assets they are more likely to experience positive outcomes and less likely to engage in risk-taking behaviors. Youth sport has
been identified as one organized activity that can be helpful in the development of
these important assets (Scales, Benson, Leffert, and Blyth, 2000).

Cultivating PYD through organized youth activities has been a growing topic
of interest since the beginning of the 21st century, yet fostering positive development through sport has been a popular topic for many years prior to the 21st century.
However, a great deal of ambiguity exists in the findings from research aimed at
determining whether or not sports build character and develops positive qualities in
youth. This ambiguity is partially due to the variance of experiences that youth have.

Jay Coakley, a prominent sport sociologist, warns that "sport evangelists" spread
a message of sport participation as a means of positive development, yet there is
little research to support this concept (2011). Clearly, the statement that "sports build
character" must be qualified by the nature of the circumstances in which they play.
For example, when an individual participates in competition where the culture
emphasizes winning above everything and devalues important concepts such as
fair play and sportspersonship, the outcomes are not conducive to character
development.

In the United States, children are specializing in sports earlier and even specializing at certain positions within those sports in order to achieve at higher levels. For some, the goal is to merit an athletic scholarship in college. For others, the

goal is to progress beyond collegiate sports and create a full-time career in athletics as a professional athlete. These goals must be carefully balanced with a focus on skill mastery, teamwork, and performance improvement. When viewed from the perspective of the youth participants, one study reveals that winning was not correlated strongly with attitudes about and enjoyment of the experience (Cumming, Smoll, Smith, and Grossbard, 2007). Critics contend that some youth sport activities are becoming money-making ventures that serve adults rather than children. Tom Farrey, in his book *Game On: How the Pressure to Win at All Costs Endangers Youth Sports, and What Parents Can Do About It*, concludes that early sport specialization filters out the weak from the strong before children have the chance to develop an appreciation for sport, and that youth sport organizations are not meeting children's need for quality sport programming (Farrey, 2008). When winning dominates the youth sport performance, the cost is often a lack of psychological and social benefits that can be associated with sport participation.

Benefits of Youth Sport Experiences

When sport experiences are tailored to the needs of youth and optimized as a means of positive development, research suggests a variety of psychological and social benefits. Psychological benefits are related to the cognitive processes of the mind (such as thinking and feeling) and the health of those processes. Social benefits refer to the interaction of individuals as members of a group or community. In sports, this might include coaches, parents, teammates, and other peers. Distinguishing between psychological and social benefits is often challenging given that they sometimes overlap. For the purposes of this entry, the combined effect of these benefits will be considered together as psychosocial benefits.

A comprehensive review of the psychosocial benefits of sport participation revealed that when comparing sport participants to nonsport participants, the most common positive outcomes were higher self-esteem, better social skills, fewer depressive symptoms, higher confidence, and higher feelings of competence (Eime, Young, Harvey, Charity, and Payne, 2013). Within five developmental domains (physical, lifestyle, affective, cognitive, and social), Bailey (2006) described the benefits of sport participation. Of particular interest to the current entry are the benefits of the affective, social, and cognitive domains that he described. In the affective domain, Bailey corroborates the association between sport and increased self-esteem and identifies enhanced perceived physical self-concept as an additional finding of sport participation.

Pertaining to the cognitive domain, relationships are identified between sport and academic performance, in that individuals who participate in sports tend to perform better in academic settings than those who are not involved in sports. Whether this is due to something inherent in sport or the added motivation of an academic eligibility requirement often delineated by schools and parents is unclear. However, when coaches and parents show interest and place value on academic performance, research suggests that sport has the potential to increase performance in this area (Hebért, 1995; Lindner, 1999).

Finally, in the social domain, Bailey suggests that, because sport is typically emotionally charged and often filled with overt opportunities to interact with others, it is a prime setting for social growth. Sport participation offers opportunities to bring individuals together from various backgrounds to work toward a common goal. However, there is also concern that perhaps the nature of sport perpetuates a culture of exclusion based on the need to possess a certain skill level in order to participate.

Notably, other specific positive outcomes have been associated with sport participation. Among PYD researchers, the five C's—caring, character, connection, confidence, and competence—have been widely accepted as evidential outcomes associated with positive development. When compared to those who do not participate in sports, those who do participate in sports programs display higher levels of confidence, competence, and connectedness (Linver, Roth, and Brooks-Gunn, 2009). Additionally, those who participated in a combination of sport and other youth development activities demonstrated greater confidence, competence, character, connection, and caring (Linver, Roth, and Brooks-Gunn, 2009; Zarrett, Fay, Li, Carrano, Phelps, and Lerner, 2009). Youth who participate in sport exhibit less suicide ideation, or suicidal thoughts, compared to nonsport participants (Taliaferro, Eisenberg, Johnson, Nelson, and Neumark-Sztainer, 2011) and less hopelessness (Taliaferro, Reinzo, Miller, Pigg, and Dodd, 2008). Further psychological benefits include increased self-knowledge (Hansen, Larson, and Dworkin, 2003) and greater psychological resilience (Bartko and Eccles, 2003). Sports are a powerful means of teaching and transmitting positive values, developing desirable attributes, and preparing youth for adulthood. However, as mentioned previously, these positive outcomes are predicated on involvement in programs that are structured for character development. Next we examine characteristics of programs that fulfill this requirement.

Characteristics of Effective Positive Youth Development Programs in Sports

Effective PYD programs, wherein character can be developed, must be carefully crafted. The intentional design of programs aimed at developing character and other desirable attributes is essential for the process of character development in sports environments. Athletes, coaches, administrators, and parents must all be contributors in this process. Research on PYD programs suggests the intentional implementation of several elements of successful programs. Subsequently, several important components to the development of positive character in youth sport are examined next.

1. Quality relationships

Fostering quality relationships in sport experiences creates the foundation for all positive experiences. In addition to healthy peer interactions in competitive atmospheres, positive adult relationships are essential to development. Youth who grow to trust and admire coaches, parents, and administrators involved in the sport realm are more willing to buy into lessons about life and character. Thus, the receptiveness to character education may be dependent on these quality relationships.

The National Research Council and Institute of Medicine (NRCIM; Eccles and Gootman, 2002) identified supportive relationships as one of eight features that will maximize positive development. According to Eccles and Gootman, ideally these relationships would be characterized by warmth, closeness, connectedness, good communication, caring, support, guidance, secure attachment, and responsiveness. Similarly, Fraser-Thomas, Coté, and Deakin (2005) acknowledge that the presence of positive relationships is critical to fostering positive youth development. They suggest that supportive parental influence is most likely when parents focus on encouragement while tempering expectations, minimizing pressure, and eliminating criticisms of athlete performance.

Evidence also suggests that coaches are most likely to develop quality relationships with athletes when coaches focus on athlete development over winning (Siegenthaler and Gonzalez, 1997). Several well-known coaches have been proponents of developing quality relationships in order to influence youth through sports. In particular, Mike Krzyzewski, men's basketball coach at Duke University, has been especially effective at creating positive relationships with his athletes. In an interview with Coach Krzyzewski in 2011, he said "If winning basketball games was the only thing—I mean, you have to win and I want to win—but there's got to be more. . . . The main thing I want a player to get from me and to carry on with is that I'm on his side. He can trust me and he will get the truth from me every time, whether he's 18 and not playing, 20 and starting, or when he's 40. If there's one person to depend on in this world, they can depend on me."

2. Opportunities for skill development

Effective PYD programs must offer opportunities to develop skills. It is not so much the actual skill that matters, but the opportunity to engage meaningfully in a challenging activity that provides success as well as failure experiences. Building sport skills are helpful in building physical competence, but psychological, social, and cultural skills may also be included in these experiences. The bottom line is that learning opportunities must be paramount in the development of youth sport programs. Therefore, it is important for coaches and parents to consider how they respond to mistakes in practices and games. When mistakes are viewed as learning experiences, opportunities for youth development flourish.

One way to offer opportunities for skill development is to avoid position specific specialization and to include a variety of sports experiences. For example, the trend in society is to specialize at certain sports at increasingly younger ages and to focus one's skill development on a single position within that sport. This can lead to burnout, injury, and unidimensional development. In contrast, allowing youth to participate at a variety of positions within a certain sport promotes perspective-taking, seeing things from another's point of view. Additionally, allowing for opportunities to try a new position creates empathy when youth rediscover how it feels to be a beginner.

3. Appropriate settings and structure

In order for youth to thrive, many PYD research groups include the necessity of appropriate settings and structure. A stable environment is vital to the overall quality of the youth sport experience. Boundaries and rules must be clear and consistent. Adults play a significant role in creating appropriate behavioral standards for sport participation. Coaches are primarily responsible for setting team rules and enforcing them. Research suggests that effective coaches more consistently reinforce team rules and standards.

However, once a solid structure and sense of discipline (combined with a sense of caring) has been established in a youth sport setting, it is valuable to foster empowerment and encourage initiative within the established structure. Larson (2000) defines initiative as the "ability to be motivated from within to direct attention and effort toward a challenging goal." Encouraging initiative may include offering leadership opportunities, promoting autonomous experiences, or designing challenging activities that require sustained engagement. In order for initiative to be present, three elements must converge—intrinsic motivation, concerted effort, and engagement over time. Youth sport is often seen as a prime environment for developing and cultivating initiative because youth typically engage in sport for fun (intrinsic motivation), and it inherently offers opportunities to strive toward difficult goals over a sustained period of time.

A key piece of appropriate structure is that the game rules, physical setting, and rule structure must all be developmentally appropriate. In other words, younger participants can benefit from more structure than older participants. The equipment may need to be adjusted for younger participants to feel successful and develop skills in a technically sound manner. For example, a 5-year-old basketball team may necessitate the use of a smaller basketball and a hoop that is lowered from 10 feet to 8 feet. This will allow coaches to teach appropriate shooting technique based on the strength and ability levels of their players.

A variety of other components, beyond the three elements of a successful PYD program that are detailed above, have been cited as important for solid sport PYD programs. Coakley (2011) explains that what is important will depend on the type of sport, the orientations and actions of peers and significant adults, how participants integrate their sport participation into the rest of their life, and what meanings are ascribed to their sport and experiences. Additionally, Fraser-Thomas, Coté, and Deakin (2005) provide a framework for PYD in sport that includes fostering the 40 developmental assets and outlines the inclusion of the developmental model of sport participation, which details developmental participation patterns in sport. Finally, Eccles and Gootman (2002) provide eight features of effective youth development programs. These features are germane to a broader context of youth organizations that includes, but is not limited to, sport. Thus, while this section has considered three elements of successful programs, it is clearly not a comprehensive list, and neither are these the only elements that must be considered.

Conclusion

The veracity of the idiom "sports build character" is difficult to unravel. Perhaps it is better to qualify the statement with sports *can* build character *if* the right elements are combined to intentionally program character education into youth sports experiences. Understanding how character is defined and what outcomes are associated with the development of character in youth sports is a hurdle that has been addressed by several researchers, yet ambiguity still exists. Sport has the potential to be powerful vehicles of character education and other PYD outcomes depending primarily on the quality of relationships developed, the availability of skill development opportunities, and the creation of appropriate settings and structure. Clearly, this issue will remain an important consideration in the future of youth sport.

Aubrey Newland

Further Reading

Bailey, Richard. 2006. "Physical Education and Sport in Schools: A Review of Benefits and Outcomes." *Journal of School Health, 76*: 397–401. doi:10.1111/j.1746-1561.2006 .00132.x

Bartko, W. Todd, and Jacqueline Eccles. 2003. "Adolescent Participation in Structured and Unstructured Activities: A Person-Oriented Analysis." *Journal of Youth and Adolescence, 32*: 233–241.

Benson, Peter L. 1997. *All Kids Are Our Kids: What Communities Must Do to Raise Caring and Responsible Children and Adolescents.* San Francisco: Jossey-Bass.

Bredemeier, Brenda Jo, and David Light Shields. 1986. "Game Reasoning and Interactional Morality." *The Journal of Genetic Psychology, 147*: 257–275.

Coakley, Jay. 2011. "Youth Sports: What Counts as 'Positive Development'"? *Journal for Sport and Social Issues, 35*: 306–324. doi:10.1177/0193723511417311

Cumming, Sean. P., Frank L. Smoll, Ronald E. Smith, and Joel R. Grossbard. 2007. "Is Winning Everything? The Relative Contributions of Motivational Climate and Won-Lost Percentage in Youth Sports." *Journal of Applied Sport Psychology, 19*(3): 322–336. doi:10.1080/10413200701342640

Eccles, Jacquelynne, and Jennifer A. Gootman. 2002. "Features of Positive Developmental Settings." In Jacquelynne Eccles and Jennifer Appleton Gootman (Eds.), *Community Programs to Promote Youth Development.* Washington D.C.: National Academy Press.

Eime, Rochelle M., Janet A. Young, Jack T. Harvey, Melanie J. Charity, and Warren R. Payne. 2013. "A Systematic Review of the Psychological and Social Benefits of Participation in Sport for Children and Adolescents: Informing Development of a Conceptual Model of Health through Sport." *International Journal of Behavioral Nutrition and Physical Activity, 10*(98): 1–21. doi:10.1186/1479-5868-10-98

Farrey, Tom. (2008). *Game On: The All-American Race to Make Champions of Our Children.* New York: ESPN Books.

Fraser-Thomas, Jessica L., Jean Côté, and Janice Deakin. 2005. "Youth Sport Programs: An Avenue to Foster Positive Youth Development." *Physical Education and Sport Pedagogy, 10*: 19–40. doi:0.1080 = 1740898042000334890

Gould, Daniel, and Sarah Carson. 2008. "Life Skills Development through Sport: Current Status and Future Directions." *International Review of Sport and Exercise Psychology, 1*: 58–78.

Gould, Daniel, Karen Collins, Larry Lauer, and Yongchul Chung. 2007. "Coaching Life Skills through Football: A Study of Award Winning High School Coaches." *Journal of Applied Sport Psychology, 19*: 16–37. doi:10.1080/10413200601113786

Hansen, David M., Reed W. Larson, and Jodi B. Dworkin. 2003. "What Adolescents Learn in Organized Youth Activities: A Survey of Self-Reported Developmental Experiences." *Journal of Research on Adolescence, 13*: 25–55.

Hébert, Thomas P. 1995. "Coach Brogan: South Central High School's Answer to Academic Achievement." *Journal of Advanced Academics, 7*: 310–323. doi:10.1177/1932202X9500700104

Larson, Reed W. 2000. "Toward a Psychology of Positive Youth Development." *American Psychologist, 55*: 170–183. doi:10.1037/0003-066X.55.1.170

Lerner, Richard M., Jason D. Brown, and Cheryl A. Kier. 2005. *Adolescence: Development, Diversity, Context, and Application (Canadian ed.).* Toronto: Pearson.

Linder, Koenraad J. 1999. "Sport Participation and Perceived Academic Performance of School Children and Youth." *Pediatric Exercise Science, 11*: 129–143.

Linver, Miriam R., Jodie L. Roth, and Jeanne Brooks-Gunn. 2009. "Patterns of Adolescents' Participation in Organized Activities: Are Sports Best When Combined with Other Activities?" *Developmental Psychology, 45*: 354–367. doi:10.1037/a0014133

National Research Council and Institute of Medicine. 2002.

Scales, Peter C., Peter L. Benson, Nancy Leffert, and Dale A. Blyth. 2000. "Contribution of Developmental Assets to the Prediction of Thriving among Adolescents." *Applied Developmental Science, 4*: 27–46. doi:10.1207/S1532480XADS0401_3

Shields, David L., and Brenda Bredemeier. 1995. Character Development and Physical Activity. Champaign, IL: Human Kinetics.

Siegenthaler, K. L., and G. Leticia Gonzalez. 1997. "Youth Sports as Serious Leisure." *Journal of Sport and Social Issues, 21*: 298–314. doi:10.1177/019372397021003006

Taliaferro, Lindsay A., Barbara A. Reinzo, M. David Miller, R. Morgan Pigg, and Virginia J. Dodd. 2008. "High School Youth and Suicide Risk: Exploring Protection Afforded through Physical Education and Sport Participation." *Journal of School Health, 78*: 545–553.

Taliaferro, Lindsay A., Marla E. Eisenberg, Karen E. Johnson, Tobin F. Nelson, and Diane Neumark-Sztainer. 2011. "Sport Participation during 'Adolescence and Suicide Ideation and Attempts.'" *International Journal of Adolescent Medicine and Health, 23*: 3–10.

Zarrett, Nicole, Kristen Fay, Yibing Li, Jennifer Carrano, Erin Phelps, and Richard Lerner. 2009. "More Than Child's Play: Variable- and Pattern-Centered Approaches for Examining Effects of Sports Participation on Youth Development." *Developmental Psychology, 45*: 368–382. doi:10.1037/a0014577

Coach Training and Education

Millions of kids participate in organized sports every year, from recreational programs to travel teams. The quality of these experiences—how much fun these young athletes have, how much they learn and develop, and whether they decide to return for another season—typically hinges on one overriding factor: their coach. Good coaches who understand their roles and what working with kids in sports is truly all about can make a positive difference in a child's life, while those ill-prepared for the wide-ranging responsibilities that accompany the position can cause horrific damage by smothering fun, wrecking self-esteem, and chasing kids away from sports forever.

Coaching kids in sports is a massive responsibility filled with challenges every step of the way: working with kids with incredibly diverse personalities and skill levels, orchestrating practices, managing game day responsibilities up to and including in-game strategic decision making and play calling, communicating with parents, and the list goes on. Thankfully, for the majority of youngsters pulling on colorful uniforms these days and heading to fields, courts, and rinks in their communities, there has been a seismic shift across the youth sports landscape that is helping to make their experiences memorable for all the right reasons. Long gone are the days (at least for a lot of the country's programs) of recreation agencies ushering in anyone willing to coach and simply handing them a whistle, a bag of equipment, and a roster of kids to call to schedule the season's first practice. An ever-growing number of recreation agencies are insisting that their volunteers are trained before turning over a group of impressionable children to their care. And some of the country's most well-known coaches have taken notice.

In an interview with the authors, legendary Duke University basketball coach Mike Krzyzewski was asked to reflect on coach training and education for youth sports:

I applaud the extra time and effort that these people give all over the world, on our military bases, and in our community centers to help the youth of the country. When they are coaching they should realize it's not about winning and losing. Obviously, you want them to be competitive, but mainly it's about developing a sense of values, a sense of teamwork, what it is to be on a team, what it is to show support, what it is to help one another, what it is to fail and then succeed, and what it is to help youngsters try their best. To me, if they can get the message across that if you try your best you are a winner and if you consistently try your best you will see improvement. So, they should keep it simple, and it should be fun. Kids should have fun learning those values.

This reflection by Krzyzewski provides a perfect perspective for coach training and education, as it is critical for coaches to understand that winning is not the main goal in youth sports.

Training Takes Off

In 1981, the National Youth Sports Coaches Association (which has since evolved into the National Alliance for Youth Sports) arrived on the youth sports scene as the first not-for-profit association offering training programs for volunteer coaches involved in youth sports. "When I founded the organization it would have been very easy for people to turn down the idea of volunteers being trained because it hadn't been done in the previous 40 years that youth sports had been around," says Fred Engh, founder and president of the National Alliance for Youth Sports (NAYS). "It just proves that the overwhelming majority of people really do care and they want to see what is best for children in sports" (interview with authors). This spirit, as exemplified by its founder, served the organization well in promoting the idea of coach training and education to recreation programs around the country.

Recreation agencies slowly began to accept that these first-of-their-kind training programs offered by the National Youth Sports Coaches Association and later the National Alliance for Youth Sports wouldn't scare most would-be coaches away. In addition, they increasingly adopted the perspective that the better prepared their mostly volunteer coaches were, the more enjoyable the experience would be for all involved. This in turn would increase the likelihood that the youth would return to play again the next season. As the quality of coaching improved and word spread, what started as a novel idea is now standard operating procedure for an ever-increasing number of youth sport programs that have embraced coach training to strengthen their programs and increase the likelihood that their participants have a safe, fun-filled, and rewarding experience.

Over the years, organizations like the Positive Coaching Alliance and for-profit groups like Human Kinetics emerged to follow in the footsteps of NAYS by offering their own coach-training resources. In addition, most of today's national youth sports organizations like Little League and AYSO Soccer have coach training as part of their programs. And now, through the emergence of online learning, today's ultra-busy parents and guardians who volunteer to coach youth teams in their communities (while juggling full-time jobs and family life) can complete a variety of trainings online from the comfort of home—and at their own pace, too.

Conquering Challenges

Whether coaches are working with an under-8 girl's soccer team or a youth football team of 13- and 14-year-olds, they are going to encounter a variety of challenges throughout the course of a season. Coaches have to know how to effectively communicate with youngsters who have vastly different personalities, backgrounds, talents, and skill levels, and they must possess sound methods for dealing with sometimes meddling and unruly parents, as well as opposing coaches crossing the line of acceptable behavior. Beyond these communication issues, they also have to acquire nuts-and-bolts skills such as basic first-aid knowledge and an understanding of how to design fun, effective, and safe practices that bolster learning and skill development.

For youth sport coaches, keeping their own ambitions in perspective is important. "Do you want to be remembered for being 12–0 in your 8-and-under youth league?" asks St. Louis Cardinals manager Mike Matheny. "Or, do you want to be remembered by those kids who you had an opportunity to impact that you made a difference—you taught them something they're going to carry with them for the rest of their life and go on and pass on to multiple others?" (interview with authors). Training programs are a first step in helping coaches to separate their own ambitions from the needs of the children they oversee.

Training programs help today's volunteer coaches meet the demands of young athletes and equip them with the knowledge and resources to help them have richly rewarding experiences. Here's a sampling of the objectives and outcomes associated with quality youth sport coach-training programs:

- **Helps them develop a coaching philosophy that focuses on kids and meshes with the program:** A volunteer coach's philosophy should be crafted around fun, good sportsmanship, skill development, and safety. This is often easier said than done, since good intentions can be washed away once the season begins and scoreboards, league standings, and championship trophies enter the picture. By having a clearly defined philosophy, coaches will be less likely to lose focus of what their priorities are—which is the kids and what is best for them.

- **Keeps their focus on all the kids:** Training programs remind coaches that they must maintain their focus on all kids—not just those who run faster, jump higher, or catch better—and that it is imperative that all youngsters feel valued and appreciated for their contributions to the team, regardless of how big or small they may be.

- **Assists them with learning the proper techniques of the sport and how to teach them:** As kids progress in sports they crave knowledge and want to play for coaches who can help them learn, improve, and see progress in the sport. Being a coach involves a lot of different aspects, and the ability to teach skills is a big one. A 2004 *Sports Illustrated for Kids* survey of 1,000 youth found that 95 percent said that the quality they most value in a coach is the ability to help them improve their skills. "Volunteer coaches have to be caring," says Alan Trammell, the World Series MVP for the Detroit Tigers in 1984. "You have to look at each young person, whether male or female, and you might be teaching the same thing and saying basically the same message; but, you might have to say it a little differently, or say it with a little different twist, and to me that's coaching. People respond to things a little bit differently, and comprehend things a little bit differently when they're sad, so I think that's what good coaching is: looking at the young person and trying to help them" (interview with authors).

- **Enables them to be more effective teachers and communicators:** One of the most important characteristics of being a good coach is being able to teach. This means possessing the ability to present information clearly and correctly, and offering young athletes feedback on how well they are executing the skills being worked on. Good coaches must be able to identify both efficient and inefficient performances, and follow those performances up with enthusiastic comments when the athlete is performing really well, and helpful and uplifting words of encouragement if the child is struggling. "I think one of the biggest things that coaches can do is always encourage, and keep encouraging kids," says Memphis Grizzlies guard Mike Conley Jr., recipient of the NBA's 2014 Sportsmanship Award. "Let them know that everybody goes through slumps and everybody has some games that are off, but as long as you stay confident, as long as you stay motivated, you'll break out of it in no time" (interview with authors).

- **Helps understand the importance of players having fun:** In a 2004 *Sports Illustrated for Kids* survey, 64 percent of the kids said they would rather play on a losing team for a coach they like than on a winning team for a coach they didn't like. When asked why they played organized sports, only 48 percent of the respondents said winning was the reason, while 92 percent said having fun is more important ("What makes a good coach," 2004).

- **Keeping control of emotions at all times:** It happens all too often in youth sports—coaches yelling at umpires or engaging in arguments with parents. Occasionally, these disputes even escalate to the point that punches are thrown, 9-1-1 calls are made, and the ugly details are played out for all to see on the evening news. And lost amid all the drama of the fighting is that the children on both teams who were looking forward to their game that day were subjected to a front row seat of adult behavior at its worst. Training programs help coaches understand that they are role models and how important it is for them to keep their emotions in check at all times. The National Alliance for Youth Sports conducted a 2008 study of more than 2,000 parents that found that 53 percent said they had occasionally seen a coach arguing with another coach, official, or parent; and 7 percent of respondents reported they had seen this happen often. Additionally, 12 percent of parents said they had occasionally witnessed a coach in a physical confrontation with another coach, official, or parent; and 16 percent said they had seen it happen at least one time.

- **Exhibiting fairness to all players, all the time:** An overwhelming majority of today's volunteer coaches—experts estimate the figure to be around 85 percent—coach teams on which their own sons or daughters participate. Coaching your own child can be tricky at times, but if it is handled properly it can be an extremely rewarding experience for both the coach and child. It's a natural tendency for some coaches to show preferential treatment toward their own children, perhaps by providing them with extra playing time, giving them more attention during practices, or putting them in charge of special tasks. On the other hand, some coaches have the opposite reaction toward their children and will go out of their way to avoid displaying preferential treatment.

- **Modeling good sportsmanship all season long:** Training programs remind coaches that win-at-all-cost philosophies and poor sportsmanship drain the fun out of a child's sports experience. They also help remind the coach that his or her behavior toward opposing players, coaches, and officials will be emulated by young players. A Purdue University study found that 83 percent of girls and 70 percent of the boys polled indicated their coach was the most important influence in whether they would take part in aggressive acts or break the rules of the sport they were playing. "I don't know the records of my teams during my youth sports participation," says Orel Hershiser, a World Series MVP and Cy Young Award winner. "But I can tell you that I must have learned a lot as a young boy about manners, sportsmanship and all the different values. But I don't have any idea what my record was" (interview with authors).

- **Prepares coaches for dealing with a myriad of issues:** Today's coaches must be well versed in many areas that in the past didn't receive much focus. Issues like bullying, and coaching children dealing with mental health challenges, reinforce how important it is that volunteers are trained to handle the many challenges that can present themselves during the course of a season.

- **Helps keep young athletes safe:** Although injuries are a part of youth sports and can't be eliminated, the chances of injuries occurring can be greatly reduced in leagues that have trained coaches. Volunteers who are not trained in teaching the proper techniques of a sport can put their young athletes at unnecessary risk of either injuring themselves or opposing players. For example, a coach who doesn't understand the proper way to tackle, or isn't able to communicate to players the proper way to tackle, opens the door to not just youngsters being injured but also lawsuits. Additionally, training can provide coaches with a better understanding of how to recognize serious injuries like concussions that require players to immediately leave the field, court, or rink, as well as how to tend to less serious injuries such as sprains and strains that nonetheless require care.

The ultimate goal of a quality youth sports coach-training program is to spark a desire in prospective and continuing coaches to learn more and ultimately grow as both a coach and a mentor.

The Case for Mandatory Training

As the youth sports landscape continues to evolve, many observers believe that the importance of volunteer training has become more widely recognized. A study by NAYS in 2012 found that 88 percent of recreation agencies have volunteer-based organizations running the youth sports programs in their communities on the fields that they oversee. This is a significant shift from the late 1990s and early 2000s, when many programs were administered through recreation agencies like the local parks department by recreation professionals. This was especially true with programs for younger children.

This shift has resulted in a change in the quality of these sports programs. In that same NAYS study in 2012, 82 percent of recreation professionals cited coach training as a requirement for the programs that they personally ran, but less than half (48 percent) held the volunteer groups utilizing the public fields to that same standard. The result is that many volunteer-based groups do not require or even offer training to volunteer coaches. Meanwhile, the general public in most communities assumes that the recreation agency that oversees the athletic facilities is responsible for what happens on those fields, courts, and rinks. But the truth is that they are far removed from the everyday decisions that go into running these very complex leagues and sometimes, multisport organizations.

In communities across the United States highly trained and educated teachers and administrators teach in and oversee both public and private schools. Education and training are required due to the important role that these individuals play in the development of the nation's children. Yet, when school ends, many parents load up their cars daily and deliver their children to mostly well-meaning but often untrained adults who happen to have signed up to coach their child. An interesting analogy is that most adults took math in high school. Some went on to take additional math courses at the college level. Does taking those classes 5, 10, or even 20-plus years ago qualify an adult to teach math to a group of 7- and 8-year-old children? Of course not, but that's what we assume in today's youth sports environment.

Although some might be skeptical of government involvement, legislation may very well be necessary to hold youth sports groups accountable for the quality of what is happening on their fields. Yes, volunteers should have their backgrounds screened, which seems to be the minimum effort required in most communities. But, shouldn't these adults have a basic grasp of all the other elements that make for a good coach?

Making a Difference

It has become evident that the majority of volunteer coaches want to do well; they want to be knowledgeable in all the different facets of coaching kids; and they want to steer their players to success and guide their teams to rewarding seasons. Offering training programs hasn't been a deterrent to volunteers stepping forward. In fact, it has been just the opposite in most communities.

Training programs have given volunteers increased confidence in their own abilities to provide quality coaching and guidance to youth. In the mid-1990s, Northern Kentucky University conducted a study on volunteer coach training and its impact on coaches, and found that an overwhelming majority were in favor of training. Of coaches who had not received any type of training, 78 percent said that the requirement of a training program would not discourage them from volunteering; and 85 percent said they would voluntarily attend a certification clinic if provided the opportunity to do so (National Youth Sports Research and Development

Center, 2000). Furthermore, of the coaches who had been trained, 85 percent said that a certification program had increased their skills and confidence in coaching children; and 86 percent of these coaches said they would voluntarily attend another certification clinic even if they were not required to do so.

Coaching youth sports is about making connections, establishing communication, and figuring out how to be a mentor, role model, teacher, confidant, and even a father or mother figure for some kids. At their best, training programs help push volunteers to excel in these diverse roles and be that special coach that kids love playing for and learning from.

Quality coaches make an impact. "I had so many good coaches growing up," says former Major League Baseball player Adam LaRoche. "And it's funny now at age 34 there are still a lot that I stay in contact with. These are coaches that I had when I was 12 and 13 years old that had a real impact on my life. Most of the ones I'm in contact with now are coaches who were not necessarily the best coaches baseball-wise but just about life in general and about teaching how to be a good person" (interview with authors). That's the power of coaching—when it's done the right way. Training programs enable volunteer coaches to gain valuable knowledge, become confident instructors, and equip them, in some cases, to have a life-defining impact on their young players.

John Engh and Greg Bach

Further Reading

Engh, Fred. 2002. *Why Johnny Hates Sports: Why Organized Youth Sports Are Failing Our Children and What We Can Do about It*. New York: Square One Publishers.

Matheny, Mike (with Jerry B. Jenkins). *The Matheny Manifesto*. New York: Crown Manifesto.

National Alliance for Youth Sports. 2012. *Facility Usage Survey*. Accessed July 23, 2015, at http://www.nays.org/default/assets/File/Recommendations-for-Communities—National-Alliance-for-Youth-Sports.pdf.

"National Alliance for Youth Sports Nationwide Study." 2008, Spring. *Sporting Kid Magazine*, 10–15.

National Youth Sports Research and Development Center, Northern Kentucky University. 2000. *Youth Sport Coach Certification & Training Survey*. Accessed July 23, 2015, at http://www.instituteforsportcoaching.org/wp-content/uploads/2011/02/Value-of-Quality-Trained-Sport-Coaches-White-Paper-2010.pdf.

Poppinga, Brady. *The True Spirit of Competition*. Raleigh, NC: Lulu Publishing.

Skolnick, Ethan J., and Andrea Corn. *Raising Your Game*. Bloomington, IN: iUniverse.

Thompson, Jim. 2007. *Positive Coaching in a Nutshell*. Portola Valley, CA: Balance Sports Publishing.

"What makes a good coach." 2004, November. *Sports Illustrated for Kids*, 5.

College Scholarships and Recruiting

When considered at its most basic, the recruitment of youth sport athletes is about hope. Athletes, encouraged by messages to work hard and reach beyond their limits, dream of playing in college and, in some cases, in the pros. To be recruited represents the next step in fulfilling those dreams.

For youth sport athletes, the recruitment process has changed greatly over time. The idea of the college coach making a visit to the local high school to watch an athlete play in a game continues to exist. Increasingly, however, that mode of in-person recruiting is being replaced with athlete showcases, camps, combines, and tournaments. Representing the marketplace of college recruits, those events draw dozens, sometimes hundreds of college coaches. Lining sidelines and watching from the stands, coaches work much like gold miners, panning for the gold of athletic talent.

The evolution of travel teams and elite club teams has altered the focus of recruiting, redirecting it in some cases away from high school teams. Innovations in technology, such as the wide availability of digital recordings and social media, have transformed the strategies coaches use to scout, identify, and communicate with athletes. The result is a mix of contradictions, with the top 1–2 percent of athletes receiving lavish amounts of attention from coaching staffs. The remaining pools of athlete prospects find themselves in the circumstance of having to figure out how to get noticed.

College Recruiting: An Overview

In the world of college sport, the process used to identify talented athletes, assess the level of their skills and potential, develop relationships with them, and persuade them to sign with a particular program is generally called recruiting. In the marketplace for players, the components of recruiting include scouting, performance evaluation (otherwise known as analytics), selling, and buying. Interestingly enough, two parties engage in the selling and buying process. The coaches sell their school with the intent of getting selected players to agree to play for their program. When a coach makes an offer to a player, there is an investment in that player. Athletes, on the other hand, are also selling their skills, engaging in self-promotion to rise to a level where a college coach will recognize them and want to recruit them. Athletes, when they accept offers, are expected to buy into the programs they join. Although the elements of recruiting remain constant, the intensity and dimensions shift somewhat depending on the level of a player's talent and the caliber of college program that the coach represents. In the United States, there is considerable variability among colleges and universities in terms of the philosophy and approach taken to running athletic programs, with a cascading designation or divisional structure. Within the National Collegiate Athletic Association (NCAA) (the sport governing body that oversees the majority of college and university athletic programs in the United States), there are three major divisions—Divisions I, II, and III.

The principal distinctions across divisions reflect differing views on the awarding of athletically related grants-in-aid (e.g., athletic scholarships) and the degree to which winning is emphasized. Further separations in divisions occur depending on whether a school sponsors football at all or, if football is sponsored, at what level. Thus, within the NCAA's highest level, Division I, schools are further separated into what are called football powers or FBS institutions (Football Bowl Series schools); mid-level FCS institutions (Football Championship Series), and non–football playing institutions.

Reflective of these differing philosophies, the allocation of athletic scholarships is greatest in Division I institutions and much less in Division II. Select Division I institutions, such as the elite academic institutions comprising the Ivy League (Harvard, Yale, Princeton, Penn, Columbia, Cornell, Dartmouth, and Brown), and Division III institutions (80 percent of which are private) have chosen not to offer athletic scholarships. This stance reflects their belief that the practice of doing so adversely affects the relationship of the athlete to the institution, as well as the arrangement between academics and athletics.

Institutions that view athletic programs as a critical piece of their marketing strategies and identities sponsor elite-level programs that are designed to garner large television audiences, draw mass numbers of spectators to stadiums and arenas, and form the basis for lucrative corporate partnerships. Such high-profile athletic programs serve as the "front porch" of a college or university; in other words, athletic programs provide curb appeal that make members of the public pause to watch. The festive atmosphere of the college sport environment, which encompasses the games themselves as well as the tailgating and social opportunities that arise around events, and the opportunities to express affinity for and loyalty to a particular institution, showcase the university and aid in marketing and branding efforts. There is a general belief among many that the creation of that atmosphere translates into benefits for institutions in the form of increased funding support, student applications for admission, and fund-raising.

Given the intense scrutiny that comes with televised events and coverage across digital media platforms, competition for top recruits is high. The stakes are high for coaches as well, who face the prospect season in and season out of piecing together successful programs that will continue to serve as sources of pride for their institutions and fans and are regarded as worthy investments for corporate interests.

Even as the greatest pressures to produce and win are located in the upper level programs, the desire to find the best player talent exists at every level. For athletes, they want to be able to fulfill their promise and potential and to be matched with programs that will bring out the best in them. For coaches and institutions, they want to field the best teams they can within the limits of what they can afford financially and the philosophical approach they have to college sport (some programs want winning teams, others are more educationally focused). Thus, regardless of level, the anchor of a college and university program is the recruited athlete, the young men and women who college sport insiders refer to as the "lifeblood" of the college sport system (Brady, Kelly, and Berkowitz, 2015).

Brief History of Recruiting

Since the earliest years of college sport, those involved—athletes, coaches, alumni, boosters, and fans—have had an unflagging interest in locating and landing top talent to play on their athletic teams. From the mid-1800s through the 1950s, a class of athletes for hire known as "tramps" or "ringers" would travel the college circuit, sometimes without enrolling in the schools they were playing for, to lend support to win-hungry programs. From those early years forward, the three key components of college recruiting—athlete eligibility, academic status, and compensation of the most talented athletes—have been the primary focus of regulation and controversy. Fraught with contradictions and ambiguities, each of those areas reflects long-standing disagreements between and among schools regarding the balance between amateurism and professionalism (if amateurism in fact actually exists); academics and athletics; and commercialism and exploitation.

In the 1980s, prompted by political pressure, college sport authorities started to negotiate a national standard of minimum academic eligibility for athlete recruits. The outcome of that discussion, which lasted nearly a decade, was the implementation of a minimum grade point average of 2.5 (on a 4.0 scale) in a core curriculum of 11 academic courses. Following revelations in the early 1990s that some college athletes were much like the tramp athletes of previous eras, playing on college teams and receiving suspect degrees despite the fact that they either could not read or were functionally illiterate, those standards would be adjusted, eventually leading to a sliding scale high school grade point average. In 1994, the NCAA Eligibility Clearinghouse (now called the NCAA Eligibility Center), was created to review high school transcripts and placement scores to verify their legitimacy. The movement in the direction of monitoring the academic credentials of athletes gave rise to a number of accountability mechanisms. The Student Right to Know Act of 1990 requires colleges and universities to report the graduation rates for athletes who have received athletic scholarships.

NCAA Rules Pertaining to Academic Eligibility

As of the time of this writing in 2015, NCAA rules to determine athlete academic eligibility (core courses, grade point average in core courses, and test scores) are in flux once again. Standards became more stringent for high school athletes who anticipate enrolling in an NCAA member institution after August 1, 2016.

Recruited high school athletes are classified according to the degree they meet the academic requirements as set forth in NCAA regulations. For those who satisfy the requirements as stated, they are referred to as *qualifiers*. A qualifier is eligible to practice, to compete, and to receive an athletic scholarship. A recruit may be designated as an *early academic qualifier* when he or she satisfied 14 core courses with a 3.0 GPA or higher within six semesters while earning a minimum 900 or greater combined SAT score or 75 ACT sum score. For a high school athlete who enrolls on or after August 1, 2016, and who does not meet all of the requirements, he or she may be designated as an *academic redshirt*, falling short of the 2.3 grade point average in core courses. The potential to receive an academic redshirt hinges on where an athlete's academic credentials fall on a sliding scale (the lower the grade point average, the higher the combined SAT or ACT score must be). The practice of *redshirting* occurs when a recruit receives an athletic scholarship and is permitted to practice but not play in games. In order for academic redshirts to practice in their second quarter or semester of their first year in college, they have to pass eight quarter hours or nine semester hours. Other athletes whose grade point average falls below a 2.0 are considered *nonqualifiers* who are prevented from receiving athletically related aid and practicing for the first year of their college experience.

The Cycle of Recruiting

In theory, an athlete becomes a prospective recruit under NCAA rules once he or she has started classes for the ninth grade. In an attempt to protect athletes from being inundated with attention from multiple coaching staffs, the rules are designed to provide space for athletes and coaches to gather the information they need while creating buffers to ensure that coach communication with athletes is not excessive.

Nearly every aspect of coach-athlete interaction is regulated during the recruitment process with specific periods of the recruiting calendar set aside for different forms of interaction. Key terms that establish understandings regarding how coaches are to approach recruits include the following:

- Face-to-face meetings that have been prearranged and involve a conversation that goes beyond a mere greeting is referred to as a *contact.*
- During weeks or months designated as *contact periods*, coaches may watch athletes perform and communicate in person.
- Time referred to as *dead periods* bars a coach from in-person contact with a player but allows for communicating in writing and speaking over the phone.
- An *evaluation period* is time set aside to assess the academic and athletic credentials of an athlete. When an *evaluation* occurs off campus, coaches may not engage in face-to-face conversation with the athlete although phone calls and written forms of communication are acceptable. Evaluations performed on campus allow for coaches to speak with athletes directly.
- During a *quiet period* coaches are restricted from having in-person meetings with athletes and families unless they occur on campus.
- Recruits may take two types of *visits* to a specific campus. One type is an *official visit.* An athlete's expenses associated with transportation, lodging, and meals may be paid for by the host institution, and athletes may receive up to three complimentary tickets to an athletic event. An athlete may take up to four additional *unofficial visits,* with expenses paid for by the athlete and their family.

Although athletes may bear the expense of calls placed to coaches, the timing of coach-initiated phone calls to recruits is dependent on the specific sport and the calendar that has been created for those kinds of interactions. As a case in point, calls to recruits from coaches begin in men's basketball on June 15 after the sophomore year, and those calls can be unlimited. In contrast, football coaches may make one call to a recruit between April 15 and May 31 of the senior year with additional calls made on or after September 1 of the senior year.

Social Media and Recruiting

The college recruiting business is big business, with both coaches and athletes seeking ways to become known to one another, to assess each other, and to arrive at mutually beneficial agreements. Social media have helped both coaches and athletes achieve their goals in the recruiting process. In many respects, the benefits to be realized by effective social media strategies are similar for both coaches and athletes. Social media afford opportunities to create awareness, to offer a window into what is happening with a program or individual, provide the chance to communicate instantaneously, and expand the number of impressions and exposures to enhance the brands of all parties. Given the amount of information available in the public domain about recruits, coaches and their staffs may rely on social intelligence tools (data analysis tools that filter information from social media) to tailor recruiting pitches to specific athletes or groups of athletes.

Both coaches and athletes experience certain limitations with the use of social media in recruiting. NCAA rules prohibit coaches from corresponding with athletes in the public domain. As a consequence, coaches have to be vigilant that privacy settings are firmly in place.

Athletes have fewer formal limits but important concerns related to content. There are potential negative consequences for athlete recruits being active on social media if they fail to consider how their postings may be viewed by coaches. Several Division I football recruiters have tweeted about dropping prospects because of what they have posted on social media. As one wrote, "Had to unfollow/stop recruiting a young man this evening. Still amazed by what recruits tweet/retweet/ College coaches are watching" (Patsko, 2015).

The Recruitment Process Ends with a Signed Contract

For scholarship athletes in NCAA Divisions I and II, "signing days" signal the end of the recruitment process. While moments to celebrate, the signed documents represent agreements between the institution and athlete that form the basis of a contractual relationship. One document, the statement of financial assistance (which will be discussed in greater detail below) is a required document. The second one, referred to as the National Letter of Intent, can be voluntarily signed.

The National Letter of Intent (NLI) is often described as a document designed to reduce or lessen recruiting pressures on athletes. Signing a NLI sets certain things in motion. First, an athlete declares publicly and in writing that he or she is accepting an offer from a particular coach and institution. Second, the NLI stipulates that other schools must stop recruiting that athlete while the coaching staff for the selected school can communicate freely with the athlete.

In order for the NLI to go into effect, the athlete must be given a promise in writing outlining the terms and conditions of the athletic scholarship offer. Barring any issues with academic or athletic eligibility, the athlete is positioned to receive an athletic scholarship award for a minimum of one full academic year and agrees to complete a full year in residence at that institution. (See section below regarding myths about athletic scholarships. Many athletic scholarships are partial awards that cover some but not all expenses.)

Should the athletes sign the NLI, and later decide that they wish to go elsewhere, they can suffer a penalty of having to give up one year of eligibility and sit out for a year before playing for their new institution. The NLI also prevents an athlete from leaving an institution in the event that the coach who recruited them leaves and goes elsewhere. Under limited circumstances, athletes who harbor second thoughts about their decisions may request a release from their contract with a school.

Although the purpose of the NLI appears benign, there are some who see it as a means of locking athletes into agreements that are not in their best interests. One reporter, in fact, questioned whether the NLI may be the "worst contract in sports" (Dodds, 2015). In the sport of football, National Signing Day occurs three months before the traditional signing period ends. Much can happen during those three months, including a coach losing his or her job or taking a job elsewhere. Locked in with an NLI, signed agreements that prevent athletes from transferring without penalty even if their coaches leave for other schools, binds the players to conditions that may not be favorable to them and may negatively impact their career.

Myths about Athletic Scholarships

For high school athletes who have been participating in their sport and competing for many years, the end goal is often the hope of an athletic scholarship—what Greg Earhart, a swimming coach at Arizona State University, has called "the holy grail" (Holland and Schoen, 2014). For some high school athletes, there is a belief that the only way they can afford higher education is by getting an athletic scholarship. For others, the athletic scholarship represents a means of making a living as they grow professionally in their sport, anticipating the day when they can leverage their college career into a professional contract. As familiar as the concept of an athletic scholarship is, there are myths about them that can affect athletes in ways that, at a minimum, can be disappointing or disillusioning or at worst, harmful and long-lasting. Some of the more enduring myths include that athletic scholarships are prevalent and are the only way that athletes can receive assistance to attend colleges and universities; that full ride scholarships are "free rides" to college; and that athletic scholarships cannot be taken away once an athlete has been awarded one. Each of these myths will be explored in relationship to the realities.

The Myth of Athletic Scholarship Abundance

The NCAA reports that Division I and II athletic programs award $2.7 billion to more than 150,000 athletes annually. With over 460,000 athletes competing among NCAA member institutions, the vast majority (350,000) does not receive athletically related scholarship assistance. Thus, the competition for an athletic scholarship is fierce. When viewed in terms of specific sports, the prospects of receiving an athletic scholarship are put into perspective. As a general proposition, only 10 percent of high school athletes will make it onto a roster of an NCAA Division I, II, or III team. In specific sports, such as men's and women's basketball, the prospects are less than 4 percent, in football and baseball the odds are approximately 6.5 percent; and men's and women's soccer, between 6 and 7 percent. Chances to earn a scholarship are slimmer than those percentages.

The Myth of the Full-Ride Scholarship

For decades, there has been a view that if an athlete received a full athletic scholarship, he or she received a "free" education. NCAA rules set the value of an athletic scholarship at tuition, room and board, and books, a value that falls short of the full cost of attending college. As a very recent development, schools in NCAA Division I may now offer athletic scholarships that include coverage of the full cost of attendance. However, schools are not obligated to do so.

The Myth That All Scholarship Athletes Receive a Full Scholarship

NCAA rules establish two ways in which athletic scholarships are allocated, either by *head count* or *equivalency*. In sports that are designated as head count sports, a specified number of full athletic scholarships must be awarded intact. The number of awards per sport and division, by the way, changes (example: FBS football—85 scholarships; FCS football—65 scholarships). Sports classified as head count sports are basketball (men's and women's), football, women's gymnastics, tennis, and volleyball. The remainder of teams that offer athletic scholarships are referred to as equivalency sports. This means that each team, within limits set by the NCAA, can parcel out awards within certain limits. Thus, some athletes in an equivalency sport may receive a full athletic scholarship, others may receive tuition and board, and still others may receive book awards. Another feature that distinguishes athletic scholarships in equivalency sports is the question of how much a family can afford to cover for an athlete's education. The financial position of the family is taken into account in the awarding of athletic scholarships in equivalency sports.

The Myth That Athletic Scholarships Cannot Be Taken Away or Reduced in Value

Some hold to the impression that athletic scholarships, once awarded, cannot be taken away for nonperformance or injury. The key to fully understanding athletic scholarship awards is in the fine print. For recruits and their families, it is important to know up front what the athletic scholarship award covers financially, how long the award is for, and the terms and conditions that govern the award. When an athlete is extended a scholarship offer, he or she should receive a written statement from the institution with that information included.

In cases where athletic scholarships are awarded on a yearly basis, the award must be renewed, and it is at the coach's discretion to renew. Although there is a significant incentive for coaches to be sparing when choosing not to renew an award, athletes and family members should not assume that verbal promises made during recruiting, or promises they believe they heard, will be fulfilled. The operative language in most agreements is that the award cannot be withdrawn or reduced within the "term of the award." If the term of the award is for one academic year, an athlete may face the prospect of scholarship nonrenewal or reduction the following year.

To complicate matters, schools in the so-called Power Five conferences (Atlantic Coast Conference–ACC, Big Ten, Big Twelve, Pacific Athletic Conference–PAC-12, and Southeastern Athletic Conference–SEC) have started to award multiyear athletic scholarships that may cover five years of eligibility and are being referred to as "guaranteed" scholarships. Although the possibility that athletes might have a more secure athletic scholarship arrangement is significant, caution should be exercised relative to assuming that a guaranteed multiyear scholarship means that it is actually guaranteed. Recruits should be aware, however, that if an athlete, such as a *nonqualifier,* enrolls in the first year without a scholarship, the institution is not obligated to offer a multiyear scholarship to that athlete in subsequent years.

Officially, the reasons why an athlete may lose a scholarship are as follows:

- The athlete becomes ineligible either academically or athletically.
- The athlete provides fraudulent information in an application, letter of intent, or financial aid form.

- The athlete is sanctioned by a university disciplinary board for misconduct.
- The athlete voluntarily quits a team.
- The athlete violates university policy.

The official rules regarding the awarding and retention of athletic scholarships are tempered by the related practices that go on around the management of player personnel. For example, athletes and parents are sometimes surprised at the end of a season to meet with their coach and learn that they are being encouraged to transfer because things are not working out. Thus, players who thought that they had signed at one school with a belief that they would be at that school for the duration of their eligibility, and would receive a scholarship throughout that time, might have to receive a transfer waiver to seek opportunities at other schools. This may occur whether an athlete has a one-year or multiyear award.

Some athletes have also reported that they have been asked to sign medical waivers that would end their careers to make space on rosters for younger players. The medical waiver allows a program to continue to provide financial support to an athlete so that the athlete remains at the school to complete a degree. However, it effectively ends the athlete's playing career in that program.

The rules do require that athletes receive a chance to appeal a decision that takes away their scholarship or reduces its value. A school administrator from the financial aid office is expected to provide that information, but the hearings are often scheduled at the end of the academic year (in late June), at a time when it is difficult to find opportunities for the next academic year. Thus, athletes may want to pay close attention to the appeal hearing process and request an expedited one if the issue arises.

Issues Faced by Athletes and Parents in Recruitment

Because the recruiting process has so many moving parts to it, decoding what is happening or should be happening can be difficult. Some of the perennial issues athletes and parents face when navigating the recruitment process include the question of whether an athlete is being recruited or not; the meaning of a "free education"; the business of athlete recruiting; and the propriety of recruiting athletes before they get to high school.

Hope Can Be Powerful but Not Necessarily Accurate

Deciphering messages from colleges and coaches can be difficult when they are occurring through a lens of optimism and excitement. As awkward as it sounds, interest on the part of coaches can sometimes be misinterpreted by athletes and/or parents to mean something that is not intended. Recruiting occurs on a continuum from "not being recruited" (routine correspondence from college admission offices and general invitations to summer camps) to "being noticed" (college coach speaks with a high school coach about a player; personal correspondence from the coach to the athlete or request for athlete to fill out a recruiting form) to "being recruited" (college coach directly calls an athlete, schedules a specific time to come to watch an athlete play, invites athlete to campus for an official visit). Prospective athletes need to be aware of the levels of coach interest when they are being recruited.

What Free Education Actually Means

Although there is a great deal of rhetoric about the balance between academics and athletics, the plain fact of the matter is that athletes may be surprised when they arrive on campus and are counseled out of taking certain majors or told that certain majors are off limits due to the demands of their sports. Ohio State football coach, Urban Meyer, just months after his team won the national championship in 2015, spoke about how the commitments players are expected to make to their sport result in them taking majors they may not be interested in or "survival degrees" (majors that are less demanding academically). Depending on the sport and the latitude given by coaching staffs, the access athletes have to internships and study abroad programs may be reduced because of their sport participation. Numerous studies have found that excessive time spent on athletics can impact an athlete in several ways, including choice of major, grade point average, interaction with academic faculty, social interaction, and other nonathletic pursuits.

The Business of Athlete Recruiting

Families often invest considerable money in supporting the youth sport activities of their children. How much more are they expected to invest in order to ensure that an athlete will be recruited? That is an evolving question. College coaches with limited budgets have gravitated toward showcase events where they can watch hundreds of athletes over a span of 2–3 days. The economic burden associated with travel to those showcases and the registration fees to get in are typically born by the athletes and their families. The registration fees alone are often several hundred dollars per event (some estimates ranging between $500–$600 per event). Layered onto that investment are fees for recruiting advisers who advertise that they provide services to athletes that link them to coaches and colleges.

Some argue that the mysteries of the athlete recruitment process can be unlocked by athletes and families with research and persistence and that recruitment services offer nothing particularly unique to the process. Others, however, suggest that the process is sufficiently nuanced and complicated that there are advantages to working with knowledgeable advisers who have worked the system over a period of years. There are others who express concern that the athlete recruitment market is becoming defined by those who have the capacity to pay for it, leaving many talented athletes under the radar and unnoticed or having to work harder to find opportunities.

How Young Is Too Young?

Over the span of decades, college coaches have directed their attentions to recruiting younger and younger athletes. Athletes who have never played a game in high school, never taken a high school course, and never taken a college placement exam are extended scholarship offers and committing to schools long before they are even prepared to attend the college (Popper, 2014). Ben James, an 11-year old golfer, is among the youngest athletes to announce a commitment to play for a university team should he graduate from high school or turn pro before that (Ringler, 2014). The seeming inability of coaches to resist the pressures of signing talent early and gambling on the futures of the young in order to retain market position and competitive advantage has been flagged as an issue to be dealt with as are the obvious loopholes that exist within recruiting rules that allow for this to occur.

Conclusion

With each new recruitment cycle, hope springs eternal. As hopeful as the process is, it should be approached by recruits and their parents with an eye toward the realities of what the college sport business is. Basic understandings about the cycle of recruiting, the vocabulary that is used in recruiting, the contractual nature of the National Letter of Intent and the terms and conditions of an athletic scholarship, levels of coach interest, and the myths surrounding athletic scholarships are essential for prospective athletes and family members to know so that they can raise questions and consider their options with as much information as possible.

Ellen J. Staurowsky

Further Reading

Allen, Rick. 2015. *The Facts about "Guaranteed" Multi-Year DI Scholarships, June 12.* Accessed July 4, 2015, at http://informedathlete.com/the-facts-about-guaranteed-multi-year-ncaa-di-scholarships.

Ayers, Kevin, Monica Pazmino-Cevallos, and Cody Dobose. 2012. "The 20-Hour Rule: Student Athletes Time Commitment to Athletics and Academics." *VAHPERD, 22*: 22–26.

Bastie, Fred. 2015a. *Recruiting Column: How to Connect with College Coaches, June 10.* Accessed July 4, 2015, at http://usatodayhss.com/2015/recruiting-column-how-to -connect-with-college-coaches.

Bastie, Fred. 2015b. *Recruiting Column: 5 Things to Consider about Using a Recruiting Service, April 29.* Accessed July 4, 2015, at http://usatodayhss.com/2015/recruiting -column-5-things-to-consider-about-using-a-recruiting-service.

Bastie, Fred. 2015c. *Recruiting Column: The Biggest College Recruiting Myth, February 25.* Accessed July 4, 2015, at http://usatodayhss.com/2015/recruiting-column-the -biggest-college-recruiting-myth.

Berkowitz, Steve. 2015. *NCAA Increases Value of Scholarships in Historic Vote, January 17.* Accessed July 4, 2015, at http://www.usatoday.com/story/sports/college/2015/01 /17/ncaa-convention-cost-of-attendance-student-athletes-scholarships/21921073.

Brady, Erik., John Kelly, and Steve Berkowitz. 2015, February 4. "Schools in Power Conferences Spending More on Recruiting." *USA Today.* Accessed August 28, 2015, at http:// www.usatoday.com/story/sports/ncaaf/recruiting/2015/02/03/college-football-recruiting -signing-day-sec-power-conferences/22813887.

Dodds, Dennis. 2015. *Roquan Smith's Commitment Issues Pinpoint Problem with Recruiting, February 12.* Accessed July 4, 2015, at http://www.cbssports.com/collegefootball /writer/dennis-dodd/25066673/roquan-smiths-commitment-issues-pinpoint-problem-with -recruiting.

Drotar, Brian. 2015. *College Coaches Are Not Coming to Your High School Games, April 7.* Accessed July 3, 2015, at http://therecruitingcode.com/college-coaches-are-not-coming -to-your-high-school-games.

Feiner, L. 2015. *Pay-to-Play: The Business of College Athletic Recruitment, June 23.* Accessed July 4, 2015, at http://www.forbes.com/sites/laurenfeiner/2015/06/23/pay-to -play-the-business-of-college-athletic-recruitment/2.

Henry, Jim. 2015. *Henry Blog: Recruiting's Changed over the Years, February 2.* Accessed July 4, 2015, at http://www.tallahassee.com/story/sports/college/fsu/football/2015/02/02 /henry-blog-recruitings-changed-years/22779287.

Holland, Kelly, and John W. Schoen. 2013. *Think athletic scholarships are a 'holy grail'? Think again.* Accessed at https://www.cnbc.com/2014/10/13/think-athletic-scholarships -are-a-holy-grail-think-again.html.

Kirsch, Brendan. 2012. *The Hopeful.* Documentary. Accessed July 3, 2012, at http://www .imdb.com/title/tt1461432/plotsummary?ref_=tt_ov_pl.

NCAA Academic and Membership Staff. 2015. *NCAA Division I Manual—2014–2015— April Version.* Accessed July 4, 2015, at https://www.ncaapublications.com/p-4385-2014 -2015-ncaa-division-i-manual-april-version.aspx.

Patsko, Scott. 2015. *How Social Media Behavior of High School Athletes Can Negatively Impact NCAA Recruiting, February 3.* Accessed July 4, 2015, at http://highschoolsports .cleveland.com/news/article/3838474443158678075/how-social-media-behavior-of

-high-school-athletes-can-negatively-impact-ncaa-recruiting-photos-polls-national
-signing-day-2015.

Popper, Nathaniel. 2014. *Committing to Play for a College, Then Starting Ninth Grade, January 26.* Accessed July 4, 2015, at http://www.nytimes.com/2014/01/27/sports /committing-to-play-for-a-college-then-starting-9th-grade.html?_r=0.

Rahmati, Ray. 2014. *How Social Media Is Changing College Recruiting, November 3.* Accessed July 4, 2015, at https://www.spredfast.com/social-marketing-blog/how-social -media-changing-college-recruiting.

Ringler, Lance. 2014. *11-Year Old Commits to Connecticut, October 15.* Accessed July 4, 2015, at http://golfweek.com/news/2014/oct/05/junior-golf-recruiting-college-uconn-11 -commitment.

Schneider, Ray, Sally Ross, and Morgan Fisher. 2010. "Academic Clustering and Major Selection of Intercollegiate Student-Athletes." *College Student Journal, 44*: 64–70.

Snyder, Mark. 2015. *U-M's Pipkins Transferring, Says He Was Told to Retire, June 26.* Accessed July 4, 2015, at https://www.freep.com/story/sports/college/university-michigan /wolverines/2015/06/26/michigan-football-ondre-pipkins/29339503.

Staples, Andy. 2008. *Á History of Recruiting: How Coaches Have Stayed a Step Ahead, June 23.* Accessed July 4, 2015, at http://www.si.com/more-sports/2008/06/23/recruiting -main.

Taylor, John. 2014. *2015 QB Recruit Who Gave USC a Verbal When He was 13 Decommits, June 28.* Accessed July 4, 2015, at http://collegefootballtalk.nbcsports.com/2014 /06/28/2015-qb-recruit-who-gave-usc-a-verbal-when-he-was-13-decommits.

Taylor, John. 2015. *Cost-of-Attendance, Multi-Year Scholarships Approved, January 17.* Accessed July 4, 2015, at http://collegefootballtalk.nbcsports.com/2015/01/17/cost-of -attendance-multi-year-scholarships-approved.

Urban Meyer Discusses Ohio State's Real Life Wednesdays and Provides Updates on Braxton Miller, May 27. 2015. Accessed July 4, 2015, at http://www.elevenwarriors.com /ohio-state-football/2015/05/54152/video-urban-meyer-discusses-ohio-states-real-life -wednesdays-and-provides-updates-on.

Community Recreation Programs

Community youth sport programs play a key role in the lives of individual participants, families, and entire communities. As Nelson Mandela stated, "sport has the power to change the world." Millions of youth in the United States, between the ages of 6 and 17, participate in organized youth sport each year. Based on the sheer number of participants alone, youth sport creates a context that can indeed change the world.

The purpose of this entry is to give a broad overview of what is currently available in youth sport community-based programs, including different types of organizations that provide programs and some specific benefits and challenges of those types of programs. Second, this chapter provides an overview of some of the major challenges facing youth sport programs of all types. Finally, the chapter concludes with a broad overview of the associated benefits of youth sport participation.

Availability of Community Recreation Programs

Historically, not-for-profit organizations, schools, and government recreation departments provided the bulk of youth sport programs. These programs developed in the middle of the 19th century as places where young men could have something to do and stay out of trouble. Early pioneers in youth sport included the Young Men's Christian Association (YMCA), the Amateur Athletic Union (AAU), and the Boys and Girls Clubs of America. Today's youth sport landscape, however, is increasingly complicated with both additional not-for-profit organizations and an array of for-profit companies stepping into this growing marketplace. Although numerous, programs can be classified by the type of organization that manages their operations, including government (generally at the local level), not-for-profit, and commercial-for-profit. Each of these is discussed below.

Government programs, frequently referred to as public services, are funded by taxes and exist to serve the needs of the entire community. Therefore, in order to maximize the number of opportunities available for all citizens, they tend to focus on recreational level players. Although opportunities exist for advanced players, including all-star, "travel," or "select" leagues, the primary focus of most government sport programs remains on the recreational player.

There are several benefits to government run youth sport programs. Since government programs receive a large percentage of their support from tax dollars, they tend to be more affordable than commercial for-profit programs. In some cases, programs may charge only a nominal fee. Many government programs also tend to offer discounts based on financial need.

In addition, government youth sport programs play a key role in the entire community. Perhaps most importantly, these programs provide a venue for the development of future adult community leaders. Research indicates that youth in sport programs are more likely to be civically engaged in their community and experience future personal success. As such, these programs provide a potential avenue to foster a healthy future community. Further, youth sports may assist in the development of a sense of community. As a place where individuals, both youth and adults, interact on a regular basis, this setting provides the opportunity for feelings of influence, membership, need fulfillment, and shared emotional connection that are indicative of a strong sense of community.

Government run youth sport programs also face numerous challenges. For example, they are often reliant on volunteers. Historically, youth sport administrators were educators with some background in teaching and child development. Today, however, with the boom in popularity of youth sport, many programs experience shortages of parents and other volunteers willing to serve as coaches, officials, and administrators. This leads to a situation where volunteers may have little to no experience either in the sport or in principles of coaching and youth development. Organizations such as Positive Coaching Alliance (PCA) and National Alliance for Youth Sports (NAYS) have created training programs that seek to provide volunteer coaches with the necessary skills related to youth development; however, these programs represent an added commitment to already stretched volunteers.

Although government youth sport programs have traditionally charged lower fees, many programs face funding challenges during difficult economic times. This dynamic has led to a reevaluation of this funding model. A decline in property values, for example, means lower tax bases for municipalities. As property taxes represent the largest portion of local government income, programs require alternative methods to cover program costs. Thus, many programs raise registration fees, seek corporate sponsorships, add additional revenue-generating programs, and/or cut programs that rely on tax support. In these cases, government programs risk mirroring the higher fees of their for-profit counterparts.

Not-for-profit organizations exist to meet a specific need, often of a specific population or demographic group. For example, the mission of Boys and Girls Clubs emphasize their role in helping all young people, but the organization makes a special effort to establish programs in underserved areas with higher percentages of at-risk youth. As such, these programs tend to be very affordable, and often, through grants and fund-raising, may even be free. Programs through not-for-profit organizations may also operate in conjunction with a government program. For instance, a YMCA may help support a team that plays in the local government recreation program.

Not-for-profit youth sport programs offer the advantage of being mission-driven. Their goals often focus on a particular population, and they seek to maximize the benefits of youth sport participation. For example, a not-for-profit program may wish to provide youth with additional positive adult support or help build self-esteem. Further, many not-for-profit programs combine a sport program with additional life skills programming and/or education; these programs are often referred to as "plus sport." A youth program called Figure Skating in Harlem, for example, uses figure skating as a means to reach underserved girls and teach discipline, health, and fitness while also providing education programs. Prior to the figure skating component of the program, participants attend educational classes that seek to enhance study skills, promote positive social and emotional skills, introduce money management skills, and promote good health and nutrition. Numerous youth sport not-for-profit organizations similar to this program exist globally. Although each varies in what it can offer, the basic goal of using sport to improve the lives of youth remains consistent across all programs.

Not-for-profit programs also serve a valuable community function. Although the potential community benefits of these programs are comparable to government programs, not-for-profit organizations frequently target vulnerable groups within the community—groups that may need more specialized services or may not be able to easily access government programs. In this way, not-for-profit programs compliment government programs by attempting to ensure that all parts of the community have the opportunity to experience the benefits of youth sport participation.

Like government programs, not-for-profit programs often grapple with limited funding. Unlike government programs, however, not-for-profit organizations do not receive direct tax dollar support. Given that these programs also charge minimal fees, they must rely on fund-raising efforts, securing grants and donations from supportive individuals and organizations. Thus, their long-term sustainability depends on outside funding. Individual giving to not-for profit organizations has a tendency to decrease during challenging economic times, such as during the Great Recession of 2008, although it may trend upward again once the economy begins to improve. In addition, funding from foundations has remained flat. The combination of relatively flat levels of funding, rising costs, and increased needs forced not-for-profit organizations to seek additional funding or cut costs. In some cases, these cost-cutting measures included eliminating sport programs, thus creating a potential void in services for more vulnerable populations.

Challenges for Community Recreation Programs

Youth sport programs of all types share several challenges. These challenges include competition with for-profit youth sport enterprises, ensuring that the benefits of youth sports are available to all, and poor behavior from parents.

Recent years have witnessed a trend toward privatization of youth sports. This trend can create competition for services with community organizations, which impacts the ability of these groups to provide services. One outcome of this trend has been an increase in commercial for-profit youth sport organizations. As the name suggests, commercial for-profit organizations attempt to generate a profit from their sports programs. Thus, programs run by these types of organizations often cost more for registration fees, equipment, and potential travel. This does not mean that for-profit programs do not provide any benefits to their participants. Indeed, for-profit programs may be more likely to have highly trained coaches, specialized services such as private coaching, better facilities, and opportunities to compete against a higher level of competition.

For-profit youth sport programs are springing up nationwide. The benefits of these programs are clear—access to elite coaches, sport science, high-quality facilities, and the national spotlight of college recruiters. One of the largest for-profit youth sport organizations is IMG Academy in Florida. IMG offers training programs in at least nine sports including basketball, football, and lacrosse. The example of IMG, however, highlights both the benefits and the challenge of for-profit programs. On one hand, IMG boasts of the success of many of its former athletes who have continued on to athletic fame. The cost of attending IMG, however, can be staggering. For one year of boarding and training a youth athlete at IMG, the cost runs in excess of $70,000. Although IMG does offer scholarships, the cost is prohibitive for many youth and their parents who are not on scholarship. As programs such as these gain popularity, some critics suggest that they are encouraging a culture where the benefits of sport are only accessible to those with the financial means to support them.

Although participation in youth sports offers the possibility of numerous benefits, it is also the case that these benefits do not automatically emerge. The specific structure and interactions with coaches, parents, administrators, as well as the influences of the wider community, play a key role in determining whether the youth sport experience is positive or negative. Although youth sport programs offer the possibility of benefits to participants, these programs exist within a larger community context that includes families, neighborhoods, schools, churches, and more. To maximize the benefits of youth sports, it is, therefore, imperative for youth sport administrators to view youth sport participation within this larger community context.

Poor behaviors of parents, coaches, and players represent another challenge facing youth sport in all its forms, including community recreation programs. An online search quickly reveals stories of the "crazy hockey Dad" or the out-of-control helicopter parent. The reputation of competitive youth sports, and out-of-control parents, was highlighted on the cable television show, *Friday Night Tykes*, which followed a youth football league in Texas. Although these examples are more the exception than the norm, the attention that they have received points toward a growing problem in youth sport. In response, youth sport administrators have enacted strategies such as parent codes of conduct and parent trainings. In some cases, leagues have gone as far as enforcing silent game days where parents and fans are not allowed to cheer during the game. If this problem persists, youth sport administrators will be forced to continue to address the behavior of parents and volunteer coaches, thus taking away time and resources from regular league-programming responsibilities.

Negative parent behavior may be one reason for the alarmingly high rate of dropout in youth sport programs. By some estimates, nearly 70 percent of youth participants drop out of sport programs by the age of 13 (Woods, 2011). These dropouts appear to be largely attributable to negative experiences, such as having a bad coach, not having fun, or not developing skills. If youth sports are to be environments for positive benefits, it is critical that all relevant components of the youth sport experience (e.g., coaches, officials, and administrators) are equipped with the knowledge and skill set of how to produce a positive experience.

Although concussions have perhaps received the most press, overuse injuries are the most frequent type of injury in youth sport. According to the American Medical Society for Sports Medicine (AMSSM), as many as 50 percent of youth sport injuries are due to overuse (DiFiori et al., 2014). These injuries can be attributed to more intense training, frequent competition, and earlier specialization. Examples of overuse injury include knee and elbow injuries due to repetitive motions such as throwing or running.

Ensuring access and benefits to all, poor behavior of parents, rising costs, and an increase in injuries represent a few of the challenges currently facing youth sport administrators. Addressing these issues will be critical as the numbers of youth in sport programs continue to grow.

Specific Sport Trends

Although traditional team sports (e.g., basketball, baseball, football, and soccer) continue to be popular, alternative sports such as lacrosse and skateboarding are drawing an increasing number of participants. Based on current numbers, basketball, baseball, and soccer remain the most popular youth sports, each boasting approximately 5 million participants in the 6–12 age group (Sports Fitness Industry Association, 2014). In addition, football, despite recent declines, remains popular with participation well over 1 million. Despite these numbers, however, each of these traditionally popular sports witnessed substantial declines in participation in recent years. From 2009 to 2013 participation in youth football declined nearly 30 percent, baseball nearly 15 percent, soccer over 10 percent, and basketball around 5 percent. The potential good news for advocates of youth sport, however, is that these declines appear not be a complete dropout of sport, but rather a migration to different sports. In a recent year, participation in lacrosse, field hockey, swimming, rugby, and triathlons all increased more than 10 percent (Sports Fitness Industry Association, 2014). For some youth sport organizations, these trends spurred the creation of new programs such as the above, as well as alternative programs including flag football, gymnastics, ultimate Frisbee, and Australian Rules football. Although these increases represent a potential positive development, they also create additional challenges as competition for funding, resources, field space, and participants amplifies.

Potential Benefits for Youth Participants

The benefits attributed to participation in youth sports are plentiful. Although the specific program elements and experiences of each program are crucial in influencing whether outcomes are positive or negative, it is clear that sport participation may lead to a number of positive benefits. The following sections give a broad overview of potential benefits. For purposes of discussion, potential benefits will be discussed under the general categories of physical, psychological-emotional, social, life skills, and academic.

As youth sports involve physical exercise, it is natural to assume that participation also leads to physical health benefits. Although the specific sport, level of competition (recreational versus advanced), and individual effort will certainly moderate the physical benefits, existing research does support positive associations between health and participation in youth sport programs. For example, youth participants generally have increased cardio and respiratory functions, improved flexibility and mobility, and increased stamina compared to nonparticipants. Further, participants in youth sport programs are more likely to engage in healthy behaviors outside of sport including healthy eating and physical activity, and avoid negative behaviors such as alcohol and drug use. For example, one study found that female high school athletes are 92 percent less likely to be involved with drugs and 80 percent less likely to get pregnant than nonathletes (Women's Sports Foundation, 1998). In this way, participation in sports may help influence positive healthy behaviors in other areas by providing structure, positive use of free time, or simply emphasizing the importance of healthy decisions.

Youth participation in sports may also be the foundation that leads to lifetime participation, thus enhancing overall lifetime physical health. For one youth, the sport may be tennis, for another it may be basketball; however, in each case, youth have an opportunity as adults to continue healthy exercise habits they learned at an earlier age.

Youth sport participation offers a venue where youth may develop a plethora of psychological and emotional benefits. For instance, participants in youth sports may experience increases in self-esteem, including physical self-concept, positive identity development, initiative, and skills such as leadership and teamwork. Again, it is important to recognize that context matters. For instance, a youth who receives appropriate positive feedback within a sports context is more likely to develop positive self-esteem, whereas a youth who simply receives criticism and experiences disappointment in youth sports will be less likely to develop positive self-esteem.

Youth sport provides not just a physical setting but also a social setting where youth may develop social skills and positive peer relationships. Further, certain contexts may allow youth to learn about different cultures and backgrounds in a positive way. Sport participation also gives youth access to adults other than their own parents (coaches or other parents). These adults can serve as valuable role models, inspiration, and resources. Some research suggests that youth sport participation also leads to social capital—social connections that have positive, practical benefits. This social capital then leads to access to resources, such as finding a job or an internship that can benefit the youth. Finally, youth who participate in community sports are also more likely to be civically engaged in their community through volunteer service, church, or other similar activities.

Sport can also be used as a context in which to teach valuable life skills. For example, pointing out the relationship between practice and results can be used to teach youth about the value of hard work and preparation. Losing a game can be used as an opportunity to discuss the value of persistence in the face of failure. LeBron James, future NBA Hall of Famer, clearly stated, "You have to be able to accept failure to get better." In any sport, failure at some point is almost inevitable;

this provides an opportunity for youth participants to learn persistence in these situations.

Participation in youth sport programs also appears to be strongly linked to improved school academic performance. Specifically, participation in physical activity, such as sport, relates to better cognitive function in children, higher grades, increased engagement in school, and higher educational aspirations. Sport also benefits academic performance by providing a structured schedule that assists in the routines of practice and schoolwork.

Eric Legg

Further Reading

Brayley, R., and D. McLean. 2008. *Financial Resource Management* (2nd ed.). Champaign, IL: Sagamore Publishing.

Brenner, J. S. 2007. "Overuse Injuries, Overtraining, and Burnout in Child and Adolescent Athletes." *Pediatrics: Official Journal of the American Academy of Pediatrics, 119*: 1242–1245.

Coakley, J. 2014. *Sports in Society: Issues and Controversies* (11th ed.) Boston: McGraw-Hill.

DiFiori, J. P., H. J. Benjamin, J. S. Brenner, A. Gregory, N. Jayanthi, G. L. Landry, and A. Luke. 2014. "Overuse Injuries and Burnout in Youth Sports: A Position Statement from the American Medical Society for Sports Medicine." *British Journal of Sports Medicine, 48*: 1–15.

Dixon, M. A., and J. Bruening. 2011. "Youth and Community Sport." In P. Pederson, J. Parks, J. Quarterman, and L. Thibaults (Eds.), *Contemporary Sport Management* (4th ed.) Champaign, IL: Human Kinetics.

Dorsh, T. (In Press). "Family Financial Investment in Youth Sports." *Family Relations.*

Engh, F. 1999. *Why Johnny Hates Sports: Why Youth Sports Are Failing Our Children and What We Can Do about It.* Garden City Park, NY: Avery Publishing Group.

Farrey, T. 2008. *Game on: The All-American Race to Make Champions of our Children.* Bristol, CT: ESPN.

Fraser-Thomas, J. L., J. Cote, and J. Deakin. 2005. "Youth Sport Programs: An Avenue to Foster Positive Youth Development." *Physical Education and Sport Pedagogy, 10*: 19–14.

Fraser-Thomas, J. L., J. Cote, and J. Deakin. 2008. "Examining Adolescent Sport Dropout and Prolonged Engagement from a Development Perspective." *Journal of Applied Sport Psychology, 20*: 318–333.

Legg, Eric, Mary Sara Wells, and Jack P. Barile. 2015. "Factors Related to Sense of Community in Youth Sport Parents." *Journal of Park & Recreation Administration, 33*: 73–86.

National Center for Charitable Statistics (NCCS). 2013. *Charitable Giving in America: Some Facts and Figures.* Accessed August 6, 2015, at http://nccs.urban.org/nccs/statistics /Charitable-Giving-in-America-Some-Facts-and-Figures.cfm.

National Council of Youth Sports (NCYS). 2008. *Report on trends and participation in organized youth sports: Market research report—NCYS Membership Survey,* 2008 ed. Accessed July 21, 2015, at http://www.ncys.org/publications/2008-sports-participation -study.php.

Rimer, S. 2002, January 9. "Rink Manager Says Hockey Father Overpowered His Victim." *New York Times,* 14.

Sports Fitness Industry Association. 2014. *2014 Sports, Fitness and Leisure Activities Topline Participation Report.* Accessed July 21, 2015, at https://www.sfia.org/press/632.

Weiss, M. R. 2008. "'Field of Dreams': Sport as a Context for Youth Development." *Research Quarterly for Exercise and Sport, 79*: 434–449.

Women's Sports Foundation. 1998. *Sport and Teen Pregnancy.* Accessed August 5, 2015, at http://www.womenssportsfoundation.org.

Woods, R. 2011. *Social Issues in Sport* (2nd ed.). Champaign, IL: Human Kinetics.

Competitive Balance

Sally (age 11) looks up at the scoreboard in the gym as the time on the clock clicks ever so slowly toward 00:00. She wants to believe the shouts of encouragement from her coach and parents in the bleachers, but instead, she lowers her head in shame. The scoreboard reads 65–9.

Sally thinks to herself, "At least it's finally over. No more blowouts. No more worrying about kids laughing at me and my teammates behind our back at school." The clock reads 00:00. This miserable experience is finally behind her!

For youth sports professionals, such scenarios are all too familiar. Competitive balance or *parity* in youth sports, meaning in its negative context an imbalance of talent/ability levels, is an important issue that impacts youth enjoyment and has the potential for far greater impacts on participation levels and organizational success.

To begin discussion on competitive balance in youth sports, it is important to start with a firm basis in child development and utilize developmental standards relative to organized youth sports leagues. Competition should be introduced to youth in a developmentally appropriate manner. However, many youth sports leagues around the country fail to adhere to the standards that have been established by reputable youth sports associations such as the National Alliance for Youth Sports (NAYS) and the Positive Coaching Alliance (PCA).

Youth sports associations have been instrumental in developing guidelines and standards for youth sports. In the *National Standards for Youth Sports* guidelines developed by NAYS (2017), for example, the organization urges leagues for youth ages 11 and over to place a high priority on "proper grouping and selection procedures to ensure fair and equitable teams." With some children at age 11 being introduced to full competition for the first time (i.e., complete with scores, statistics, standings, playoffs, championships, and all-star recognition), the issue of maintaining a competitive balance assumes greater importance than leagues for younger children, which typically do not place as high an emphasis on scoreboard results. The potential negative impacts of failing to ensure a certain level of competitive parity among older youth can be significant, from both personal and sociocultural standpoints.

Many youth sports administrators have heard something resembling the following questions at some time or another:

- How could you possibly allow a team to blow out another team so badly?
- Why is that coach allowed to stockpile players and dominate the league every year?

But one of the problems associated with youth sports environments is that opinions relative to the purity of sports sometimes override our common sense. As a result, youth sports administrators do not always hear and are not always challenged by these questions. Instead, parents and coaches simply accept that in sports some teams will dominate, and so they do not challenge the underlying organization of leagues and teams.

The advantages and disadvantages of the round robin scheduling format are a significant consideration in this regard. Round robin scheduling forms the basis for almost every youth sports league in the country, as well as many collegiate intramural programs. One of the disadvantages in round robin scheduling that can potentially lead to forfeitures and lack of interest or enjoyment from participants is competitive balance. A strategy to offset the disadvantage of a competitive imbalance is divisional leveling (i.e., segmented by talent or ability level). In most cases, this works pretty well, but program coordinators have been forced to put in place measures that prevent "ringers" (i.e., those with higher ability levels playing in inappropriate divisions) and/or teams trying to purposefully "play down" a division in order to dominate by competing at a level below their actual skill level. Many youth sports administrators do not have the ability, for one reason or another (most commonly due to participation numbers), to implement the divisional leveling strategy in their leagues. Therefore, competitive balance can become a huge issue with certain coaches taking aggressive steps to stockpile their teams with talent and dominate the leagues in which they compete. Ironically, the people utilizing this competitive advantage often are the same people who will inevitably cry foul and argue loudest when strategies are implemented to offset a competitive imbalance. If enjoyment is the primary motivation for "kids" young and old, competitive imbalance may very well be the leading barrier to having fun through youth sports.

Time and time again, research has shown that enjoyment is the overriding reason that people of all ages participate in sports. As if the work of countless researchers over the years was not enough, coaches, parents, and administrators have received further verification from youth themselves. Peter Barston, a 15-year-old from Darien, Connecticut, wanted to see for himself whether youth sports researchers were accurate in their assignment of "fun" as the prevailing reason for participation (Hyman, 2010). After collecting survey data from many of Darien's sport leagues, Barston concluded that enjoyment was indeed the dominant reason for participation. Mark Hyman, author of the *New York Times* article highlighting Barston's work (and an established youth sports expert himself), wrote, "Adults may lean toward turning children's games into an approximation of professional sports. But ask young players what they want, and the answer can be disarmingly simple" (Hyman, 2010).

If competitive imbalance diminishes enjoyment, it is both necessary and appropriate to take steps toward enhancing parity and competitive balance. That leads us to the doorstep of practicality and implementing measures that might help offset a competitive imbalance. Before doing so, it is important to consider the steps that have historically been taken across all levels of sports to address the issue of competitive balance. Here are several that immediately come to mind:

- **Youth sports**: The 10-run mercy rule has long been a staple in baseball and softball (even as high as the high school and intercollegiate levels). After a set number of innings, the game is halted if a team is ahead by 10 runs or more. Even in Major League Baseball (MLB), the unwritten rule is that teams no longer steal bases after they are ahead by 10 runs or more.
- **Intercollegiate athletics:** The National Collegiate Athletic Association (NCAA) implemented divisional leveling (Divisions I, II, and III) and further broke down Division I to level the playing field further (Football Bowl Subdivision [FBS] and Football Championship Subdivision [FCS]). At an individual sport level, wrestling has rule provisions that halt a match if one person is ahead by 15 points or more.
- **Professional sports:** Leagues such as the National Football League (NFL) and the National Basketball Association (NBA) have salary caps and revenue-sharing practices aimed at enhancing parity and thereby creating more excitement (i.e., closer and more meaningful games). In comparison, Major League Baseball (MLB) does not utilize these practices and has been widely criticized for allowing large-market teams to have an unfair competitive advantage over small-market teams.

So, competitive balancing or enhancing parity is not without precedence. Surely the first person who proposed a 10-run rule in youth baseball was met with criticism, but it is now an accepted rule throughout many levels of the sport. As mentioned, the rule is even utilized sparingly by the NCAA.

Youth recreational sports leagues have taken other steps to help level the playing field and further enhance the enjoyment of participants as well. Below are a few practical examples with ideas for potential improvement and/or implementation in youth sports:

1. **Skill assessment:** Many youth sports leagues already employ some form of skill assessment to ensure that the most accomplished players (and the ones that are less advanced developmentally) are evenly distributed among all the competing teams. Leagues can also take further steps to ensure fairness by having staff or other volunteers assess skills (rather than would-be coaches). When coaches do so, some observers believe that it creates unnecessary pressure on youth and subconsciously promotes a professional sports mentality (i.e., advanced scouting).

2. **Redraft every year:** The arguments against redrafts are varied and in some cases viable. But, ultimately, a redraft helps with two issues central to youth ages 11–14 in particular. First, it addresses the current issue of competitive imbalance and prevents teams from stockpiling talent year after year (if you have a *dynasty* in youth sports leagues, you likely have a problem). Second, it addresses the prevalent issue of cliques. It's true that kids prefer to play on teams with their friends, but this practice can sometimes exacerbate issues involving bullying and social ostracization. By redrafting, clique problems are reduced and youth are exposed to—and given the opportunity to make friends with—more children their age.

3. **Prevent coach recruitment:.** In conducting a redraft, do not allow managers to prestock their teams by signing up parents as coaches in order to have that parent's star player on their team. Many organizations such as Little League International have detailed guidelines to guide these practices, but some coaches and parents will try their hardest to circumvent even the most stringent of guidelines.

4. **Pool play as an alternative to divisional leveling:** Divisional level was discussed earlier in the entry, but many youth sports leagues do not have the participant numbers and/or the resources to handle multiple divisions for the same age group or cohort. Therefore, similar to some international competitions, pool play could be implemented. This would involve teams playing a set number of games in the first half of league play and then being reorganized by win-loss record for the second set of games. This would in effect serve as a leveling function and potentially allow for more competitive games in the second half of league play.

5. **Resets:** We need to look no further than pickup or informal games for inspiration. When games get out of hand in pickup games, what is done? In

many cases, it's either a reset (i.e., "Let's play best 2 of 3"), or if others are waiting, strategies are put in place to speed up the game. For organized youth sports, the strategy to "run it back" and play "best 2 of 3" is simply not plausible due to time and facility constraints. However, resets can easily be implemented in any sport. When the score gets to a certain level (and it should be one where a comeback is improbable), the score is simply reset. If there's time left on the game clock or for the preestablished time limit, a reset can keep both teams engaged. This can even be a quality alternative to the traditional 10-run rule in baseball.

Ultimately, it should be communicated that no strategy is going to be successful unless organizations develop a culture of respect surrounding competition and receive buy-in from league stakeholders—coaches, parents, and participants.

Youth sports administrators should recognize that implementing competitive balance measures in a unilateral fashion may result in severe backlash from those stakeholders that are so critical to a league's success. But if leagues educate coaches and parents about the benefits of implementing parity measures, engage with and listen to youth participants, and maintain an open dialogue between coaches, parents, officials, and administrators, youth sports professionals can ultimately do more toward promoting their organizational mission and maintaining a league where competitive balance contributes to overall enjoyment.

The vast majority of youth sports organizations have mission statements that firmly support the notion of competitive balance. Why? Because most youth sports organizations have stated missions that align with child or youth development rather than overt competition or a win-at-all-costs attitude, such as the mission statement for Little League, Incorporated, one of the most popular youth sports organizations:

> Through proper guidance and exemplary leadership, the Little League program assists youth in developing the qualities of citizenship, discipline, teamwork and physical well-being. By espousing the virtues of character, courage and loyalty, the Little League Baseball and Softball program is designed to develop superior citizens rather than stellar athletes.

The phrase that sticks out in this mission is the final four words: ". . . rather than superior athletes." Yet, one could make a case that Little League has lost participants in the last 10–15 years to the Cal Ripken League due to the perception of an overly competitive environment rather than a developmental focus—one no doubt magnified by an increasingly more publicized Little League World Series. However, although overt competitiveness and the creation of rising stars may be public perception, it is not the league's mission. The focus should be, as stated in the mission, "to assist youth in developing the qualities of citizenship, discipline, team-work and physical well-being." That mission seems very clear, and maintaining competitive balance helps to do just that. But, doing so will naturally lead to some criticism that must be addressed.

Youth sports administrators who have implemented measures to counteract problems with competitive balance have been met with a new round of questioning:

- Why do we coddle today's youth and insulate them from the realities of life and competition?
- Where would Kobe Bryant be today if he was not allowed to be a star and dominate his opponents?

These are important questions for youth sports professionals to anticipate. Weathering the backlash that can ensue after competitive balance measures are implemented is a paramount consideration. Unfortunately, sometimes the loudest voices in the room are not always those who care deeply about sport being a positive experience for all children. Some in the general population would have us believe that children these days are coddled, rewarded, and praised too effusively in today's youth sport world. In some cases, they may absolutely be correct. However, in many youth sports organizations, the people organizing leagues genuinely care about the well-being of the participants in their programs. They are not trying to remove losing; they are not trying to isolate children from experiencing success and understanding failure. On the contrary, most are trying to organize environments where youth development is the key to success. Yet, where does the popular sentiment and accompanying criticism arise? It's due in part to the generational notion that all those who come after us are flawed in some way or another. That message resonates almost universally and is cyclical.

Each and every generation wants better for their children, and then ironically, since that *better* is not what is experienced; the children are sometimes criticized for being too soft or too lazy. This notion is supported by Alfie Kohn in *The Myth of the Spoiled Child: Challenging the Conventional Wisdom about Children and Parenting* (2014). Kohn breaks down the popular but misguided sentiment that each and every successive generation of children are spoiled and/or coddled. Participation trophies have become an oft-cited example of this misperception. Many people believe that participation trophies have become standard for all youth sports leagues. On the contrary, in the *National Standards for Youth Sports* (2017) developed and published by NAYS, participation tokens (e.g., trophies, medals, and certificates) are only recommended for the younger developmentally appropriate age groups (8 and under).

As some people decry that competition has been diminished in today's youth sports world, private club sports organizations have never been more popular at any point in our country's history. Many of these club sports or travel teams are designed to refine and highlight the skills of high-level youth athletes and promote a higher level of competition among teams. So, if a young Kobe Bryant were to time travel to today's era, he'd find an environment wherein high-level competition and the ability for him to dominate would perhaps be even more magnified than it was when he was in high school.

The last 50 years of the sport industry have seen an enormous increase in the salaries that professional athletes garner, and that overwhelmingly powerful motivating factor, combined with the rising costs of a college education, make the allure of an intercollegiate athletic scholarship (a stepping stone to professional sports stardom in most instances) even more pronounced for parents. Yet, as Bill Pennington pointed out in highlighting that only partially funded athletic scholarships are available for many athletes in nonrevenue sports, "parents often look back on the many years spent shuttling sons and daughters to practices, camps and games with a changed eye. Swept up in the dizzying pursuit of sports achievement, they realize how little they knew of the process" (Pennington, 2008).

NCAA president Myles Brand agreed with this general sentiment, stating that "the youth sports culture is overly aggressive, and while the opportunity for an athletic scholarship is not trivial, it's easy for the opportunity to be over-exaggerated by parents and advisers" (Pennington, 2008).

Even if disagreement persists as to the extent or cause of the problem of over-competitiveness in youth sports settings, everyone agrees that sport has the potential to be a healthy outlet, a setting where our nation's youth grow, prosper, and develop. Yet, intentionality in creating those healthy environments is key to that success. If professional sports and intercollegiate athletics can agree that competitive balance is important to ensuring success in their leagues, why can't youth sports do the same? By implementing commonsense measures designed to ensure that organizational missions are being promoted above and beyond misguided popular sentiment or an overly competitive mentality of dominance, youth sports organizations will foster enjoyment in the youth they are serving.

P. Brian Greenwood

Further Reading

Gould, Daniel, and Linda Petlichkoff. 1988. "Participation Motivation and Attrition in Young Athletes." In Frank L. Smoll, Richard A. Magill, and Michael J. Ash (Eds.), *Children in Sport* (3rd ed., pp. 161–178). Champaign IL: Human Kinetics.

Hyman, Mark. 2010, January 30. *A Survey of Youth Sports Finds Winning Isn't the Only Thing.* Accessed May 10, 2016, at http://www.nytimes.com/2010/01/31/sports/31youth.html.

Kohn, Alfie. 2014. *The Myth of the Spoiled Child: Challenging the Conventional Wisdom about Children and Parenting.* Boston: Da Capo Books.

Little League, Incorporated. 2016. *Why We Are Relevant.* Accessed May 2, 2016, at http://www.littleleague.org/Little_League_Big_Legacy/About_Little_League/Why_We_Are_Relevant.htm.

National Alliance for Youth Sports. 2017. *National Standards for Youth Sports, 2017.* Accessed December 28, 2017, at https://www.nays.org/resources/nays-documents/national-standards-for-youth-sports.

Pennington, Bill. 2008, March 20. *Expectations Lose to Reality of Sports Scholarships.* Accessed January 18, 2016, at http://www.nytimes.com/2008/03/10/sports/10scholarships.html?_r=0.

Perez, Braulio, and Chris Ryan. 2015, December 22. *Report: Cape Atlantic Girls Basketball President Says 101-Point Blowout Bad for All.* Accessed July 28, 2016, at http://highschoolsports.nj.com/news/article/-2820080589402697653/report-cape-atlantic-girls-basketball-president-says-atlantic-city-blowout-bad-for-everyone.

Positive Coaching Alliance. 2016. *Better Athletes, Better People.* Accessed August 1, 2016, at http://www.positivecoach.org.

Powell, Robert Andrew. 2004. *We Own This Game: A Season in the Adult World of Youth Football.* New York: Grove Press.

Seefeldt, Vern, Martha Ewing, and Stephan Walk. 1992. *Overview of Youth Sports Programs in the United States.* Washington, D.C.: Carnegie Council on Adolescent Development.

Concussions

Media coverage of concussions has grown exponentially in the 21st century due to multiple lawsuits and acts of violence by former professional athletes. However, the concept of long-term consequences from sports-related brain injuries is not new; it was first introduced in 1927 by Michael Osnato and Vincent Giliberti. The following year, Harrison Martland (1928) coined the term *punch drunk syndrome* in relation to boxers. In 1949, Macdonald Critchley first used the term *chronic traumatic encephalopathy,* or CTE, which is still widely used today. The early research into this field was based mostly on boxing, as it was the most popular sport at the time with obvious increased risk for head injury. More recently, however, injuries relating to American football have been driving research and news stories.

A lawsuit accusing the National Football League (NFL) of not warning players of the risk of brain injury, as well as of hiding damages of said brain injuries, was settled in April 2015. This suit, coupled with multiple reports of former NFL players committing suicide, has pushed American football to the forefront of the discussion. Although football carries obvious risks of head injury, it is not the only sport with serious implications. Many other recreational activities, including popular youth sports like soccer, basketball, hockey, and baseball, carry a risk for traumatic brain injury. This problem is not confined to professional or even collegiate athletics. For example, tackling in football, heading the ball in soccer, or chasing loose balls in basketball is required regardless of level of competition. Although the intensity of play is certainly a factor, the risk of concussion is inherent to sport.

Based on this pervasive risk, concern about acute and long-term ramifications of sports-related concussions (SRCs) has risen accordingly. The sporting and health care communities have responded with an emphasis on education and awareness at all levels. The Centers for Disease Control and Prevention (CDC), Pop Warner, Major League Soccer, the National Football League, and other youth and professional sport associations have spearheaded the effort with multiple campaigns and resources for athletes, parents, coaches, and health care providers. These campaigns have led to an increase in presentation for treatment. From 2001 to 2009, annual emergency room visits for traumatic brain injuries rose from 153,375 to 248,418 in persons younger than 19 engaged in sporting or recreational activity (CDC, 2015a). Hopefully, more education and awareness will continue to lead to more treatment and prevention of long-term deficits.

One of the earliest attempts to clarify and explain many of the uncertainties clouding the concussion debate took place at the First International Conference on Concussion in Sport (ICCS), which was held in Vienna, Austria, in 2001. A group of world-renowned experts in many different disciplines related to concussions released concise recommendations, including return-to-play guidelines and sideline assessment procedures. When the fourth ICCS conference was held in Zurich, Switzerland, in 2012, recommendations continued to expand and evolve.

Defining Concussions

Finding a clear definition for concussion is a long-standing problem. One 2014 systematic review of concussion studies between 2001 and 2012 found 50 different concussion definitions. Consensus groups have been assembling to alleviate this problem. As defined at the Consensus Statement on Concussion in Sport in 2012, a concussion is a brain injury caused by biomechanical forces that could be from a direct blow anywhere on the body (McCrory et al., 2013). It is on the spectrum of traumatic brain injury (TBI) and has also been known as mild TBI or mTBI. However, debate continues as to whether these words are purely interchangeable. Semantics aside, this injury with resulting neural damage has several common features, including, but not limited to neurologic impairment that, usually, has a rapid onset and rapid recovery; acute clinical symptoms based on functional, *not* structural, abnormalities; or a set of clinical physical, behavioral, cognitive, and/or emotional signs and symptoms.

The vagueness of these features may not even seem to be a definition, but it highlights the case-by-case difference in presentation: a fundamental principle in understanding concussions in youth. Instead of a rigid set of criteria, the bigger picture should focus on a set of clinical symptoms that tend to display similar duration (rapid onset and recovery) and pathophysiology (functional abnormalities). Unfortunately, for all involved, concussions are, by their nature, transient and variable.

Presentation

Because of previously listed defining characteristics, the athlete often does not know that he or she should be seen by a medical professional. Therefore, the importance of the observer's role cannot be overstated, and education is a prerequisite for an effective evaluation. The individual who identifies the injury is as variable as the injury itself. This identifying individual could be anyone, including other athletes, coaches, parents, and sports officials. This highlights the importance of education for all involved at the youth sports level to ensure the presence of capable observers who have the athletes' health interests in mind. Any play associated with acceleration, followed by deceleration of the head, should raise suspicion. There are two types of this movement of the head: rotational and linear. Forces from rotation generally cause more damage than those from linear motion. Keeping with the historical boxing reference, a jab versus a hook is a useful analogy. The rotational force from a hook punch knocks out the opponent more often than the linear force from the jab. This same concept can be applied to other sports to monitor for potential head injuries.

After identifying these movements of the game, the observer must also be able to monitor for signs that raise suspicion for brain injury as well as to inquire regarding symptoms. A "sign" is an objectively observed finding indicative of a medical condition, and a symptom is subjectively felt by the patient and, therefore, requires self-reporting. However, the distinction is not always this clear, especially for signs involving cognition or emotion.

The Centers for Disease Control and Prevention (CDC) Heads Up (2015b) program distinguishes symptoms into four different categories. Concussion signs are often more dramatic and well documented than symptoms, and they can also be divided into four categories. There is often overlap between these signs and symptoms. Table 1 is meant to serve as a general guide.

Table 1 Signs and Symptoms of Concussion

	Symptoms	**Signs**
Cognition	"Foggy" Drowsy	Confusion Concentration difficulty Memory difficulty
Emotion/behavior	Mood labiality Nervousness Anxiety	Changes in behavior
Sleep	Insomnia Changes in sleep patterns	Insomnia
Physical	Headaches Neck pain Nausea Blurred vision Double vision	Loss of consciousness Amnesia of events Seizures Convulsions

A well-known sign, loss of consciousness, is commonly associated with concussion. However, loss of consciousness, as a requirement of diagnosis, is one of many myths surrounding this injury. This is particularly true in the youth athlete. A recent study focused on this topic and found that 11 percent of high school athletes presented with concussion versus 34 percent of college athletes (Daneshvar, Nowinski, McKee, & Cantu, 2011). This 11 percent only includes those diagnosed with a concussion and does not take into account those that went undiagnosed due to subtle signs and symptoms that went unrecognized. Therefore, athletes observed with the signs or reporting the symptoms shown in Table 1 should be taken seriously. They should not "walk it off" or "rub some dirt on it," as this type of injury is not comparable to playing through musculoskeletal pain. It is not a sign of weakness or a lack of toughness to suffer from a concussion.

Diagnosis

Diagnosis starts with observation at presentation, as previously mentioned. Once an athlete's injury, signs, or symptoms have been identified as high risk, then a sideline evaluation by a trained medical professional is required. This begins with a neurologic or cognitive assessment. Cervical spine injury must also be ruled out, and the patient should not be left alone due to the risk of deterioration, such as changes in vision, worsening headache, or decreased consciousness. Serial exams can monitor for any changes as some symptoms can evolve over minutes to hours (McCrory et al., 2013) Although invaluable, these exams are subjective, and objective standardized sideline tests are available. For example, the third edition of the Sports Concussion Assessment Tool (SCAT-3; 2015) provides a three-page document developed by the ICCS and approved by many organizations, such as the International Olympic Committee and the Federation International Football Association (FIFA). This test comes with administration instructions as well as return-to-play guidelines. It gives a numeric scoring system encompassing a detailed sign-and-symptom evaluation as well as a detailed history. If the athlete is 12 years of age or less, then there is a pediatric specific SCAT-3 (McCrory et al., 2013). If the sideline assessment is abnormal or if there is still a high suspicion for concussion, an urgent evaluation at an emergency room or medical office is warranted.

However, many youth sports teams do not have trained sideline personnel for the evaluation and management of suspected head injuries. This again highlights the importance of informed parents, coaches, and athletes. If athletes have any of these signs or symptoms, they should be taken to a physician or emergency department for evaluation.

Other modalities common to a doctor's office, such as magnetic resonance imaging (MRI) or computed tomography (CT or CAT scan), are not useful for the diagnosis of a concussion. In a concussion, the damage is functional and not structural; the current imaging techniques cannot identify functional abnormalities. However, these tests are commonly utilized if there is concern that the patient may have suffered a concomitant brain bleed or a skull fracture. Overall, there is no single entity that can diagnose or exclude a concussion. Multiple tools and multiple participants are required for an accurate and timely diagnosis.

Treatment

Treatment should begin immediately after a diagnosis is made and requires a multidisciplinary approach. If a concussion is suspected, then the athlete should not be allowed to return to play until he or she has cleared the sideline assessment, regardless of the level of competition (McCrory et al., 2013). This strategy decreases the risk of second impact syndrome (SIS), a condition in which an athlete sustains a second head injury before the symptoms of the first head injury have resolved (Cantu, 1998). However, even a minor second impact while the brain is vulnerable can lead to coma, and this mechanism is currently unknown. In 2006, Mori, Katayama, and Kawamata reported mostly men with a mean age of 17.9 playing football (71 percent) and boxing (14 percent) suffered from SIS (Mori et al., 2006). These young men are playing high-intensity, high-risk sports with a culture of toughness that creates a perfect scenario for SIS.

Physical and cognitive rest have been the mainstay of acute concussion treatment for years, but there are no current evidence-based recommendations for duration or type of rest. Other conservative measures used to treat specific symptoms include establishing regular sleep patterns; understanding helpful coping strategies such as remaining calm or not getting frustrated if short-term memory is not fully restored immediately; professional counseling; and avoidance of caffeine, alcohol, and nicotine (Meehan, 2011). As a general rule, a patient should resume normal cognitive activity, school, and social life before resuming normal physical activity. Also, serial monitoring is necessary to detect worsening symptoms, such as headache, nausea and vomiting, slurred speech, confusion, agitation, restlessness, etc. (McCrory et al., 2013). These require immediate and more intense evaluations by a medical professional because they can indicate a more serious brain injury.

Medication can also be used in the treatment of concussions in the acute and chronic setting. When considering pharmacologic treatment, two questions must

Table 2 Graduated Return to Play Protocol

Rehabilitation Stage	Function at Stage	Objective of Stage
No activity	Physical and cognitive rest	Recovery
Light aerobic exercise	Walking, stationary bike, swimming. No resistance training.	Increase heart rate
Sport specific exercise	Simple: running, skating	Increase kinematic activity
Noncontact participation	Complex: passing and route running. May begin resistance training.	Increase coordination and cognitive factor of sport
Full contact	Normal training	Preparation for return to play
Return to play	Normal match play	

be raised: Have the symptoms exceeded the normal recovery period, and are the treatment benefits going to outweigh the negative treatment side effects (Meehan, 2011)? Treatment is symptom-specific and varies depending on the patient. Acetaminophen or Tylenol is the drug of choice for acute headaches, but the use of chronic medication depends on the nature of the headaches. Other symptoms commonly treated are dizziness, fatigue, nausea, sleep disturbances, depression, anxiety, and cognitive slowing. The symptoms are often intertwined, and treating one may relieve another. If the symptoms improve with medication, that does not necessarily mean the patients are fully recovered. However, they may be able to recover more comfortably. Therefore, proper pharmacologic management requires a unique assessment of all symptoms and plan for each case.

ICCS recommends phases for return to play following a sports-related concussion. Each phase should be completed in 24 hours, and the patient must remain asymptomatic to advance to the next phase. This process should last roughly one week. If a patient experiences symptoms during a transition, then there should be no activity for 24 hours with the patient downgraded to the stage below. Additionally, an athlete should not return to play while still taking a medication as it could mask signs or symptoms of neurologic injury from a second impact. Table 2 is based on these guidelines.

Prognosis

Following these treatment guidelines generally leads to a favorable prognosis. The majority of athletes recover spontaneously in only several days (Johnston et al.,

2004). In a study led by Michael Collins in 2006, 50 percent of athletes returned to play in one week, and 83 percent returned to play by three weeks (Collins, Lovell, Iverson, Ide, and Maroon, 2006). In 2003, another study reported that some of the collegiate football players included recovered within 24 hours and 91 percent had recovered by seven days (McCrea et al., 2003). However, some residual effects remain, and they may not be readily observable. Some signs and symptoms may persist for 30–45 days, and others may persist for years (Brooks et al., 2000; Iverson, Gaetz, Lovell, and Collins, 2004).

Multiple modifiers are associated with the prognosis for concussions. Compared to adult and collegiate athletes, younger patients have longer duration of recovery and worse outcomes (Field, Collins, Lovell, and Maroon, 2003; Giza, Griesbach, and Hovda, 2005). In a 2007 study (Boden, Tacchetti, Cantu, Knowles, and Mueller, 2007) focused on high school versus collegiate football players, researchers proposed possible explanations for this disparity that could be applied to other sports as well:

- A less developed brain could lead to a lower injury threshold.
- A thinner skull provides less protection.
- More medical staff at collegiate events, which leads to improved diagnosis and treatment.
- Worse technique.
- Poor body control due to developing coordination.

Decreased neck strength has also been proposed, as it leads to more force being transmitted to the brain. This is especially important for sports with the highest risk of concussion, including football, hockey, and soccer.

Along with age considerations, ICCS proposed other concussion modifiers, as shown in Table 3.

Following a concussion, symptoms may persist for three months or more. This condition is known as post-concussion syndrome (PCS). In a study targeting post-concussion syndrome, researchers found that patients with personal and/or family history of mood disorders, psychiatric illness, and migraine headaches were at an increased risk of PCS. They also noted an increased risk with delayed symptom presentation (Morgan, Zuckerman, Lee, King, Beaird, Sills, and Solomon, 2015). The study hypothesized that delayed symptom presentation may have resulted in athletes not being removed from play, thus raising the likelihood the athletes suffered repetitive neurologic injury. These findings highlight the importance of preseason physicals and exams to discover pertinent medical history as well as the importance of training individuals to identify high-risk plays and/or players at every level possible. The researchers also grouped the symptoms into four domains similar to those previously mentioned: somatic/physical, cognitive, emotional, and sleep.

Table 3 Concussion Modifiers

Factors	Modifier
Symptoms	Number, severity, duration (>10 days)
Signs	Prolonged loss of consciousness
Sequelae	Convulsion
Temporal	Frequency of repeated concussions Interval between repeated concussions Time from most recent brain injury
Threshold	Repeated concussions with progressively less impact Slower recovery
Age	Less than 18 years old
Comorbidities	Migraine Mental health disorders: depression Learning disability and ADHD Sleep disorder
Medication	Psychoactive drugs and anticoagulants
Activity	High risk or high level of competition

As a three-month duration is required for diagnosis, some of the symptoms seen in PCS are not observed in the acute presentation of concussion and include cognitive slowing, exercise intolerance, changes in reaction times, and emotional changes. If concussions are not managed properly, the likelihood of developing chronic post-concussion syndrome (CPCS) is higher. Symptoms of PCS include:

- Headache
- Dizziness
- Irritability
- Depression
- Impaired attention
- Poor memory
- Executive dysfunction (Harmon et al., 2013; Kelly and Rosenberg, 1998)

Chronic traumatic encephalopathy (CTE), a serious potential long-term complication associated with concussions, has been covered extensively in recent media. CTE is distinguished from PCS by a slow but progressive development of symptoms.

There is a latency period of years to decades with a subtle onset of symptoms, which include irritability, impulsivity, aggression, depression, short-term memory loss, and increased risk of suicide (Stein, Alvarez, and McKee, 2014). This neurodegeneration is associated with an abnormal accumulation of tau proteins (Tartaglia et al., 2014). The temporal and insidious symptom onset is further complicated because many of the above symptoms, including depression and anxiety, are common to all forms of TBI (Johnston et al., 2004). However, although they are often linked in popular media, the mechanism of the progression from concussion to CTE remains speculative and warrants further research (Ling, Hardy, and Zetterberg, 2015).

Prevention

Due to the potential serious long-term effects and the difficult diagnosis, prevention is preferable to treatment of concussions. However, as previously mentioned, risk is inherent to every level of every sport and at every age. Is it possible to change the sport or change the rules to decrease this risk of concussion? Resistance will obviously be met when attempting to change sports that have become deeply ingrained into our society. Athletics, as a whole, has a culture surrounding it, and each sport also has its unique niche of a culture. Some of these focus on mental and physical toughness, playing through injury or pain, and intense play. Such attributes often make for a great athlete, but they also subtly hinder self-reporting and must be addressed in order to make gains in concussion awareness and treatment. Also, many sports feature a regular "flow" of play. Prolonged or increased stoppages in play are needed for better examination, but there is concern that the "flow" of sports could get disrupted.

If the sport itself cannot be changed, what can be done once the game or event has begun? Helmets meant to decrease forces imparted on the head are an obvious tool that can be employed in concussion prevention. They are being used in some of the sports with the highest concussion risk, including football, hockey, lacrosse, and even soccer. However, concerns abound that an increase in helmet technology and padding has led to a false sense of security among athletes. This leads to increased severity of hits and increased severity of force transmitted to the head, a paradox commonly referred to as risk compensation (Hagel and Meeuwisse, 2004). There have been discussions regarding decreasing the amount of padding in football helmets to prevent the use of the head as a weapon, but tackling and style of play would have to be greatly altered. The benefit of that change might not be worth the negative impact.

Although helmets are not as commonly associated with soccer as football, they have been introduced in some settings in an attempt to reduce concussion incidence. Although not yet a requirement to play, it has been reported that headgear provided protection against concussions during a single season in 2006, and researchers recommended helmets for types of players who would benefit the most: goalkeepers, children, and players who have previously suffered a concussion (Delaney et al., 2008).

Researchers have also noted that virtually all sports, with the exception of cheerleading and gymnastics, have more concussions in games than in practice. Cheerleaders and gymnasts are learning a risky skill perfected for competition, while most other sports compete with less intensity in practice than in a game (Daneshvar, Nowinski, McKee, and Cantu, 2011). Cheerleading and gymnastics are also started at a very young age and are very popular in the United States. However, limiting the number of practices or the amount of contact in practice would decrease the potential head injuries. Pop Warner, a multistate organization for youth football, has recently made rule changes limiting the amount of time for contact drills in a practice (Farrey, 2015). Some observers believe, however, that this presents a Catch-22: decreased time practicing technique leads to worse technique in highly competitive games, thus leading to an increased risk of injury. Although this may work for very young children in Pop Warner, it may not be as feasible for high school and/or collegiate athletes. However, training more could also decrease risk. Increasing neck and core strength could potentially decrease concussion risk as research has demonstrated, in a biomechanical assessment of head impact in high school football (Broglio, 2009). In a similar move, in 2016 the organization U.S. Club Soccer set forth rules for restricting youth players from heading the soccer ball. Specifically, heading the ball is banned in the age group 11 and under and is restricted for 12- and 13-year-olds. This raises the question: When will players learn proper technique for heading the ball and for challenging for the ball? At age 14, when they are about to enter high school and the level of competition is much higher? Changing rules regarding high-risk plays such as tackling and heading the ball may prevent earlier exposure but could also lead to more accidents from poor technique later. There is no easy answer.

There are also preventative measures that do not involve competition. As previously mentioned, preparticipation history and physical exams are another method to prevent concussions. They identify athletes at higher risk and provide opportunities for educating parents and athletes alike about concussions. Advocates assert that this direct connection with the athletes could potentially lead to higher self-reporting and a quicker diagnosis. The government has also become involved, with many states passing legislation involving sports-related concussions.

In 2006, a 13-year-old boy named Zackery Lystedt returned to play after his concussion was improperly managed, and he suffered a severe head injury playing football. The state of Washington passed the Zackery Lystedt Law in 2009 organized around three core elements: annual education of athletes and parents, mandatory removal from play of athletes suspected of being concussed, and required clearance by a designated health-trained professional before returning to play (Harvey, 2013). All 50 states and Washington, D.C., passed legislation between July 2009 and January 2014 (Gibson, Herring, Kutcher, and Broglio, 2015). These laws focus on secondary rather than primary prevention; they change how concussions are managed, before and after they occur. Like the Lystedt Law, most of these laws focus on three main elements to varying degrees: education, removal from play, and evaluation and clearance to return to play (Harvey, 2013). Most of these laws are relatively new, and the ramifications may not be evident for some time.

Finally, what can parents, coaches, and athletes do to reduce vulnerability to concussion? Although mandated by many state laws, education and awareness are paramount in concussion prevention and treatment. The CDC Heads Up program is widely distributed, and the website contains separate tabs for parents, athletes, and coaches, as well as online training. This program exemplifies the required multidisciplinary approach; everyone must be involved to properly manage this subtle and potentially devastating injury. It is a great resource for further reading and learning about current concussion knowledge for all readers. This information is readily accessible and free on the CDC website at www.cdc.org.

Future of Concussion Diagnosis and Treatment

There is still much to learn about every aspect of concussion diagnosis and management, as well as general brain function and cognitive process. Moving forward, the importance of self-reporting should be reinforced starting with our youth athletes and continuing with increased public education and awareness. Current effective programs and campaigns must be continued. Also, there needs to be a focused and intentional change in the culture of sports to address underreporting of concussion symptoms.

Diverse research avenues requiring diverse methods of data collection and experiment design highlight the most important aspect of concussion diagnosis and treatment: the multidisciplinary approach. Everyone involved must make a focused effort to work together to prevent the dangerous complications of traumatic brain injury in youth sports.

William Melton and J. Benjamin Jackson III

Further Reading

Boden, B. P, R. L. Tacchetti, R. C. Cantu, S. B. Knowles, and F. O. Mueller. 2007. "Catastrophic Head Injuries in High School and College Football Players." *American Journal of Sports Medicine, 35*(7): 1075–1081.

Broglio, S. P., J. J. Sosnoff, S. Shin, X. He, C. Alcaraz, and J. Zimmerman. 2009. "Head Impacts during High School Football: A Biomechanical Assessment." *Journal of Athletic Training, 44*(4): 342–349.

Brooks, W. M., C. A. Stidley, H. Petropoulos, R. E. Jung, D. C. Weers, S. D. Friedman, et al. 2000. "Metabolic and Cognitive Response to Human Traumatic Brain Injury: A Quantitative Proton Magnetic Resonance Study." *Journal of Neurotrauma, 17*(8): 629–640.

Cantu, R. C. 1998. "Return to Play Guidelines after a Head Injury." *Clinical Sports Medicine, 17*(1): 45–60.

Centers for Disease Control and Prevention (CDC). 2015a. Nonfatal traumatic brain injuries related to sports and recreation activities among persons aged < 19 years—United States, 2001–2009. Accessed May 30, 2015, at https://www.cdc.gov/mmwr/preview/mmwrhtml/mm6039a1.htm.

Centers for Disease Control and Prevention (CDC). 2015b. *HEADS UP to Youth Sports.* Accessed May 30, 2015, at http://www.cdc.gov/headsup/youthsports.

Collins, M., M. R. Lovell, G. L. Iverson, T. Ide, and J. Maroon. 2006. "Examining Concussion Rates and Return to Play in High School Football Players Wearing Newer Helmet Technology: A Three-Year Prospective Cohort Study." *Neurosurgery, 58*(2): 275–286.

Critchley, M. 1949. Punch-Drunk Syndromes: The Chronic Traumatic Encephalopathy of Boxers. Hommage a Clovis Vincent.

Daneshvar, D. H., C. J. Nowinski, A. C. McKee, and R. C. Cantu. 2011. "The Epidemiology of Sport-Related Concussion." *Clinical Sports Medicine, 30*(1): 1–17, vii.

Delaney, J. S., A. Al-Kashmiri, R. Drummond, and J. A. Correa. 2008. "The Effect of Protective Headgear on Head Injuries and Concussions in Adolescent Football (Soccer) Players." *British Journal of Sports Medicine, 42*(2): 110–115.

Farrey, T. 2015. *Pop Warner to Limit Practice Contact.* Accessed May 30, 2015, at http://espn.go.com/espn/story/_/id/8046203/pop-warner-toughens-safety-measures-limiting-contact-practice.

Field, M., M. W. Collins, M. R. Lovell, and J. Maroon. 2003. "Does Age Play a Role in Recovery from Sports-Related Concussion? A Comparison of High School and Collegiate Athletes." *Journal of Pediatrics, 142*(5): 546–553.

Gibson, T. B, S. A. Herring, J. S. Kutcher, and S. P. Broglio. 2015. "Analyzing the Effect of State Legislation on Health Care Utilization for Children with Concussion." *Journal of the American Medical Association Pediatrics, 169*(2): 163–168.

Giza, C. C, G. S. Griesbach, and D. A. Hovda. 2005. "Experience-Dependent Behavioral Plasticity Is Disturbed Following Traumatic Injury to the Immature Brain." *Behavior Brain Research, 157*(1): 11–22.

Hagel, B., and W. Meeuwisse. 2004. "Risk Compensation: A Side Effect of Sport Injury Prevention?" *Clinical Journal of Sport Medicine, 14*(4): 193–196.

Harmon, K. G., J. Drezner, M. Gammons, K. Guskiewicz, M. Halstead, S. Herring, et al. 2013. "American Medical Society for Sports Medicine Position Statement: Concussion in Sport." *Clinical Journal of Sport Medicine, 23*(1): 1–18.

Harvey, H. H. 2013. "Reducing Traumatic Brain Injuries in Youth Sports: Youth Sports Traumatic Brain Injury State Laws, January 2009–December 2012." *American Journal of Public Health, 103*(7): 1249–1254.

Iverson, G. L, M. Gaetz, M. R. Lovell, and M. W. Collins. 2004. "Cumulative Effects of Concussion in Amateur Athletes." *Brain Injury, 18*(5): 433–443.

Johnston, K. M., G. A. Bloom, J. Ramsay, J. Kissick, D. Montgomery, D. Foley, et al. 2004. "Current Concepts in Concussion Rehabilitation." *Current Sports Medicine Reports, 3*(6): 316–323.

Kelly, J. P., and J. H. Rosenberg. 1998. "The Development of Guidelines for the Management of Concussion in Sports." *Journal of Head Trauma Rehabilitation, 13*(2): 53–65.

Kristman, V. L, J. Borg, A. K. Godbolt, L. R. Salmi, C. Cancelliere, L. J. Carroll, et al. 2014. "Methodological Issues and Research Recommendations for Prognosis after Mild Traumatic Brain Injury: Results of the International Collaboration on Mild Traumatic Brain Injury Prognosis." *Archives of Physical Medicine and Rehabilitation, 95*(3 Suppl.): S265–S277.

Ling, H., J. Hardy, and H. Zetterberg. (2015). "Neurological Consequences of Traumatic Brain Injuries in Sports." *Molecular and Cellular Neuroscience, 66*(Pt. B): 114–122.

Martland, H. (1928). "Punch Drunk." *Journal of the American Medical Association, 91*: 1103–1107.

McCrea, M., K. M. Guskiewicz, S. W. Marshall, W. Barr, C. Randolph, R. C. Cantu, et al. 2003. "Acute Effects and Recovery Time Following Concussion in Collegiate Football Players: The NCAA Concussion Study." *Journal of the American Medical Association, 290*(19): 2556–2563.

McCrory, P., W. H. Meeuwisse, M. Aubry, B. Cantu, J. Dvořák, R. J. Echemendia, et al. 2013. "Consensus Statement on Concussion in Sport: The 4th International Conference on Concussion in Sport Held in Zurich, November 2012." *Journal of the American College of Surgeons, 216*(5): e55–e71.

Meehan, W. P. 2011. "Medical Therapies for Concussion." *Clinical Sports Medicine, 30*(1): 115–24, ix.

Morgan, C. D., S. L. Zuckerman, Y. M. Lee, L. King, S. Beaird, A. K. Sills, and G. S. Solomon. 2015. "Predictors of Postconcussion Syndrome after Sports-Related Concussion in Young Athletes: A Matched Case-Control Study." *Journal of Neurosurgery, 15*(6): 589–598.

Mori, T., Y. Katayama, and T. Kawamata. 2006. "Acute Hemispheric Swelling Associated with Thin Subdural Hematomas: Pathophysiology of Repetitive Head Injury in Sports." *Acta Neurochir Supplement, 96*: 40–43.

National Football League. 2015. *NFL Concussion Settlement.* Accessed May 30, 2015, at https://www.nflconcussionsettlement.com.

Osnato, M. 1927. "Postconcussion Neurosis—Traumatic Encephalitis." *Archives of Neurology & Psychiatry* :181–211.

Sports Concussion Assessment Tool (3rd ed.). 2015. Accessed May 30, 2015, at http://bjsm .bmj.com.

Stein, T. D., V. E. Alvarez, and A. C. McKee. 2014. "Chronic Traumatic Encephalopathy: A Spectrum of Neuropathological Changes Following Repetitive Brain Trauma in Athletes and Military Personnel." *Alzheimer's Research & Therapy, 6*(1): 4.

Tartaglia, M. C., L. N. Hazrati, K. D. Davis, R. E. Green, R. Wennberg, D. Mikulis, et al. 2014. "Chronic Traumatic Encephalopathy and Other Neurodegenerative Proteinopathies." *Front Human Neuroscience, 8*: 30.

U.S. Club Soccer. 2016. *Implementation Guidelines for US Soccer's Player Safety Campaign: Concussion Initiatives and Heading for Youth Players.* Accessed July 10, 2016, at http://usclubsoccer.org/2016/03/14/implementation-guidelines-for-u-s-soccers-player -safety-campaign-concussion-initiatives-heading-for-youth-players.

Coping with Failure

Since the early 2000s, a plethora of literature has been written exploring the theoretical downsides of the self-esteem movement. Many of these authors hypothesize that the emphasis on repeatedly telling children how great they are and focusing coaching and parenting practices on creating positive and happy experiences has led to some significant downsides in preparing youth to become successful adults. Critics have expressed concern that in this attempt to create positive experiences, many adults have created opportunities for children and youth to continually achieve success without having to experience failure. Although this is likely to make youth happy in the moment, unfortunately, current research suggests that this is harmful to their long-term development. Children who do not learn to overcome failure tend to be more unprepared as young adults when failure inevitably occurs in their lives. Adults working with children, therefore, must demonstrate some responsibility in ensuring that programs serve the young athletes by preparing them for this aspect of adulthood. Researchers are thus urging parents, coaches, and other adults to consider the role of learning from failure in youth sport.

Sport presents a unique arena in life in that it is specifically designed to produce winners and losers. Youth sports thus provide a *potential* opportunity for children to learn how to win well and lose well. Furthermore, at the youth level, sport should offer a setting in which this learning can take place in a safe and natural environment. If the experience is designed for there to be an overall winner, then naturally, those who do not win have the opportunity to learn and grow from the experience. In addition, the fact that a single youth sporting event tends to have a minimal impact on an individual child's future means that the learning and growth can occur in a time and place that will prepare them for larger and more crucial life events such as college, the job market, or marriage, when the consequences of failure will likely be significantly greater. Critics assert, though, that the same societal trends that have pushed parents toward forcing success in numerous settings such as schools have also infiltrated youth sport in a way that pushes these programs, for example, to provide trophies to all participants simply for registering, despite the potential learning opportunities these policies sacrifice. This entry will explain the benefits of failure in both the short and long term, especially as it relates to youth sport, and then discuss how best to implement failure as a learning experience in youth sport programs.

Benefits of Failure

The process of failing at some goal or objective, both in general and more specifically in the sport world, provides youth with the opportunity to learn to overcome challenges and setbacks in the pursuit of success. Persistence and perseverance are crucial skills to being successful adults, and young athletes are less likely to learn these skills if all they experience are easy accomplishments. These skills are best learned through overcoming significant obstacles such as failure. It is a process that provides growth to the individual and makes him or her more likely to succeed in the future.

Researchers assert that people who never have the opportunity to fail as children grow up increasingly unprepared for college and the real world due to a lack of resilience and coping skills. Protecting youth from ever experiencing failure does damage in multiple ways. It not only prevents them learning necessary skills for success, it can potentially lead them to perceive themselves in a more damaging light. Lessons that children might learn through failure include appropriate coping skills, consequences to choices, how to strategize, motivation to improve, and many other lessons that can have a positive impact throughout their lives. By living in a world in which they are protected from failure, however, there are also a number of lessons that may be learned, which are not as positive. By eliminating the failure experience, children may grow to believe they need to be protected, that they lack the skills to handle anything but success. Their lack of confidence in their own abilities to overcome failure can be detrimental to their ability and willingness to face obstacles in the future. For example, if a youth runner is continuously rewarded for performances despite continuously placing last, he or she may start to believe that the rewards are given because he or she is not capable of doing any better. In this case, the athlete might perceive himself or herself as not having the potential to succeed and drop out of the sport altogether, thereby eliminating the chance to improve or gain the benefits of long-term sport participation. The end result of all this is that removing failure from children's lives may make them happy in their current state, but it will most likely make their lives significantly more difficult in the future.

In 2008 researcher Carol Dweck utilized the concepts of mindsets to describe how this process works. Essentially, children are likely to have one of two types of mindsets that influence their beliefs about their abilities and potential. Individuals with a fixed mindset tend to believe their abilities are set or predetermined. These people see themselves as being either good at something or not. Talent, whether in terms of intelligence, athletic ability, or in any other area, is more innate than learned and consequently; failure is seen as a lack of skill and not an opportunity for growth. Individuals with a growth mindset, however, tend to believe that all people have the opportunity to improve themselves in any area through practice and experience. In the case of individuals with a fixed mindset, failure is viewed as a development tool, an opportunity to improve from where you were before, as it is only through failure that one determines what does not work.

The reality of life is that everyone experiences failure at some point. The concept of mindsets suggests that it is not merely the opportunity to fail that is important, but also how one approaches these failures after they have occurred. For the most part, a growth mindset is seen as more beneficial to long-term success because these types of individuals tend to be more willing to learn and overcome challenges in their lives. In the long run, people who put forth effort into overcoming challenges are more likely to be successful in life and in sport than those who stop at initial failure and assume they cannot accomplish the goal or task.

Failure in Sport

Sport presents an essential opportunity for youth to grow and develop in numerous ways, but it may be one of the most opportune places to develop a growth mindset due to its competitive nature. Sport participation by definition involves a multitude of failures. There are failures in learning and demonstrating new skills, failures in practices, failures to reach specific individual and team goals, and especially failures in competition due to the fact that at most 50 percent of the people in a competition will win while that number is significantly lower in tournaments and individual sport competitions. For the most part, successful athletes will have some inherent ability but will also be the ones who repeatedly and consistently treat failure as a learning opportunity rather than a permanent indicator of ability level. The best athletes, according to researchers, have to struggle at some point. Learning early on that success is an inherent trait rather than earned, on the other hand, can stop young athletes from reaching their full potential.

For example, in the sport of swimming, in every race there are stroke judges with the job of making sure the athletes participate using the correct technique and follow a multitude of rules throughout the race. Even one minor infraction can lead to the athlete being disqualified (a DQ). Young athletes in particular will typically receive a multitude of DQs during the beginning of their athletic careers. In swimming this is seen as a part of the learning process. Following the race, swimmers learn what they did wrong, then use practice to try to correct the mistake, and hopefully in the next race, or within the next few races, correct their technique in ways that result in improved performance. As swimmers become more experienced, they have fewer and fewer DQs. The overall culture within the sport of swimming sees the process of DQing young athletes with a growth mindset. Because this type of failure is seen as an opportunity for growth and improvement rather than an unnecessary setback, the young athletes become better swimmers in the long run.

An additional reason young athletes should not be made to feel badly about failure is because it may help with development of skills and techniques. When these athletes are pressured to continuously win and not "mess up," they may be afraid to become creative in their skill development. Learning to be a successful athlete can be hindered by the stress of trying to get everything exactly right, thereby undermining an athlete's current and future performance. This can be seen in some ways in the American approach to soccer. Children in the United States who play soccer often start games at a young age and may be on competitive teams near the beginning of elementary school. In other countries, however, competitive training does not start until much later. Until that point, children are more likely to play with their skills rather than complete specific drills. The absence of pressure on winning allows them to focus on their footwork and creativity without too much pressure to win from parents, coaches, and other adults. In terms of international elite competition, American soccer players who grew up in the American system of competition tend to not be as successful as players who were more creative and learned how to improvise in a more relaxed environment. Consequently, one could infer, that the lack of pressure to win provides greater opportunity to develop skills and techniques because there is less stress over what will happen if they do not work. Trying new ways to approach a problem in sport should not make young athletes nervous to make a mistake. It should make them eager to learn what will happen and, therefore, when youth sport provides the freedom to fail, these young athletes also have the freedom to be flexible, to improvise, and to become stronger, better athletes.

Appropriate Inclusion of Failure in Youth Sport

If it is clear that failure should be a central part of the youth sport experience, the question remains how it should be used to create the most benefit for young athletes. Obviously, setting up children to intentionally fail is not what is being advocated. There are plenty of natural opportunities in youth sport to learn from failure, making forced failure unnecessary and ethically questionable. But youth sport administrators, coaches, referees, and other concerned adults can be trained in how to employ the natural elements of failure in sport to the benefit of all those involved.

The easiest way to do this is by allowing the natural consequences of one's actions to occur. Lack of practice, improper nutrition, not enough sleep, disagreements with teammates, and a number of other factors can lead young athletes to perform poorly. In these cases, it is important that the significant adults in their lives allow them to fail as a result of their choices rather than step in and save the day in some way. Otherwise, these habits are not likely to improve. Similarly, young athletes should feel encouraged to try new techniques or skills within reasonable safety parameters. Often there is more than one way to go about accomplishing a goal or a task, and the freedom to fail means the freedom to experiment.

Although sometimes failure in sport is the natural consequence of choices made by an athlete, at other times it is simply the result that occurs. At these times it is important for significant adults in a young athlete's life to acknowledge the loss, help him or her use appropriate coping skills, and develop a strategy to lessen the likelihood of a loss next time. It is not appropriate in these situations to blame the referee, the coach, or another player. Dwelling on excuses does not help the athlete overcome the obstacle. It may be that a referee made a bad call at the end of the game, but the fact is referees do make bad calls. Sometimes they go against you, and sometimes they are in your favor. That is outside of the athlete's control. What is in his or her control is his or her own performance and figuring out a way to perform his or her best, regardless of outside influences.

Perceived biases of significant adults also play a role in whether young athletes will learn from their athletic failures or give up. Youth sport professionals should keep in mind that their own personal beliefs regarding failure will do less to influence their young athletes than those athletes' perceptions of the adults' beliefs. In other words, regardless of whether a coach or parent personally believes that failure is a constructive opportunity, if a child thinks that the coach or parent believes failure is an indicator of inability, he or she is more likely to adopt that mindset and act accordingly. Simple questions at the end of a game can lead to these perceptions. If a parent who missed a game, for example, sees the young athlete and first asks "did you win?," this gives the perception to the child that the most important result of the game is winning, not skill development, teamwork, fun, or any other potential area of development. Consequently, that child may then start to focus on avoiding loss as the most important outcome rather than what the parent actually believes is important, and somehow a parent who wants to promote a growth mindset in his or her child has unintentionally done the opposite. As youth sport professionals and parents, it is crucial to remain aware of how our words and actions are perceived by youth, not how they are intended, as they attempt to help youth develop appropriately through sport participation.

Finally, youth sport professionals also need to be aware of how they are providing feedback in more subtle ways. For example, praising young athletes for their accomplishments by saying that they are intelligent, athletic, or simply good at something is likely to lead those children toward a fixed mindset. They will hear that they have an ability, and when they fail to perform another time, they may fall victim to assumptions that they are no longer as capable or athletic. Instead, it is more appropriate to use feedback related to effort, perseverance, and hard work. Even better, the feedback should be focused on these areas and be constructive in some way. Providing vague statements such as "good job" is not useful in helping children learn exactly what was done well and how. Instead, for example, it would be better to compliment them on the number of times they practiced to improve, and the specific attributes you saw improving as a result. This type of encouragement should lead them more toward a growth mindset where they become energized and determined when they struggle with something difficult and are consequently more likely to use the failures they face in sport to their advantage.

Conclusion

Youth sport professionals have an opportunity and a responsibility to help their young athletes develop in a way that they become successful adults, not merely athletes. The way failure in sport is approached by these professionals can play a significant role in that development. Experiencing failure through sport is one tool that can result in promoting growth mindsets, which can generalize across a number of areas that are beneficial to youth. Therefore, it is important for youth sport programs to be designed and implemented in ways that use failure as an opportunity to learn how to overcome challenges and thrive in the face of difficulty.

Mary Sara Wells

Further Reading

Dwek, C. S. 2008. *Mindset: The New Psychology of Success: How We Can Learn to Fulfill Our Potential.* New York: Random House.

Farrey, T. 2008. *Game on: The All-American Race to Make Champions of Our Children.* New York: ESPN Books.

Lahey, J. 2015. *The Gift of Failure: How the Best Parents Learn to Let Go So Their Children Can Succeed.* New York: Harper Collins.

Marano, H. E. 2008. *A Nation of Wimps: The High Cost of Invasive Parenting.* New York: Random House.

Wilson, C., J. Sibthorp, and D. Richmond. 2016, February. "Freedom to Fail, Space to Grow." *Parks and Recreation Magazine,* 16–18.

Development of Youth in Mind and Body

A key element in creating quality youth sport programs is making sure they are designed to fit the needs of participants. This means more than just ensuring that the program reaches its goals and objectives. Perhaps more importantly, these programs also need to be designed in a way that helps young athletes meet the desired goals and objectives in a way that is developmentally appropriate physically, cognitively, and psychosocially. If not, there is potential to cause more harm than good in terms of both the health of the young athletes and their long-term participation. Young athletes are not merely miniature adults. Their bodies, minds, and emotions are continuing to develop long into young adulthood in ways that are not always visible. Unfortunately, as adults it is at times difficult to remember where we were at that stage of development because where we are now seems so natural. In addition, youth sport leagues are often run and/or coached by volunteers, typically parents, who have a background in the sport but may have less experience in the field of child development. Although often these volunteers are parents who have children in the program and may understand their development, these well-intentioned coaches might not have a full picture of where their children fit in with the norm for that age group, and consequently, might have higher or lower expectations for what their teams can reasonably be expected to accomplish. By contrast, individuals who have a greater understanding of the different physical, cognitive, and psychosocial developmental stages youth experience are better equipped to create well-designed youth sport programs that maximize the benefits for their young participants.

Key to discussing development is pointing out that physical, cognitive, and psychosocial development are generally described in terms of the average individual. This means that when describing where a 7-year-old is physically, the description is of the average 7-year-old, not a specific individual. However, every child is unique and, therefore, each young athlete will likely be somewhat more advanced in some areas and somewhat less advanced in others. Youth sport professionals should design their programs for what is typical of the age, but adaptations may be necessary based on the specific capabilities of the individuals with whom they are working.

A second important note to discuss when dealing with the topic of development is a reminder that development cannot be forced. Much as one cannot ask a child to grow faster or taller, one cannot also ask that child's brain or optic nerve to develop more quickly than it is currently doing. So while it is good to help a child reach his or her limits of capability so that he or she is prepared to make advancements when the child has developed more fully, asking the child to reach beyond that point will simply lead to frustration for all involved. For example, asking a child to understand abstract concepts before her brain has developed that capability will likely lead to frustration for coaches, parents, and other adults providing such instruction. Meanwhile the child is also likely to grow frustrated for multiple reasons, from an inability to understand how to accomplish what is being demanded, to a sense that her efforts are not being recognized or appreciated.

Physical Development

Physical development refers to the physiological changes that occur in regard to individuals' abilities and growth over the course of their lives. It is very easy to see the connection between physical development and youth sport. By definition, every sport requires physical skill and movement at some level. The most obvious types of physical development occur in attributes such as height and size. It is easy to see that youth playing basketball, for example, may need to use a smaller ball or use a lower basket because they have smaller hands and are not as tall. In addition, several other physical attributes are less obvious and so natural to adults that they forget at some point they were not born that way. Consequently, it is important to remember that we need to recognize all ways physical development can impact the young athlete in order to design the most appropriate youth sport programs for participants. Attributes such as balance, eyesight, gross and fine motor skills, and heat tolerance can all play a role in sport performance and are not fully developed when most children first enroll in youth sport programs. For example, when children first enroll in youth sport programs around the age of 5, in addition to being simply smaller, they also have other differences in comparison to a fully grown adult. These differences include an optic nerve that is not fully developed, making tracking balls more difficult; changing height and weight along with incomplete inner ear development, which may make balance an issue; and heat tolerance that is not fully functioning, making it difficult for them to determine when they are overheated. Each of these will have an impact on a child's ability to learn and play most sports. Further explanation on these concepts will be given later in the entry.

Cognitive Development

A second aspect of child and youth development that plays a role in sport is cognitive development. Cognitive development refers to a person's growth over the course of the life span in his or her intelligence and ability to process thought, learn, and solve problems. Cognitive development occurs over a very long time frame often until a person is in his or her twenties. Consequently, understanding where a young athlete is in the cognitive development process should have an impact on all youth sport programs. Although somewhat less obvious to sport performance than physical development, it would be very difficult to argue that cognitive abilities do not play a role in athletic performance. Based purely on cognitive development, it would be unrealistic to assume that the same teaching techniques would work as well for a 15-year-old as a 5-year-old because their brains are simply capable of different things. This is particularly true in areas such as the capability to understand abstract thought, attention spans, and learning styles. Thus, for example, children at younger ages will learn better if you guide them through the motions repeatedly rather than simply telling them how to perform a skill and will likely need additional breaks and changes in activities to keep their minds from wandering off. More depth to these ideas will be provided in later sections of this chapter.

Psychosocial Development

A final developmental area that should be a concern of youth sport professionals is psychosocial development. Psychosocial development refers to how individuals' emotional, moral, and social abilities grow and change throughout their lives. Athletic performance has an impact on young athletes in terms of their overall self-concept and requires them to withstand a certain amount of stress, both of which are impacted by where they are in their psychosocial development.

Now that we understand the different types of development and how they relate to youth sport, it is important to see how these areas apply to the youth with whom professionals will be working in a youth sports setting. To do this, we will be covering the following age groups: young children (ages 2 to 7), childhood (ages 7 to 11), and adolescence (ages 11 to 18). Although development issues occur throughout an individual's lifetime, we will only be covering the stages of life through adolescence as these are the stages that most apply to youth sport.

Young Children

Young children are at early stages of development in all three areas (physical, cognitive, and psychosocial), which can have a major impact on their sport participation. Physically, children in this age group tend to have energetic bursts, and they are still developing balance, visual skills, and large and fine motor skills. They also have a tendency to lack aerobic capacity, flexibility, and heat tolerance. This means that youth sport programs should have opportunities for them to demonstrate short bursts of speed rather than extended cardiovascular activity. In other words, it may be more beneficial for youth sport organizers to put together a short 1-mile fun run associated with an adults' 5K rather than expecting young children to run the full 3.1 miles. Balance is related to multiple factors such as inner-ear development and growth spurts that change a child's center of gravity. Coaches and others should be patient with children of this age and realize that if they are tripping and falling a lot, it is not necessarily a sign of inability but may be a temporary result of the fact that the child recently grew an inch and is adapting to the change. Youth sport professionals should also keep in mind that due to their development of balance and inability to track a ball related to optic nerve development, complex tasks such as running up to a moving ball and kicking it can become extremely frustrating, especially for the younger children of this age group. This is the reason a sport such as tee-ball works well. There is no need to track the ball in addition to other complex coordinated movements. Sports that focus more on gross motor skills may also be more appropriate as these skills tend to develop more quickly than fine motor skills. Finally, as their heat tolerance is not fully developed, youth sport professionals need to schedule water breaks in order to help their participants cool down and hydrate, as they likely will not initiate this on their own until they are far hotter and thirstier than they should be.

Cognitively, children at this age are concrete thinkers with an inability to understand abstract ideas. They do not completely understand rules but are creative and curious. They tend to have a very physical learning style and have difficulty processing complex skill building. All these factors play a significant role in how a coach or facilitator might teach a particular sport to young athletes in this age group. For example, if teaching a new stroke in swimming, it would behoove the instructor to first teach the kick, then the arms, before the two are combined. Rather than explaining to the young swimmer how to move his or her legs, the instructor should physically move them as he or she is describing it so that it is a more concrete idea in the child's mind. And making it fun will help the lesson stick, such as calling a "streamline" a "superman."

Psychosocial development also plays a role in learning sport skills, and in this age group children tend to be sensitive, egocentric, and crave approval. They also do not typically have well-developed stress-processing skills. This means that teaching children of this age group requires providing significant amounts of approval from the instructor, taking care to point out specifically what the child is doing correctly, often in terms of reminding him or her how it felt when his or her body performed the task. In addition, because they cannot handle or understand stress at the level of someone older, it is beneficial for their learning and performance to be soothing and supportive rather than harsh and abrasive in both teaching the skill and in providing feedback on performance.

Childhood

Once children are approximately at age 7 and until they are around 11, they are in the childhood stage of life. Physically, much like in early childhood, they are still developing and in the lower stages of aerobic capacity, flexibility, and heat tolerance. However, they are improving in their coordination and focus and also might be in the early stages of puberty. This means that they will likely be able to be more efficient and demonstrate complex skills and can practice for longer periods of time without getting overly tired. Puberty factors in significantly for youth sport professionals as some children will develop more quickly than others, creating a wide variety of body types all within the same age group. Consequently, youth sport professionals should make sure, for example, that in the sport of football that an underdeveloped 9-year-old is not matched up against a highly developed 11-year-old for obvious safety reasons.

Cognitive development in childhood has improved, and children in this age group are able to better solve problems and follow rules and directions. Although they may not necessarily be efficient at processing complex skills, they are more likely to be able to use a visual learning style than those in young childhood. This provides an opportunity for coaches and other instructors to use a less hands-on approach to instruction and instead provide demonstrations from teammates or adult leaders. In addition, in game or competition situations, young athletes may start to develop ideas on how to resolve particular issues facing them, and coaches can expect more compliance to rules than when working with even younger athletes.

Athletes in the childhood stage of development are somewhat similar to their younger counterparts in terms of their stress-processing skills and are similarly focused on adult approval. They do, however, now have the ability to have more realistic comparisons to others and improved sharing abilities. The combination of all these factors makes it necessary for coaches and others working with this age group to be particularly careful when placing their athletes in overly competitive situations. Children in this age group may find it particularly impactful on their self-confidence and self-worth. Much like younger children, they seek and value the approval of adults, and because they are better able to compare how they are doing to their peers, they may see a perceived failure as a sign not of a momentary issue but as a more global symbol of their self-worth. This is not to say that coaches and other youth sport professionals should never allow children to be challenged; rather, they should be aware of this potential issue in order to confirm to their athletes that performance on the field, good or bad, does not reflect their value as human beings, otherwise they may be less willing to take risks and challenge themselves in the future.

Adolescence

Once youth are between the ages of 11 and 18, they are considered to be in adolescence. At this point physically, most are undergoing puberty and have a corresponding regression of balance and coordination as they adjust to their changing bodies. Their endurance and strength can now become more developed with practice, but they also have a tendency to be overly flexible. Much as with younger children whose bodies are changing rapidly, adolescent athletes might have temporary setbacks in their ability to perform complicated tasks based on growth spurts. This simply takes patience to get through as their bodies adjust. Now that endurance and strength can be built up through practice, it now becomes beneficial to institute longer practices and introduce strength training to the routine, both of which would have had a minimal impact prior to this point. Finally, flexibility is another issue somewhat related to puberty. Hormones may cause ligaments to relax, creating heightened flexibility among youth of this age group. Although this seems like a good thing, coaches and others working with children in this group should be careful not to push the athletes too far as doing so could potentially result in injuries such as a dislocated shoulder.

Adolescents have reached higher levels of cognitive development specifically as it relates to logic, strategy, perspective-taking, and abstract thought. This can have a positive impact on their involvement in game planning, understanding complex ideas, and their ability to understand instructions. Coaches can now explain how a skill should be performed with the expectation that the athlete will understand rather than needing to go through the process of physical demonstrations that can still help in the case of minor tweaks to performance. It also means that abstract ideas such as a zone defense in basketball can be understood and performed by a team more easily rather than the simpler defensive concepts of man-to-man.

Finally, in terms of psychosocial development, adolescents are very different than those young athletes in childhood and young childhood. One of the more stark differences is in the new importance placed on peer perceptions, which now typically supersede the approval of adults. This has an impact on both learning and performance, as instead of trying to impress parents, adolescents are more likely to try and impress their friends. In addition, the issue of self-image and identity plays more of a role with young athletes in this age group. Young athletes who place significant value on their image or identity as an athlete may be more likely to act in both positive and negative ways that enhance that image. On the other hand, adolescents who are less tied to their image or identity as an athlete may be more likely to drop out of youth sport at this point in order to focus their energies on other activities that better support how they want to perceive themselves. Parents, coaches, and administrators who see the value in sport for all adolescents at some level should be cognizant of this issue in order to adapt programs in a way that both promotes positive identity formation and helps maintain participation for those who are less tied to being seen as an athlete. By doing so, youth who may otherwise drop out can continue to receive the many benefits of youth sport participation.

Conclusion

It is quite clear that young athletes vary widely in their abilities and needs, and consequently it is important to design programs appropriately. The information on youth physical, cognitive, and psychosocial development is vast, and the implications of that information on youth sport adaptation and performance are valuable for any youth sport professional. Although not comprehensive, the information in this chapter presents an introduction to the ways these professionals can better design their programs to meet the needs of their young athletes, thereby creating an improved experience for all involved.

Mary Sara Wells

Further Reading

Crain, W. 2000. *Theories of Development: Concepts and Applications* (4th ed.). Upper Saddle River, NJ: Prentice Hall.

Keating, D. P. 2004. "Cognitive and Brain Development." In R. M. Lerner and L. Steinberg (Eds.), *Handbook of Adolescent Psychology* (pp. 45–84). Hoboken, NJ: Wiley.

Stricker, P. R. 2006. *Sports Success Rx! Your Child's Prescription for the Best Experience: How to Maximize Potential and Minimize Pressure.* Elk Grove Village, IL: American Academy of Pediatrics.

Economic Impact of Youth Sports Tournaments

Sport plays a significant role in the lives of millions of youth who participate recreationally and competitively each year. As a society, we believe sport teaches youth valuable life lessons because it simulates many aspects of life. J. W. Keating once stated that competition is not an end in itself; it is simply a means to a socially desirable end (Keating, 1978). Although sports are valued in large part because they provide the socially desirable end of personal development of the individual athletes, entire communities can benefit from sport as well. Many communities have turned to youth sport tournaments as a means of economic development for the area. There are many benefits for communities that organize youth sport tournaments. In the current state of youth sport participation and attitudes toward sport, many communities are in the position to provide youth sport tournaments and reap those benefits. However, it is important for communities wishing to offer youth sport tournaments for the purpose of economic development to understand the status of sport participation, attitudes toward sport, factors that can affect the economic impact of sport tournaments, and how to maximize the economic impact of sport tournaments.

Sport Participation and Youth Sport Attitudes

A lot of youth participate in sport. In 2008 the National Council of Youth Sports (NCYS) reported that there were approximately 44 million youth sport participants across the United States. According to a 2013 ESPN study, an estimated 21.5 million children (boys and girls) participated in sports. Since 2012, however, studies have found a modest but persistent decrease in youth sports participation.

Although many children are growing up playing sports, the structure of sports participation has changed over the years. Youth once played pickup style games with children in the neighborhood, but sport has become increasingly organized and rigidly structured for youth. Leagues have been formally developed. Competitive travel teams are now commonplace, and adults have placed strict rules on how youth play sport. Additionally, attitudes toward sport have changed. There is a trend in youth sport toward an emphasis on the "performance ethic," resulting in programs increasingly focusing on competitive excellence and sport specialization at a younger age for athletes (Coakley, 2014). Youth are encouraged to focus on a single sport so that they can master it, and specialized performance-based training is often sought out for young children.

Parents frequently evaluate success in the same manner as coaches; success is based on winning (Petlichkoff, 1992). With increased sport specialization at young ages, greater emphasis on organized competitive leagues, and attitudes of winning, there is greater demand for tournaments, for which parents are willing to spend money. Communities can fill that demand by offering youth sport tournaments, and communities can enjoy numerous benefits in their region by doing so.

Benefits of Youth Sport Tournaments for the Community

Many communities already have much of the necessary infrastructure and resources to host youth sport tournaments. Therefore, events can often be held without requiring much additional public investment. The benefits of hosting youth sport tournaments for the community are varied. For instance, sport tournaments can attract visitors from outside of the local community who are likely to spend money in the local region. In many cases, these tournament experiences become extended vacations because tourists often schedule additional days prior to tournaments and after tournaments to sightsee, explore the region, and visit local attractions. As a result, sport tournaments may introduce people to communities that otherwise they may not have visited. When they have a positive experience, they may return in the future, bring others to the region, and spread positive word-of-mouth about both the sporting event and the region in general, which can positively impact the region in the long term. In some cases, tournament experiences may even attract athletes to the region whose families eventually relocate to the area.

As communities develop and maintain successful youth sport tournaments from year to year, they can gain recognition, develop their reputation, and improve their image in the eyes of those who are not local residents. Large, high-profile events can lead to public relations and media coverage that further foster positive awareness of the community and can generate additional tourism. In addition to tangible financial benefits, there are several intangible impacts that stem from communities hosting youth sport tournaments. Communities that are able to gain support for youth sport tournaments from the local residents and local businesses can build their sense of community around these events. Sport tournaments can increase volunteerism, create excitement in a community, and nurture a sense of team spirit within a community (Duy et al., 2014).

Economic Impact

Although there are a number of benefits to a community from running youth tournaments, it has been suggested that sport tournaments generate little economic activity and that youth sport has little economic impact because spectators have relationships with the participants, and consequently, spend more time at the tournament itself and less time out in the community (Andreff, 2011). On the other hand, there are also many studies that suggest that youth sport tournaments can have a positive economic impact for communities. The economic impact of youth sport tournaments can fluctuate due to a number of factors, and the results of economic impact analyses rely on assumptions that may or may not be justified, which can dramatically influence the results of economic impact studies.

In order to get a sense of influential assumptions as well as the factors that often cause the economic impact of youth tournaments to fluctuate, it is important to understand how the economic impact of youth sport tournaments is analyzed. To begin, what is economic impact? It is the consequences of new money that enters the host community and flows through the region (Jago and Dwyer, 2013). Economic impact is the "net economic change in a host economy that results from spending by visitors from outside the community" (Crompton, 2010, 27).

In general, economic impact analysis is reasonably straightforward; however, in practice, it can be quite challenging. For example, tournament organizers can determine the number of participants based on registration records. However, it is important to determine how many of the participants are visitors as opposed to locals from the community. Visitors bring new money into the economy, whereas locals simply transfer money throughout the economy. It would be misleading to report the economic impact of a tournament if the results included the spending patterns of locals because that money would not be new money that was attracted to the region by the tournament. In addition to determining the number of visiting participants, tournament organizers need to determine the number of nonparticipant visitors. Because the participants in youth sport tournaments are children, family members and friends often accompany them. Tournament administrators can determine the number of visitors as well as their average spending through a simple questionnaire. However, in order to clearly distinguish visitors from locals, and to discern new money that is spent in the local economy, it is important for the boundaries of the local economy to be clearly defined prior to collecting this information.

Total economic impact involves direct, indirect, and induced effects of visitor spending. Direct effects are the effects from the first round of visitor spending in the local economy. For instance, visitors arrive in the community and spend money on a meal at the local pizzeria. The pizzeria then uses that money to pay employees, purchase pizza ingredients, pay utility bills and rent, and so on. These are direct effects from visitor spending. But when new money recirculates throughout the local economy, indirect effects come into play as well. Indirect effects are the subsequent rounds of spending between organizations for goods and services after the first round of spending. For example, if the local pizzeria received the initial visitor spending, but then had to purchase supplies (e.g., cheeses, meats, and soda drinks) from a local supplier, and the supplier then purchased its own supplies (e.g., additives for cheeses) from another local supplier, these effects would be the indirect effects of visitor spending. Induced effects, meanwhile, are the effects of local purchases by employees who received wages from businesses that were impacted directly or indirectly from visitors. For example, an induced effect would be when an employee who is paid wages in part by the new money from visitor spending then spends that money in the local economy for food and entertainment.

Indirect and induced effects are often collectively referred to as secondary effects of spending. When new money is injected into the local economy directly by visitors, it is spent and then respent multiple times creating new economic activity that generates new business, employment, and income. With each successive round of spending, some money leaks out of the local economy to other regions or into savings, for example. Multipliers, or multiplier coefficients as they are sometimes called, are values that are used to represent the frequency with which new money is circulated through the local economy. The larger the multiplier value, the more often new money circulates through the local economy before it has entirely leaked out of the economy. Multipliers vary from one region to another depending on the community's size and business structure. In general, the larger the local region is, the larger the multiplier, because it is likely to have less leakage than smaller regions. Large regions are more likely to have more businesses and resources located within their boundaries, so purchases between organizations are more likely to stay within the local economy. Because multipliers depend on the community's size and business structure, there is no universal value to be used for all sport tournaments. This presents a challenge to those who conduct economic impact analyses, as they must determine an appropriate multiplier to use in calculations. An inappropriately large multiplier will artificially inflate the results of economic impact analyses, which will make it appear as though a tournament had a greater economic impact than it actually did. An overly conservative multiplier will not fully capture the magnitude of the economic impact of a tournament. Tournament administrators who conduct economic impact analyses must be cautious in using appropriate multipliers and not abuse multipliers in their calculations or results interpretations. Because of the complexities of multipliers, it may be best for administrators to simply focus on getting accurate estimates of the number of visitors, visitor spending, and direct effects and to avoid using multipliers altogether (Crompton, 2010).

Economic impact analyses are useful for communities because they can help determine changes in economic activity in the local economy in terms of sales, personal income, and employment. More specifically, they can help determine how much visitors spend in the area, how much income visitors generate for households and businesses in the area, and the impact of visitor spending on jobs in the local region (Stynes, n.d.c). Economic impact analyses can demonstrate positive contributions to the goal of economic development, which can generate positive perceptions of youth sport tournaments in the minds of legislators, local businesses, and the residents of the community (Crompton, 2010). If economic impact studies demonstrate positive impacts, they build the reputation for the tournaments, help provide justification for holding youth sport tournaments in the community, and communities may be able to generate additional public funding for youth sport tournaments. Furthermore, positive economic impacts may help youth sport gain support from local businesses and the community (Williams and Riley, 2003).

Strategies for Maximizing Economic Impact of Youth Sport Tournaments

Understanding how youth sport tournaments may impact a community's economy provides insight into how sport administrators can foster more positive economic impacts in the region. There are a number of strategies that administrators can take in order to maximize the economic impact of youth sport tournaments, including marketing effectively to nonlocals, engaging with visitors, extending the average length of stay by visitors, ensuring a well-run tournament for a positive experience, and making sure local businesses are aware of tournaments.

Economic impact is determined based on the amount of spending by nonlocal visitors. A tournament that generates a positive economic impact will have a high proportion of out-of-town visitors. As a first step to maximizing the economic impact of youth sport tournaments, it is important for those involved with marketing youth sport tournaments to not only market to locals but also to attract athletes and "travel" teams from leagues that are outside of the local area to the extent that the marketing budget will reasonably allow. Tournament administrators can identify and use relatively low-cost digital marketing strategies that will allow them to connect with target markets outside of their immediate geographic region.

As tournament administrators expand their reach to participants outside of the local community, they might attempt to expand the size of the tournament by increasing the number of teams or individuals who can participate in the event (Smith, 2012). One strategy for expanding the size of the tournament is to target a wider range of participants. This might mean hosting a tournament geared toward moderate competitive levels, as opposed to hosting only elite competitors, in order to allow a broad range of participants to enter the tournament. This could require organizing several brackets to accommodate multiple skill levels and ensure competitive balance in the tournament. Tournament administrators need to evaluate and secure sufficient facilities (e.g., fields, courts, or pools) depending on the size of the tournament so that the participants, spectators, volunteers, and staff have a positive experience with the event. The existing sports infrastructure in the community may or may not allow for tournaments to be expanded.

Once participants, coaches, families, and other visitors arrive to the tournament region, tournament administrators should be sure to make out-of-town visitors feel welcome in the community (Smith, 2012). This can begin at registration and check-in. It is helpful for tournament staff to actively engage with out-of-town visitors by sharing information and ideas about the region including restaurants, parks, trails, museums, shows, and other attractions that the community may have to offer. In order to make sure visitors are welcomed appropriately, the community could appoint a dedicated tournament concierge or provide information in registration packets to help orient them to the region, provide maps and brochures, and make visitors feel welcome.

By welcoming visitors to the region as well as the tournament, the tournament organizers can foster awareness of what the community has to offer and can encourage visitors to get out in the community and enjoy themselves. When visitors learn about the community and interact with all that it has to offer, it is more likely that they will spend more money into the community's economy. Perhaps even more importantly, when visitors learn about the region and have a positive first experience with the community, it's more likely that the experience will lead to future return visits.

In addition to expanding the size of the tournament, one of the most efficient methods for increasing the economic impact of a tournament is to extend the average length of stay by visitors (Crompton, 2010). Tournaments that are organized over multiple days of competition as opposed to single-day tournaments will extend the stay for many out-of-town visitors. However, many families use tournament outings as vacations that include nontournament activities. In order to encourage visitors to do this, communities can showcase their region by promoting local attractions that visitors may be interested in experiencing on the days before or after the tournament. Then visitors can turn their sport tournament experience into a vacation that goes beyond the tournament itself. Tournament organizers could schedule leisure time between tournament games so that visitors can explore the region. They could even consider scheduling local activities into the tournament schedule for teams to participate in together during the tournament. For example, large swim meets are often scheduled with younger swimmers taking part in the morning session and older swimmers racing in the afternoons. This leaves time during the day for athletes and their families to engage in local activities if they are provided with information on where to find them. For instance, administrators might arrange for a tournament team night at a community attraction. Whether tournament administrators choose to plan elements such as these into the tournament schedule or to simply advertise the region to visitors, tournament confirmation e-mails and reminders, tournament resources, and other promotional collaterals provide opportunities for administrators to inform travelers of local attractions that they can consider exploring while in the region.

A multiday tournament with a lot of participants and a welcoming environment may be great, but at the core of the event is the tournament itself. In order to maximize economic impact and keep visitors coming back year after year, the tournament must be well organized and well run. It is important for registration to be simple, tournament rules to be clearly communicated, and games to start on time. Facilities need to be in good condition. Fields and courts need to be properly marked and have appropriate safety precautions in place. There needs to be adequate space for spectators, food available nearby, and clean restrooms. Officials and referees need to be well trained, and tournament administrators should carefully consider the tournament environment.

Recently, there has been concern that sportsmanship is on the decline (Engh, 2002). There seems to be a growing trend toward unsportsmanlike and unruly behavior among athletes, spectators (Battikh et al., 2011), and even among coaches, who should be teaching both how to win and how to be a good sport. Tournaments can bring out the best and the worst of sportsmanship in players, coaches, and spectators, but often youth sign up for sports primarily for fun (Petlichkoff, 1992). If the youth who are participating do not have fun and other visitors do not enjoy their visit, it is less likely that they will return in the future. Administrators can have a positive impact on sportsmanship by training referees (Arthur-Banning, Paisley, and Wells, 2007) and structuring tournaments for positive sportsmanship (Wells et al., 2005; Wells et al., 2006). They set the structure of the tournament, define objectives, designate policies, hire referees, specify spectator rules, create expectations, and make sure that everyone is trained appropriately for establishing the tournament environment and maintaining it by being prepared to handle issues that may arise. The sporting environment is just one of many elements of the experience that tournament administrators should closely monitor in order to ensure that everyone has a positive experience and wants to return.

Lastly, tournament administrators should make sure local businesses are aware of the tournaments so that they can support them and accommodate participants accordingly. Tournaments can place extra demand on local businesses. For instance, restaurants may see unusually high volumes of customers who arrive suddenly after games end. It is important that they can plan to have additional staff and sufficient food so that they do not run out of popular items or make customers experience exceedingly long wait times, thus dissatisfying customers and perhaps missing out on the revenue that could have been gained if they were prepared for the excess demand. Additionally, tournament participants and their families need to be able to find accommodations, parking, and transportation around the community. It is very important for tournament administrators to work with local businesses to ensure a successful tournament for competitors, spectators, and the community (Smith, 2012).

If communities have the resources and infrastructure in place to host youth sport tournaments, doing so can have a positive economic impact on the community. By strategically planning tournaments to attract out-of-town visitors, engaging with visitors and encouraging them to stay for multiple days, highlighting and promoting the region's attractions, preparing the community for tournaments by informing local businesses and securing their support, and by ensuring a well-run tournament for a positive experience, communities can maximize the economic impact of youth sport tournaments in their region. When communities effectively manage the complete youth sport tournament experience successfully, communities can benefit in the short term as well as the long term. The number one method of marketing for youth sport organizations is positive word-of-mouth (NCYS, 2008). If administrators create youth sport tournaments that foster positive experiences for the players and the families, it is likely that not only will coaches, families, and participants want to return to those tournaments, it is likely that those who are satisfied with their experience will spread positive word-of-mouth that could draw in new participants and visitors in the future.

Preston J. Tanner

Further Reading

Andreff, Wladimir. 2011. "Sports Accounting." In Wladimir Andreff and Stefan Szymanski (Eds.), *Handbook on the Economics of Sport*. Northampton, MA: Edward Elgar Publishing.

Arthur-Banning, Skye G., Karen Paisley, and Mary Sara Wells. 2007. "Promoting Sportsmanship in Youth Basketball Players: The Effect of Referees' Prosocial Behavior Techniques." *Journal of Park and Recreation Administration, 25*: 96–114.

Battikh, S., A. Cerimele, S. Dafilou, D. Dhanurendra, S. Gillooly, J. Marshall, et al. 2011. *Marketing Positive Fan Behavior at the Pennsylvania State University.* Unpublished manuscript.

Cela, A., C. Kowalski, and S. Lankford. 2006. "Spectators' Characteristics and Economic Impact of Local Sports Events: A Case Study of Cedar Valley Moonlight Classic Soccer Tournament." *World Leisure Journal, 48*: 45–53.

Coakley, J. 2014. *Sports in Society: Issues and Controversies* (11th ed.). New York: McGraw-Hill Education.

Crompton, J. L. 2010. *Measuring the Economic Impact of Park and Recreation Services.* National Recreation and Park Association. Accessed at http://www.nrpa.org/uploaded Files/nrpa.org/Publications_and_Research/Research/Papers/Crompton-Summary.PDF.

Daniels, M. J., and W. C. Norman. 2003. "Estimating the Economic Impacts of Seven Regular Sport Tourism Events." *Journal of Sport Tourism, 8*: 214–222.

Dawson, P., and P. Downward. 2011. "Participation, Spectatorship and Media Coverage in Sport: Some Initial Insights." In W. Andreff (Ed.), *Contemporary Issues in Sports Economics: Participation and Professional Team sports* (pp. 15–42). Northampton, MA: Edward Elgar.

Duy, T. A., D. Cole, J. Hurley, and J. Naber. 2014. *The Economic Impact of Sporting Events in Lane County.* Accessed at http://economics.uoregon.edu/wp-content/uploads/sites/4/2014/12/Naber_Cole_Hurley_Thesis.pdf.

Engh, F. 2002. *Why Johnny Hates Sports: Why Organized Youth Sports Are Failing Our Children and What We Can Do about It.* Garden City Park, NY: Square One.

Higham, J. 1999. "Commentary—Sport as an Avenue of Tourism Development: An Analysis of the Positive and Negative Impacts of Sport Tourism." *Current Issues in Tourism, 2*: 82–90.

Jago, L., and L. Dwyer. 2013. "Events and Economics." In R. Finkel, D. McGillivray, G. McPherson, and P. Robinson (Eds.), *Research Themes for Events* (pp. 68–77). Boston: CAB International.

Keating, J. W. 1978. *Competition and Playful Activities.* Washington, D.C.: University Press of America.

Madrigal, R. 1995. "Cognitive and Affective Determinants of Fan Satisfaction with Sporting Event Attendance." *Journal of Leisure Research, 27*: 205–227.

May, R. A. B. 2001. "The Sticky Situation of Sportsmanship: Contexts and Contradictions in Sportsmanship among High School Boys Basketball Players." *Journal of Sport & Social Issues, 25*: 372–389.

National Council on Youth Sports. 2008. *Report on Trends and Participation in Organized Youth Sports.* Accessed at http://www.ncys.org/pdfs/2008/2008-ncys-market-research -report.pdf.

Petlichkoff, L. M. 1992. "Youth Sport Participation and Withdrawal: Is It Simply a Matter of Fun?" *Pediatric Exercise Science, 4*: 105–110.

Rosentraub, M.S., and D. Swindell. 2009. "Doing Better: Sports, Economic Impact Analysis, and Schools of Public Policy and Administration." *Journal of Public Affairs Education, 15*: 219–242.

Smith, S. B. 2012. *Game on! The Impact of Youth Sports on a Regional Economy.* Accessed at http://tcchamber.org/wp-content/uploads/2012/10/YouthSportsReport.pdf.

Stynes, D. J. (n.d.a). *Economic Impact Concepts.* Accessed at https://www.msu.edu/course/prr/840/econimpact/concepts.htm.

Stynes, D. J. (n.d.b). *Multipliers.* Accessed at http://www.msu.edu/course/prr/840/econimpact/multipliers.htm.

Stynes, D. J. (n.d.c). *Economic Impacts of Tourism.* Accessed at https://www.msu.edu/course/prr/840/econimpact/pdf/ecimpvol1.pdf.

Wells, M. S., Gary D. Ellis, Karen P. Paisley, and Skye G. Arthur-Banning. 2005. "Development and Evaluation of a Program to Promote Sportsmanship in Youth Sports." *Journal of Park and Recreation Administration, 23*: 1–17.

Wells, M. S., Gary D. Ellis, Skye G. Arthur-Banning, and Mark Roark. 2006. "Effect of Staged Practices and Motivational Climate on Goal Orientation and Sportsmanship in Community Youth Sport Experiences." *Journal of Park and Recreation Administration, 24*: 64–85.

Williams, W., and K. Riley. 2003. "Using Economic Impact Studies to Gain Support for Youth Sports from Local Businesses." *Journal of Physical Education, Recreation & Dance, 74*: 49–51.

Women's Sports Foundation. 2008. *Go Out and Play: Youth Sports in America.* Accessed at http://www.ncys.org/pdfs/2008/2008-go-out-and-play-report.pdf.

Forced Exertion

Run, run, run! Stop and puke, if you have to, then keep running! You guys are going to learn one way or another that goofing off during my practice is not tolerated.

For some who engaged in team sport environments in this country, whenever they attempt to run for fitness, they hear some offshoot of these words reverberating in their minds. A large percentage of the American population spent some part of their childhood and/or adolescence engaged in team sports, and most value the life lessons forged through youth sports. However, those experiences may in some cases have also left them with negative psychological associations with cardiovascular exercise. This negative association is largely due to a culture in the United States where some coaches have persisted in utilizing cardiovascular exercise as punishment and/or as a compulsory (and sometimes even demeaning) element in team sports environments. This practice of *forced exertion* continues as a coaching strategy today. This entry will examine this long-held, deeply ingrained practice and discuss the changing tide of public opinion due to the associated negative impacts. It will also explore alternatives in order to empower coaches and youth sports administrators to continue the momentum toward fostering more healthy youth sports environments.

Whether they take the form of "suicides" in basketball, "stadiums" in football, or "gassers" in soccer, lacrosse, or other sports, cardiovascular training under the guise of these drills is widely utilized in team sports. The daunting and negative connotation of labeling an exercise as "suicides" aside, there is nothing inherently wrong with any of these forms of exercise. The potential harm lies in the way they are framed in relation to the sport. Cardiovascular exercise should absolutely be integrated into every team sports practice irrespective of level or orientation (e.g., recreational, youth, interscholastic, club, and/or competitive), yet the pervasive practice of the past has been to frame cardiovascular training in a compulsory and/or punitive sense. For example:

Compulsory

At the end of practice, a basketball coach gives the following directive: "Girls, now it's time for suicides. If every team member doesn't make it in the 5 minutes that we have allotted for 10 full suicides, everyone runs an additional mile."

Punitive

A football coach starts practice with the following: "Guys, your energy yesterday was lackluster, so today I'm going to give you a reason to be dragging. Everyone give me five stadiums and then line up for stretches. That'll teach you to loaf around on my practice field!"

In both of these examples, many coaches of the past would have also likely stood nearby and rather than shout encouragement, they would instead utilize fear-based motivational tactics that promote the underlying compulsory and/or punitive framework associated with the strategy.

For mainstream team sports in the United States, such as football, baseball, and basketball, most former youth and interscholastic athletes of generations past will attest to the fact that forced running or cardiovascular exercise, not only as punishment but integrated into practice in a compulsory manner, was simply the way things worked. Legendary coach Paul "Bear" Bryant's grueling 10-day football camp for Texas A&M football players in 1954 has become the stuff of lore and even prompted a best-selling book that was made into a television movie, *The Junction Boys*. This notion of "survival" and "never quitting," regardless of the circumstances, formed the basis for team sports conditioning for much of the last century. Jason Halsey, associate director for Campus Recreation at UNC-Chapel Hill, who grew up playing youth sports in Mount Pleasant, South Carolina, in the 1980s, offered affirmation:

I never thought twice about being forced to run as part of basketball or football practice. We ran for teammates missing free throws at the end of practice in basketball. We ran for teammates who missed blocks or tackles in football. Running as punishment for a lack of focus or ability to execute was a common, almost everyday experience. You knew it was coming, you accepted it; and, it became as much a part of practice as drills or scrimmages (interview with author).

It is clear that forced exertion has long been integrated into the daily routine of many team sports, but that culture is slowly beginning to change with the realization of potential consequences—from negative associations with exercise that could impact lifelong fitness to health risks associated with overexertion. Overexertion is defined as placing too much exertion on one's self, to the point that strain or injury results. Particularly for youth sports settings where development and enjoyment should be the focal point, overexertion can be problematic.

Due predominantly to the obesity epidemic that has negatively impacted the United States for the better part of the last 40 years, considerable attention has been given to youth sports as a vehicle for fostering healthy lifestyles. Naturally, that attention has led to people questioning the cultural practices associated with our youth sports environments. Research has shown youth sports participation to be predictive of sports and fitness involvement as young adults (Perkins, Jacobs, Barber, and Eccles, 2004). Further, Rasmussen and Laumann (2014) found exercise during adolescent years to be predictive of both positive moods and exercise as an adult. Yet, there is also evidence that adolescents who are forced to exercise are more likely to not engage in physical activity as adults (Taylor, Blair, Cummings, Wun, and Malina, 1999). Unfortunately, the question of negative association with exercise as punishment promotes methodological issues, as it must be either longitudinal (i.e., track youth sports participants over a lifetime) or retrospective (i.e., looking back on one's youth sports experience). Longitudinal research is costly and time-consuming, and retrospective research promotes reliability issues. Irrespective of these issues, if a person develops a negative association with an activity due to compulsory and/or punitive exposure to that activity in his or her childhood, it seems clear that the individual's likelihood of engaging frequently in that activity as an adult would be diminished. Although these research findings are certainly compelling and should be enough to promote commonsense reform, it unfortunately often takes high-profile tragedy or extreme circumstances to enact change when practices such as these are so deeply ingrained.

When 15-year-old Max Gilpin collapsed and died of a heat stroke during a high school football practice in Louisville, Kentucky, in 2008, he became 1 of 140 heat stroke–related deaths in youth football in the United States from 1960 to 2014 (National Center for Catastrophic Sport Injury Research, 2014). Yet Gilpin's death actually marked a seminal moment in youth sports history, as the head coach of the team, Jason Stinson, was charged with reckless homicide and wanton endangerment for overseeing the grueling running-for-punishment session that ended in Gilpin's death (Popke, 2012). Stinson's trial marked a clash between ingrained and evolving thought patterns relative to forced exertion in youth sports. Defense attorney Alex Dathorne summarized the ingrained side in stating during his closing argument: "You've got a man looking at prison time for being a football coach. Jason Stinson, on August the 20th, of 2008, did absolutely nothing different than every coach in this county, in this Commonwealth, in this country, was doing on that day" (Lake, 2010). Stinson's trial was believed to be the first time a high school football coach was charged and placed on trial for actions related to forced exertion during team sports. He was ultimately found not guilty, but the trial helped to shape public discourse by publicizing the potential health risks associated with running or exercise for punishment. Although the case of Max Gilpin rises to the extreme, there are many health risks associated with overexertion, from muscle fatigue to exhaustion and dehydration, and other heat-related diagnoses. Growing awareness of these risks have led sports organizations to speak out with greater frequency against such punitive actions—and against running for punishment specifically.

Canadian sport organizations have led the way in connecting the international movement toward banning the physical punishment of children by applying the principles to youth sports settings. Several notable organizations in the United States have followed suit, including SHAPE America (Society of Health and Physical Educators) and the National Association for Youth Sports (NAYS), in recognizing the potential negative by-products associated with running for punishment. These organizations have developed official position statements against the practice. The official position statement from SHAPE America came in 2009 and reads as follows:

> The Society of Health and Physical Educators opposes administering or withholding physical activity as a form of punishment and/or behavior management.

Similarly, NAYS (2016) has the following position statement posted on their website:

> Using running, or any physical activity, as a punishment is never appropriate in youth sports. Using running, as punishment for children, should be prohibited for the following reasons: (1) Negative associations with running; (2) Health risks. (*Note: NAYS goes on to explain these negative associations and potential health risks.*)

These statements send a clear message regarding running for punishment, and it is an important first step in counteracting a culture that has long regarded it as an accepted practice.

In the associated documentation of its position statement on exercise for punishment, SHAPE America contributors go on to highlight the important ramifications associated with a failure to understand and implement policies designed to diminish the associated practices. Most notably, some states consider exercise as a form of punishment as corporal punishment, and corporal punishment is illegal in most states. Further, the state boards of education in California and Hawaii have weighed in and prohibit either withholding or utilizing exercise as a form of punishment. Brooke de Lench, a child rights and protection advocate and executive director of the MomsTeam Institute and Smart Teams, reflects on the issue:

> Abuse, or witnessing abuse, in a sports setting can turn off a child to exercise and participation in sports, preventing the development of a healthy adult lifestyle. It can adversely affect a child's ability to learn, increase the likelihood that the child will engage during adolescence in unhealthy behaviors, including suicidal behavior, and delinquent and aggressive behaviors. It has also been linked to adverse health outcomes in adulthood, including mood and anxiety disorders and diseases (interview with author).

If truly committed to a healthier youth sports environment for children and adolescents (to include interscholastic and intercollegiate athletes), advocates say that organizations must begin to consider an outright ban on forced exertion in recognizing the *compulsory* orientation associated with many youth sports settings. Consider the Gilpin case as a starting point for discussion.

Max Gilpin's death could have occurred without any notion of punishment whatsoever. Yes, Stinson was punishing his team for not listening to him on that fateful day in 2008, but he just as easily could have instigated the grueling regimen at the end of practice without any associated punishment. We need to look no further than the testimony of Jeff Gilpin, Max Gilpin's father, who expressed pride for the determination exhibited by his son, "'I underestimated this kid, big-time. His heart. Can you imagine the fortitude it took to keep running out there?" (Lake, 2010) We might shift that orientation to imagine the fear Max may have felt inside— the fear of letting down fellow teammates, the fear of disappointing his father, and/ or the fear of retribution or further punishment from his coach. As Judith McMullen stated, "The line is not always clear between encouragement, whether from coaches or other players, and abusive conduct that pushes a young athlete to dangerous extremes" (McMullen, 2014, 187). However, if coaches are empowered to recognize that framing youth sports settings differently can both foster positive development and serve to mitigate many of the issues that coaches deal with on a daily basis, the evolution will continue.

Ron Ensom and Joan Durrant (2010) utilized *consent* and *intent* as the two crucial elements that coaches and youth sports administrators should consider in determining whether their supervision of youth sports settings rises to be punitive in nature, and these criteria can also be utilized in a more general sense for assessment of forced exertion. Through *consent*, it should be recognized by all parties that no one should be participating in a youth sport against their will. Whether it's the tall female pressured to play volleyball or basketball, a father's legacy in baseball, or a football-driven community in the deep South, some youth do not feel in control or perhaps are not in control of their decisions relative to participation in sports. By listening to youth, and empowering them to make their own decisions, parents and coaches enhance the potential for a more intrinsically motivated participant. *Intent*, as denoted by Ensom and Durrant, "reflects the crucial distinction between demanding performance of an activity intended to cause physical discomfort/pain or humiliation in order to punish, and requiring performance of an appropriate training activity that has associated physical discomfort/pain to build athletic ability (endurance, strength, speed)" (Ensom and Durrant, 2010, 43). The combination of these two criteria is crucial to the notion of removing forced exertion from youth sports settings, yet we will never do so fully unless administrators and coaches are convinced of the value through concrete examples.

Another key to changing the culture relative to forced exertion is the athletes themselves. If youth athletes are positively encouraged to recognize the notion of shared responsibility in their own fitness, rather than framing cardiovascular training as compulsory or punitive, coaches can successfully shift from their traditional orientation as authoritarians to one that is more aligned with being a mentor, a facilitator, and/or a motivator. This shift has successfully been implemented in many business and school settings, and there is no reason why youth sports settings should be any different. The problem with businesses struggling with this concept of employee motivation is similar to one that might be encountered on the practice field. There is a tendency, whenever a change in culture occurs, to throw our collective hands in the air and wish for simpler times. Those "simpler" times in the case of business or youth sports, when bosses or coaches lost their temper in screaming and yelling and doling out punishment, are for the most part a thing of the past. Yet, for many coaches, a "thing of the past" is all they know.

The importance of youth sport programs being designed to facilitate positive experiences and enduring involvement cannot be underestimated, but unfortunately, many volunteer and paid coaches alike have only their prior experiences in athletics from which to build. When faced with difficult situations, such as athletes not trying their hardest, not listening or paying attention, and/or getting in trouble at school or in the community, the common historical practice of forced exertion as either a means for punishment or integrated into practice in a compulsory manner is often the only "solution" for coaches. Yet, there are many strategies that can be employed that ultimately help a coach shift from compulsory and punitive to voluntary and positive. Here are a few coaching strategies designed to facilitate that successful shift (each example may be tweaked depending on the age and level of the sport):

1. **Communicate the importance:** Youth sport athletes at all levels must be convinced that cardiovascular exercise is an important component of

success in sport and life. Do not simply assume they understand this element. If resources are available, bring in an expert to speak to them about the subject.

2. **Listen and value the individual as well as the team:** Many youth sport coaches were involved with team sports when it was decidedly one-way in terms of communication ("my way or the highway!"), but it does not have to be so. Coaches need to listen to and value each and every member of the team. Communicate that each individual is in charge of one's own body and one's own fitness, and everyone is different along those lines. By doing so, each individual is empowered to make decisions and values his or her own personal fitness.

3. **Integrate rather than end:** Coaches have long left cardiovascular exercise as the last item on the daily practice agenda, and in so doing, have both subconsciously sent the wrong message and set themselves up for a compulsory or punitive orientation (i.e., if practice did not go well, if athletes are dragging, etc.). Instead, integrate cardiovascular exercise into the daily routine and rather than long periods of athletes standing in line or being inactive, make practice active and engaged and think about how to implement sustained movement throughout drills. By doing so, the subconscious message is that cardiovascular exercise matters and is integral to success.

4. **Make it fun!** This last element cannot be underestimated. Rather than dreading cardiovascular exercise, shift the orientation to one where elements that athletes enjoy (i.e., competition in making it a game) are enhanced through cardiovascular training. Resist the temptation that many coaches have fallen victim to in this regard in making the losing team run more, as it defeats the purpose. During cardiovascular-oriented sessions or competitions, also resist the temptation to yell generally, as it creates an environment that could lead athletes to feel confined. Instead, be jovial and encourage each through specific praise.

In addition to these commonsense strategies, youth sports organizations have been instrumental in developing solutions and strategies for coaches to help enhance motivation of athletes and promote more positive youth sports settings.

One such organization is the Positive Coaching Alliance (PCA). The PCA's "Power of Positive" guiding principle for coaches provides both an underlying philosophy and a practical strategy for implementation on a daily basis:

Encouraging athletes with positive reinforcement helps them hear and heed the necessary corrections. With that winning combination of truthful, specific praise and constructive criticism, athletic performance improves and so do the chances that kids stick with sports longer and learn all the valuable life lessons inherently available through organized competition.

This guiding principle is one that fosters a healthy youth sports setting across all domains, which is a key component to changing the culture related to physical fitness through team sports.

Youth sports can be a perfect venue to promote lifelong fitness and wellness; yet it does not simply happen by virtue of the setting alone. Coaches must be trained to foster positive experiences, and when empowered to utilize alternative means and frame cardiovascular exercise as positive rather than negative, the healthy mission that should be conveyed through youth sports programming can be realized.

P. Brian Greenwood

Further Reading

Children's Hospital of Eastern Ontario. 2004, September 29. *Joint Statement on Physical Punishment of Children and Youth.* Accessed July 22, 2016, at http://www.cheo.on.ca/en/physicalpunishment.

David, Paulo. 2005. *Human Rights in Youth Sport: A Critical Review of Children's Rights in Competitive Sports.* London: Routledge.

Dent, Jim. 1999. *The Junction Boys: How Ten Days in Hell with Bear Bryant Forged a Championship Team.* New York: St. Martin's Press.

Ensom, Ron, and Joan Durrant. 2010, Summer. "Physical Punishment of Children in Sport and Recreation: The Times They Are A-Changin'." *Coaches Plan, 17*(2): 43–44.

Lake, Thomas. 2010, December 6. "The Boy Who Died of Football." *Sports Illustrated.* Accessed July 24, 2016, at http://www.si.com/vault/2010/12/06/106012866/the-boy-who-died-of-football.

McMullen, Judith G. 2014. "Addressing Abusive Conduct in Youth Sports." *Marquette Sports Law Review, 25*(1): 181–205. Accessed July 28, 2016, at http://scholarship.law.marquette.edu/sportslaw/vol25/iss1/9.

MomsTeam Institute of Youth Sports Safety. *Protecting the Health and Safety of the Whole Sports-Active Child.* Accessed September 26, 2016, at http://www.momsteaminstitute.org.

National Alliance for Youth Sports. 2016. *Using Running as Punishment.* Accessed June 26, 2016, at https://www.nays.org/resources/more/position-statements/using-running-as-punishment.

National Center for Catastrophic Sport Injury Research. 2014. *Annual Survey of Football Injury Research: 1931–2014.* Accessed July 21, 2016, at https://nccsir.unc.edu/files/2013/10/Annual-Football-2014-Fatalities-Final.pdf.

Perkins, Daniel F., Janis E. Jacobs, Bonnie L. Barber, and Jacqueline S. Eccles. 2004. "Childhood and Adolescent Sports Participation as Predictors of Participation in Sports and Physical Fitness Activities during Young Adulthood." *Youth and Society, 35*: 495–520. doi:10.1177/0044118x03261619

Popke, Michael. 2012, October. *Blog: Running for Punishment Does Nobody Any Good.* Accessed July 26, 2016, at http://www.athleticbusiness.com/athlete-safety/blog-running -as-punishment-does-nobody-any-good.html.

Positive Coaching Alliance. 2016. *The Power of Positive.* Accessed July 28, 2016, at http:// www.positivecoach.org/the-power-of-positive.

Rasmussen, Martin, and Karin Laumann. 2014. "The Role of Exercise during Adolescence on Adult Happiness and Mood." *Leisure Sciences, 33*(4): 341–356. doi:10.1080/026143 67.2013.798347

Roan, Shari. 2011, February 6. *A Growing Danger for Athletes.* Accessed July 22, 2016, at http://articles.latimes.com/2011/feb/06/health/la-he-muscle-disorder-20110206.

Society of Health and Physical Educators (SHAPE) America. 2009. *Position Statement: Using Physical Activity as Punishment and/or Behavior Management.* Accessed July 25, 2016, at http://www.shapeamerica.org/advocacy/positionstatements/pa/upload/Using -Physical-Activity-as-Punishment-2009.pdf.

Taylor, Wendell C., Steven N. Blair, Sharon S. Cummings, Chuan C. Wun, and Robert M. Malina. 1999. "Childhood and Adolescent Physical Activity Patterns and Adult Physical Activity." *Health Promotion & Behavioral Sciences, 31*(1): 118–123. doi:10.1097 /00005768-199901000-00019

Gender Identity and Inclusion

In addressing issues and policies involving transgender and intersex individuals' access to youth sports, it is useful to establish definitions for terms commonly used in relation to the issue. *Sex* is the label of male or female that is assigned to a child at birth, often on the basis of genitalia and/or chromosomes. *Gender* is the social construction of behaviors, attitudes, and feelings that are culturally ascribed to a certain sex, masculine and feminine, man and woman. *Gender identity* refers to a person's innate and deeply felt psychological identification as a man, woman, or other gender. This may or may not correspond to the sex that they were assigned at birth. *Cisgender* is a term used to describe people whose gender identity matches the sex that they were assigned at birth. *Transgender* is a term for people whose gender identity does not match the sex that they were assigned at birth. It serves as an umbrella term that includes people who are transitioning male-to-female (MTF; transgender women) and female-to-male (FTM; transgender men). It can also include those who transcend the gender binary and who may identify as gender-queer. It does not designate how individuals have or have not altered their bodies. Finally, *intersex* is a term that refers to people who are born with reproductive or sexual anatomy that that does not fit with typical definitions of the male or female binary. Gender binary refers to the social construct of gender, which consists of only two options, male or female. However, recent developments show gender lies more on a spectrum inclusive of intersex, transgender, and nonbinary gender identities. This is often a result of hormonal or chromosomal anomalies that impact how the body produces or processes steroid hormones (e.g., testosterone or estrogen) or how many sex-linked chromosomes an individual has. Some common examples of intersex conditions include Klinefelter (XXY) syndrome, androgen insensitivity syndrome, and female hyperandrogenism.

Stigmas, Stereotypes, and Statistics
of Transgender Individuals

Transgender individuals, whether they are youths or adults, face many stigmas, stereotypes, and bullying in everyday life. These challenges can be particularly acute during adolescence. According to the 2013 GLSEN National School Climate Survey, 75 percent of transgender youth feel unsafe at school (GLSEN, 2013). GLSEN is a national organization committed to creating a safer school (K–12) environment for LGBTQ students that is free of bullying and harassment. They conduct original research, develop teacher resources, work with schools and students, and partner with other national education organizations. Forty-two percent of transgender students who responded to the survey reported being prevented from using their preferred name, 59.2 percent had been required to use the locker room or bathroom of the sex they were assigned at birth, and 31.6 percent of transgender students were prevented from wearing clothing of their choice, as it was deemed inappropriate for their legal sex. The presence of these structural barriers at school not only makes the school environment less safe and hospitable for transgender students, it also propagates societal transphobia—fear of transgender individuals. If a school prevents students from presenting and utilizing resources according to their gender identity that can teach other students that not accepting them is acceptable. According to the National Transgender Discrimination Survey, of transgender and gender nonconforming individuals who were "out" as K–12 students, 78 percent reported verbal harassment in school (Grant et al., 2011).

Such sustained hostility and abuse can have an enormous impact on physical and emotional well-being. Forty-one percent of transgender individuals attempt suicide, compared to 1.6 percent of the general population (Grant et al., 2011). One in five transgender individuals report being homeless at some point in their lives, and it is estimated that 40 percent of homeless youth are LGBTQ, primarily due to family rejection and discrimination. With these numbers, it is clear that transgender youth face a plethora of stressors and issues to daily life. Youth sport activities can ease these stressors by providing transgender youth with a community in which to have fun; develop a sense of belonging; and receive the physical, emotional, and social benefits that athletic activities can provide, at their best, to all participants, no matter their sexual orientation or identity. Conversely, youth sports can add to the difficulties faced by transgender youth if they become additional sources of social rejection or harassment.

Athletes who are transgender face separate issues from gay and lesbian athletes because the issues deal directly with the gender of the athletes that sport currently relies heavily on for its organization. Youth sports are segregated by gender, sometimes starting as young as 6 years old. The locker room thus often becomes a significant site of contention as well as a stressor for transgender individuals. If students are not allowed to use the bathrooms or locker rooms that match their gender identity, they will be less likely to want to participate in the sport in question. If a student does not feel comfortable or welcome in the locker room, sport participation will likely be one of the first activities that they forgo.

Due to the assumptions of masculine superiority in sport, people who are transitioning from male-to-female face different assumptions and constraints than those transitioning from female-to-male. Transgender women are assumed to have an unfair advantage in athletics as men are viewed as naturally superior athletes, due to differences of size, strength, and the influence of testosterone. These athletes must thus fight the stigma that they are gaining an unfair advantage by competing against cisgender women. Some opponents of transgender athletes have even charged that men claim to be transgender and pretend to be women solely to gain an unfair competitive advantage. However, due to the transphobia and harassment that transgender individuals face every day, this is highly unlikely. Michelle Dumaresq faced accusations of gaining an unfair advantage in mountain biking, for example, as did Fallon Fox, who competes in mixed martial arts. In addition, even at highly competitive levels, medical transition quickly negates strength-based advantages.

Athletes who are transgender women also face accusations of being perverts and wanting to play on women's teams simply to gain access to women's locker rooms. However, the effort of transition, the social risks, and the risk to physical safety due to cultural transphobia makes this a highly unlikely scenario as well. Unfortunately, this accusation of perversion is most harmful when it comes to youth sports because parents, schools, and other leaders are all concerned with protecting their children, and particularly girls, from sexually predatory behavior. The fear of boys "infiltrating" girls' locker rooms feeds this desire to protect, but advocates for transgender youth argue that the "protection" of children often comes at the expense of transgender children who are already extremely vulnerable. The unlikelihood of a child pretending to be transgender means that this accusation can make the adults organizing the activities hesitant to be truly inclusive of athletes who are transgender without realistic rationales.

Athletes who are transgender men face significantly fewer stigmas to their participation, since society has traditionally regarded individuals that are assigned female at birth to be inferior athletes to counterparts that are assigned male at birth. Most people have trouble believing that a person assigned female at birth would be able to compete at high levels with men. However, athletes are beginning to disprove this assumption. In 2015, Chris Mosier became the first transgender man to make a national roster for the United States. He competed for USA Triathlon in the World Duathlon Championships in 2016. Schulyer Bailar was accepted to Harvard to swim for the women's side in 2015, but entered school and competed for the men's swim team with the full support of the coaching staff.

Stigmas and stereotypes around transgender athletes play a role in the athletes' willingness to participate in sport and to be out as their true selves while they participate. However, transgender athletes are becoming more visible members of the sporting community, due to an increase of societal visibility and acceptance of members of the LGBTQ community. As such it is important to consider how to support participation of all youths in a respectful manner.

Transgender Inclusion

Transgender athletes face unique circumstances when it comes to participating in sport. Due to sports' reliance on binary gender divisions for organizing teams and competitions, it can be challenging for people who identify as transgender to feel comfortable in sport settings. This is accentuated by managers not fully understanding, or being aware of, appropriate or currently accepted best practices for inclusion.

The first issue is determining the team or division in which a transgender athlete should be placed. Ideally this should be the team whose gender most closely resembles that with which the athlete identifies. This can be a complex task, depending on what stage of transition the athlete is at or if they identify outside of the binary. Personal comfort, competitive fairness, and safety perspectives all need to be taken into consideration. The athlete may not be fully out or feel comfortable playing for the gender they identify as if they are still early in the transition process or still presenting regularly as the sex assigned at birth.

Like all youth, transgender youth want to fit in and be respected in school, sport, and other social settings. In order to facilitate this, best practices according to experts on inclusive youth sports, urge athletic leagues and programs to place transgender youth on the team of the gender that they identify with and present as, particularly at younger and less competitive levels. Experts contend that prior to puberty there is no biological reason to segregate the teams by gender, and allowing an individual to play on the team they identify with serves to support the individual. Post puberty, some issues arise regarding the size and strength differential of participants. At this point, best practices for inclusion support integration on the team that the individual identifies and presents as.

Transgender Inclusion Policies

Sport organizations are currently working to create guidelines and policies for transgender athletes. These guidelines and policies differ by level. Research has shown that after one year of hormone treatment, the effect of the primary hormones has been negated. For example, after one year on androgen suppressants and estrogen supplements, transgender women no longer have the muscular strength advantages of the higher testosterone levels of men. The International Olympic Committee and a few other international sport organizations require athletes to have undergone sex reassignment surgery (SRS) and two years of hormone treatment. Recognizing the issues of access to transitioning, including costs, and the age of college students, and taking the research under consideration, the National Collegiate Athletic Association (NCAA) does not require SRS and only requires one year of hormone treatment for transgender women to be able to compete on women's teams. The NCAA only requires documentation of transgender status of transgender men (a double standard based on assumptions of male athletic advantages) to compete on men's teams. NIRSA, the governing body of collegiate recreation, recently published their own policy, which is the most inclusive. It favors allowing participation based on personal identity for intramural sports or, in the case of club sports, the rules of the sport's governing body.

At the youth and high school levels, both the Department of Education and the Department of Justice have released statements stating students should be treated according to gender identity. In 2015, the DOJ stated that:

> under Title IX, discrimination based on a person's gender identity, a person's transgender status, or a person's nonconformity to sex stereotypes constitutes discrimination based on sex. The term 'sex' as it is used in Title IX is broad and encompasses gender identity; including transgender status . . . prohibiting a student from access the restrooms that match his gender identity is prohibited sex discrimination under Title IX. There is a public interest in ensuring that all students, including transgender students, have the opportunity to learn in an environment free of sex discrimination. (Ennis, 2015)

Transgender discrimination constitutes sex discrimination and should be treated as such in terms of school actions and legal actions when discrimination occurs. Subsequently, in 2016, the DOE and DOJ released a joint statement in the form of an Office for Civil Rights Title IX Dear Colleagues letter containing guidelines for supporting transgender students (Department of Justice & Department of Education, 2016). The letter stated that discriminating on the basis of gender identity is a form of sex discrimination under Title IX and that students should have access to facilities and resources that match their gender identity. The departments also recognized that it is often challenging for students to obtain medical documents and/ or treatment. Due to these challenges, the statement noted that this documentation should not be required by schools to treat students in accordance to their gender identity. The Dear Colleague letter stated that students must be allowed to access bathrooms and locker rooms consistent with their gender identity. However, in February 2017, the DOJ and DOE rescinded this interpretation of Title IX and its protections for transgender students, asserting that it is up to states to determine if and how to include transgender students. However, there are ongoing legal battles that will determine if the courts will interpret Title IX to protect transgender students.

In respect to athletics, schools are allowed to adopt medically supported, age-appropriate requirements to accessing sex-segregated sport opportunities. These requirements for participation in sex-segregated athletics differ from state to state. States including Minnesota, Washington, and Wyoming have begun to create policies for transgender student access to athletics. The states with inclusive policies allow students to participate based on the gender identity of the student. However, many require multiple people—including parents, doctors, therapists, and friends—to verify the gender identity of a noncisgender individual before they are allowed to compete. This requirement serves to allay the fears of those who think transgender girls are claiming to be girls just to gain an advantage or access to the girls' locker rooms. This requirement can also serve as a barrier to participation when multiple verifications are required. Documentation from doctors and therapists present economic constraints for some families, and parental support of transitioning may not be present. Some states also require hormone treatment, SRS, and/or change of sex on legal documentation. However, medical treatment is costly and often requires parental consent, which many transgender teens may not have. SRS is very unlikely for high school age and younger individuals.

With respect to changing gender on legal documents (such as birth certificates or driver's licenses), the requirements for obtaining this change also vary from state to state. Different states require different levels of transition, and some do not allow residents to change their legal sex at any point. As such, requiring youth to medically transition or change legal documentation of sex can prevent students from participating according to the gender they identify with and present as. Some of the stricter state regulations may be in violation of the new Title IX guidance. For instance, in 2016 North Carolina passed House Bill 2, which restricted bathroom access to the sex designated on one's birth certificate in all public buildings. Since the North Carolina measure flouted the DOJ-DOE guidelines laid out in the aforementioned 2016 Dear Colleagues letter, which stated that students should be allowed to access bathrooms based on gender identity rather than sex assigned at birth, the Department of Justice threatened to withhold federal funding if North Carolina schools implemented this law. The DOJ and North Carolina dropped their lawsuits against each other in April 2017 after the state legislature passed House Bill 142 that replaced HB2. However, LGBTQ advocates called it a fake repeal as many of the problematic portions of HB2 remained in the new law. Experts urge recreational and youth sports authorities and administrators to consider the costs of treatment, their population's ability to access medical transition (for financial, age, and other reasons), and the ability to change legal documentation in creating their inclusion policies.

Minnesota passed its policy in 2014, after months of heated debate. The policy that was ultimately implemented requires documentation from the student's parent/ guardian, friends or teachers, and a medical professional affirming the student's gender identity. Although this is a high level of documentation, there is no explicit requirement of medical transition, either hormonal or surgical. After the adoption of the policy, the St. Paul School District issued a statement of support for the inclusive policy, asserting that "we believe that it is our moral responsibility to welcome our students' whole selves into our schools. No child should be required to check a part of themselves at the door in order to gain access to school programming, including participation in student athletics" (Payne, 2014). However, there were also vocal critics of the policy, many of whom expressed fears about cisgender boys falsely claiming they are transgender to look for competitive advantage or to gain access to the girl's locker room. Some opponents of the policy took out ads in the *Minneapolis Star Tribune* to this point. One such ad had an image of a girl on a softball field with the text: "The end of girls' sports? Her dreams of a scholarship shattered, your 14-year-old daughter just lost her position on an all-girl team to a *male* . . . and now she may have to shower with him" (Payne, 2014).

In a guide for states and high schools creating policies published for the National Federation of State High School Leagues, Pat Griffin, a professor emerita in social justice education at the University of Massachusetts, Amherst, and a long-time advocate for the inclusion of lesbian, gay, bisexual, and transgender students in college and interscholastic athletics, dismissed this argument. "It is important for policymakers to understand that transgender girls (who were assigned a male gender at birth) are not boys," she wrote. "Their consistent and affirmed gender identity as girls is as deep-seated as the gender identity of non-transgender girls." She also pointed out that the requirement of multiple points of verification "eliminates the unlikely situation where a boy pretends to be a girl to play on a girls' team" (Griffin, 2014). New York has one of the most inclusive policies. After a student notifies the superintendent of their desire to participate in interscholastic athletics consistent with her or his gender identity, the superintendent confirms the asserted gender identity with one of the following individuals: parent, guardian, guidance counselor, doctor, psychologist, or other medical professional. Once the student's gender identity is confirmed, eligibility is granted for the remainder of the interscholastic participation. It allows participation based on the identity of the student and requests that the school obtain minimal documentation of the student's gender identity, which could be a note from a parent, guardian, or medical professional. Only one piece of documentation is requested and is not required by the proposed policy.

However, in states that do not have participation policies in place, individuals do not know how their school or state sport association will treat requests for access. Both the Department of Justice and the Department of Education have put out briefs stating that discrimination against transgender individuals is a Title IX violation. The DOJ (2015) stated that, "under Title IX, discrimination based on a person's gender identity, a person's transgender status, or a person's nonconformity to sex stereotypes constitutes discrimination based on sex. The term 'sex' as it is used in Title IX is broad and encompasses gender identity; including transgender status . . . prohibiting a student from access the restrooms that match his gender identity is prohibited sex discrimination under Title IX. There is a public interest in ensuring that all students, including transgender students, have the opportunity to learn in an environment free of sex discrimination" (Ennis, 2015). Transgender discrimination constitutes sex discrimination and should be treated as such in terms of school policies and legal actions. However, this guidance was rescinded in February 2017 stating that Title IX does not protect transgender students and that states have the authority to decide if and how to protect the students. Despite ongoing court cases, this puts transgender students in uncertain territory and schools in a position of deciding how to act with very little guidance.

There are also issues of privacy when dealing with transgender students. Beyond general aspects of respecting a person's privacy, there are concerns regarding the privacy of medical information. Organizations that require any sort of medical transition, and even those that require doctor's notes asserting an individual's status as transgender, must be aware that all of this information falls under medical privacy laws. The athlete may be required to disclose the information to a director to be allowed to participate, but who that person is then allowed to share the information with is questionable. Administrators should air on the side of privacy and should work in conjunction with the athlete and their family. There is often no reason that a coach, or other players would need to know the individual is transgender unless that individual chooses to share that information. In fact, due to the high presence of transphobia in society, disclosure may actually put the athlete at more risk rather than protecting them.

Intersex Inclusion

Intersex athletes also face challenges to participation; however, this is primarily at the elite and international levels. Sex testing requires female athletes to prove that they are female and fit within culturally acceptable definitions of femininity in order to compete. However, many athletes, and most youth athletes are able to participate as the sex they are assigned at birth (or hopefully as the gender they identify with in the case of transgender athletes) without their status as an intersex individual being salient or even disclosed since this testing only occurs at the elite levels.

Intersex individuals are sometimes not even aware that they are intersex until they hit puberty or try to have children, and some may never be aware that they are intersex. For most youth athletes whether or not they are intersex will never be an issue. However, for select elite athletes, being intersex proves to be problematic, and sport is sometimes how an individual learns they are intersex. This is more likely to happen to athletes who were assigned female at birth. The IOC, IAAF, FIFA, and other international sporting organizations have policies that allow for "sex testing" if there is a question that an athlete is competing in the "wrong" gender category. This generally only happens to female athletes and primarily to those whose looks do not conform to traditional norms of Western femininity and are at the top of their sport. Sex testing was introduced out of fear that men would dress and compete as women in order to gain an unfair advantage. It continues to serve to police appropriate femininity of athletes, and it disparately impacts intersex athletes. Intersex athletes are sometimes not aware that they are intersex prior to undergoing the sex test. Intersex athletes have been disqualified from competition because it was deemed that they were receiving an unfair advantage over other women in the competition. Sex testing has taken many forms over the years, from naked parades, to gynecological exams, to chromosome testing. Currently the IAAF and IOC rules are based on hormone testing with an acceptable limit of naturally occurring testosterone set for female athletes. Female athletes who have a level above the limit must undergo treatment to reduce their testosterone levels; however, this was suspended in 2015.

In 2014 Dutee Chand, an Indian sprinter, was forced to undergo sex testing, which revealed she had female hyperandrogenism. The IAAF required her to undergo hormone treatment to reduce her testosterone levels before she could compete again. She refused and fought this decision in order to be able to compete without altering her hormones. She stated, "I want to remain who I am and compete again" (Branch, 2015). In July 2015, the Court of Arbitration for Sport (CAS) issued a ruling suspending the hyperandrogenism regulation for two years. During the two-year suspension of the rule, the IAAF must quantitatively show a direct link between hyperandrogenism and a distinct competitive advantage. If the IAAF fails to show this, the regulation will be voided (CAS, 2015). Chand and a number of other athletes snared by the hyperandrogenism regulation were allowed to compete in the interim, including the Rio 2016 Olympics, without testosterone suppression treatments.

Another high-profile controversy concerned Spanish hurdler María José Martínez-Patiño who, in 1986, "failed" a chromosome-based sex test. She was dismissed from the Spanish national team and stripped of her medals, even though she had passed a previous sex test. In 1988 the IAAF allowed her to compete again when androgen insensitivity syndrome was better understood, but she failed to make the team for the subsequent Olympics.

Conclusion

Transgender, gender nonconforming, and intersex youth face many barriers to navigating everyday life, including high rates of harassment and bullying in school, elevated risks of homelessness due to family rejection, and higher risks of being victims of hate-based violence. Sport has the capacity to be an enormous benefit to such youth, if the sport is organized in an inclusive format with policies facilitating access and organizers encouraging respect. Conversely, youth sports can be a source of additional stress and pain when organizations prevent participation or fail to provide a welcoming and inclusive environment. As more athletes like Chris Mosier and Fallon Fox participate at high levels, and as visibility of transgender individuals such as Caitlyn Jenner, Janet Mock, and Lavern Cox become more common and more socially accepted, school and sport organization policies may become more inclusive and understanding of transgender youth. Society is currently grappling with the issue of how to include transgender youth in sport in a way that is respectful of the individual and appropriate for the competitive setting they are in. Society's perspectives and treatment, and the subsequent policies around inclusion, are rapidly changing at this time.

Erin L. Morris

Further Reading

Branch, J. 2015, July 27. "Dutee Chand, Female Sprinter with High Testosterone Level, Wins Right to Compete." *The New York Times.* Accessed at http://www.nytimes.com /2015/07/28/sports/international/dutee-chand-female-sprinter-with-high-male -hormone-level-wins-right-to-compete.html?_r=0.

Ennis, D. 2015. "Department of Justice: Title IX Protects Trans Students from Discrimination." *The Advocate.* Accessed at http://www.advocate.com/politics/transgender/2015 /06/30/department-justice-affirms-title-ix-protection-trans-students.

GLSEN. 2013. *The 2013 National School Climate Survey, Executive Summary.* Accessed at http://www.glsen.org/sites/default/files/NSCS_ExecSumm_2013_DESIGN_FINAL.pdf.

Grant, J. M., L. A. Mottet, J. Tanis, J. Harrison, J. L. Herman, and M. Keisling. 2011. *Injustice at Every Turn: A Report of the National Transgender Discrimination Survey, Executive Summary.* National Center for Transgender Equality and National Gay and Lesbian Task Force. Washington, D.C. Accessed at http://www.thetaskforce.org/static _html/downloads/reports/reports/ntds_summary.pdf.

Griffin, P. 2014, November 21. *Developing Policies for Transgender Students on High School Teams.* National Federation of State High School Associations. Accessed at http:// www.nfhs.org/articles/developing-policies-for-transgender-students-on-high-school -teams.

Human Rights Campaign. (2015). *Sexual Orientation and Gender Identity Terminology and Definition.* Accessed at http://www.hrc.org/resources/entry/sexual-orientation-and -gender-identity-terminology-and-definitions.

Intersex Society of North America. 2008. *What Is Intersex?* Intersex Society of North America. Accessed at http://www.isna.org/faq/what_is_intersex.

Parents, Families, and Friends of Lesbians and Gays. (2015). *The PFLAG National Glossary of Terms.* Accessed at http://community.pflag.org/glossary.

Payne, M. 2014, December 4. "Minnesota Approves New Transgender Friendly Policy for High School Athletes." *The Washington Post.* Accessed at http://www.washingtonpost .com/blogs/early-lead/wp/2014/12/04/minnesota-approves-new-transgender-friendly -policy-for-high-school-athletes.

Sharp, B. 2015, July 16. "NY Eyes Transgender Guidelines for High School Sports." *Democrat & Chronicle.* Accessed at http://www.democratandchronicle.com/story/news/2015 /07/16/ny-eyes-transgender-guidelines-high-school-sports/30252185.

Policies

Department of Justice & Department of Education. (2016). *Dear Colleagues Letter on Transgender Students.* Accessed at http://www2.ed.gov/about/offices/list/ocr/letters /colleague-201605-title-ix-transgender.pdf.

Dutee Chand v. Athletics Federation of India (AFI) & The International Association of Athletics Federation, CAS 2014/A/3759. CAS, 2015. Accessed at http://www.tas-cas.org /fileadmin/user_upload/award_internet.pdf.

Griffin, P., and H. Carroll. 2010. *NCAA Inclusion of Transgender Student-Athletes. NCAA.* Accessed at https://www.ncaa.org/sites/default/files/Transgender_Handbook_2011_Final .pdf.

International Olympic Committee. *Policy on Transgender Inclusion.* Accessed at http:// www.transathlete.com/#!policies-by-organization/c1vyj.

Medical and Scientific Committee. 2012. *IOC Regulations on Female Hyperandrogenism.* International Olympic Committee. Accessed at http://www.olympic.org/Documents /Commissions_PDFfiles/Medical_commission/2012-06-22-IOC-Regulations-on -Female-Hyperandrogenism-eng.pdf.

Minnesota State High School League. 2015. *2015–2016 MSHSL Official Handbook.* Accessed at http://www.mshsl.org/mshsl/Publications/code/handbook/300%20Bylaws .pdf.

Shane Bennett, S., S. Bravo, J. Hill, V. McCutchan, W. Motch, and B. Turner. 2014. *Updates to Policies and Tournament Materials around Transgender Athlete Participation in NIRSA Championship Series Events.* NIRSA. Accessed at http://nirsa.net/nirsa/wp -content/uploads/here.pdf.

Transgender Inclusion Policies by Organization. Accessed at http://www.transathlete.com /#!policies-by-organization/c1vyj.

Girls in Sports

"My coach said I ran like a girl. I said if he ran a little faster, he could too."
—Mia Hamm, Team USA women's soccer

American society has traditionally trafficked in the stereotype that if someone is playing a sport "like a girl," the person is doing it in a weak and inferior manner. Girls playing sports are stereotyped as running slower, throwing softer, and competing less aggressively than boys. Yet if a girl does show uncommon strength, speed, or ability, she is criticized for being excessively masculine.

Girls have fewer opportunities to participate in sports than boys and more barriers to accessing sport programs that do exist. A gender equality gap in American youth sports is thus painfully evident. Sport administrators are obliged to make sports more accessible to girls by breaking down barriers that limit their participation. To that end, this entry focuses on the history of girls in sports, what girls' sport participation looks like today, the barriers that inhibit girls' involvement, the benefits that flow from girls playing sports, the importance of role models for girls in sports, and recommendations for sport programming that better lead to girls' growth and development as human beings.

Title IX and Girls in Sport

Title IX, enacted in the United States in 1972, proclaims, "No person in the United States shall, on the basis of sex, be excluded from participation in, be denied the benefits of, or be subjected to discrimination under any educational program or activity receiving Federal financial assistance" (U.S. Department of Education, 2015, 1). Title IX was an important milestone for girls' participation in sports. Before Title IX, girls rarely participated in organized sports programs at the elementary, high school, or college levels. Gender stereotypes prevailed and sport programs were seen as advantageous for sons but not daughters. Athletic organizations were controlled by men, which discouraged girls from becoming involved. As a result, only 3 percent of high school girls played sports prior to the passage of Title IX (Women's Sports Foundation, 2008). Those sports were largely viewed as feminine, such as cheerleading and dance. At the same time, women's athletics in colleges and universities received only 2 percent of their institutions' overall athletics budget (Women's Sports Foundation, 2008). Title IX changed that.

Title IX compliance has three different segments: (1) effective accommodation of student athletic interests and abilities (participation), (2) athletic financial support (scholarships), and (3) other program components such as equipment and supplies, scheduling of games and practice times, and access to tutoring (Title IX; Women's Sports Foundation, 2011a).

The number of girls participating in sports has grown dramatically since Title IX's enactment. Approximately two in five girls now participate in high school sports. The number of women's college and university athletic programs has also increased exponentially—more than 600 percent (Dusenbury and Lee, 2012), and women's athletic teams receive a more equitable proportion of budgets and scholarships. There are also more sport opportunities now for women once they graduate from college to compete at elite levels. Examples include the Olympics, World Championships, and professional leagues (Women's Sports Foundation, 2008).

Title IX, however, has not accomplished all that it was set out to do. For example, girls enter sports later than boys, thus delaying the benefits they could be receiving (Woods, 2011). Not only do girls start sports later, but they drop out sooner and in greater numbers (Women's Sports Foundation, 2008). Girls are not involved across multiple sports, and participation is not sustained at every age (Woods, 2011). There are also discrepancies among girls who are playing. They are predominantly Caucasian and from suburban neighborhoods (Kelley and Carchia, 2013; Sagas and Cunningham, 2014). Furthermore, schools are providing 1.3 million fewer chances for girls than boys to play sports in high school, and while one-half of the students at National Collegiate Athletic Association (NCAA) schools are women, women receive only 44 percent of the athletic participation opportunities. Financially, female athletes receive 28 percent of the total athletic budget, 31 percent of the recruiting dollars, and 42 percent of athletic scholarship dollars. Also, the number of women who coach girls' athletics has diminished as well (Title IX, 2015). Why is this?

Barriers to Girls in Sport

Many barriers (intrapersonal, interpersonal, and structural) inhibit girls from participating in sports (SHAPE America, 2014). A girl may, for example, think negatively about her body or weight and thus not feel comfortable being physically active; girls in a coed physical education class may get bypassed by the boys during activities; or girls simply may not be interested in the sport programs offered. It is important to investigate these barriers more deeply so they can be addressed and ultimately eliminated.

Intrapersonal barriers are perceptions or beliefs that affect an individual's intentions to participate (Dilworth, 2010). The internal perceptions and insecurities girls deal with significantly limit their desire to participate in sports. Girls commonly struggle with body dissatisfaction and poor self-esteem. When girls are self-conscious about their bodies, it causes them to avoid sports and physical activity (Women's Sports Foundation, 2011a). Because girls start sports later than boys, they are delayed in developing their coordination and motor skills. They think they do not possess the required capabilities for a sport, and they feel self-conscious about displaying what skills they do have. Other girls simply lack motivation or interest and want to spend their time doing other activities such as working, completing homework, or socializing with friends (Eime, Harvey, Sawyer, Craike, Symons, Polman, and Payne, 2013).

Interpersonal barriers arise from breakdowns in informal and formal social support networks and interactions between people (Dilworth, 2010). Girls often report having negative social interactions in physical education classes with others. Many girls want to participate in sports, but are worried about what boyfriends and significant others will think. Girls want to appear attractive and feminine to peers; however, there is a sweaty muscular image attached to athletic women that is not appealing to young girls. Mixed Martial Arts fighter Ronda Rousey knows all too well the feeling of being called "masculine" for her involvement in martial arts as a young girl:

> When I was in school, martial arts made you a dork, and I became self-conscious that I was too masculine. I was a 16-year-old girl with ringworm and cauliflower ears. People made fun of my arms and called me "Miss Man." It wasn't until I got older that I realized these people are idiots. I'm fabulous. (Bustle, 2015, 1)

Although Rousey persevered in her martial arts pursuits, the reality for many girls is that they drop out of sport due to these types of disparaging comments.

Girls are also greatly influenced by boys inside and outside of school. The competitive nature of physical education classes that include boys is an ongoing issue. Girls tend to be marginalized by boys in physical education classes, and many girls are left out of activities because boys do not involve them. Teachers can also worsen the situation by encouraging a largely competitive atmosphere, and by not intervening when boys do not allow girls to participate fully. Out of class, some boys reinforce gender stereotypes by actively discouraging their girlfriends from participating in sport because it allegedly makes them look "butch." Some girls may adopt the unfortunate view that "feminine" women do not participate in sport or physical activity. These views are not as commonplace as they once were, but they still exist in some households, schools, and communities (Allender, Cowburn, and Foster, 2006).

Structural barriers can also impede participation in an activity. Examples of structural barriers include inadequate equipment and insufficient access to opportunity (Dilworth, 2010). Limited sport programming also discourages girls from participating in sports. Girls, more so than boys, can be uninterested in traditional sport offerings such as football, basketball, and rugby. They want to sample from a wider variety of sports and exercise activities such as volleyball, cheerleading, and dance. Such nontraditional activities provide girls with the opportunity for fun and enjoyment while minimizing competition (Allender, Cowburn, and Foster, 2006). Other major structural barriers involve poor facilities, inconvenient travel schedules, and an absence of support services. In the majority of high school athletic programs, for example, girls' programs are still struggling for resource equity. Girls' programs tend to have lower quality facilities, fields, scheduling of games and practice times, and coaching. Community or school sport facilities may be less accessible to girls and women because of administrators' tendency to give boys and men priority in making facility schedules (United Nations, n.d.). Due to these barriers, girls are missing out on important developmental benefits from sport participation.

Benefits

There are a vast array of physical, psychological, intellectual, and social benefits gained through participation in sport (Hancock, Lyras, and Ha, 2013). Girls should be made aware of the benefits they can receive throughout their lifetime from participation in sports so they will be better able to take advantage of them (Kotschwar, 2014).

Sport promotes increased levels of activity and exercise that benefits participants physically. Obesity, for example, is a critical health issue facing youth throughout the United States. Indeed, 30.4 percent of girls are overweight or obese according to one study (NIDDK, 2012). Engaging in sports helps control and maintain a healthy weight in girls, which can help reduce obesity (Hancock, Lyras, and Ha, 2013). Participating in physical activity and sports is thus an effective prevention and health risk reduction strategy for girls. Sports participation significantly reduces the risk of developing disease and illnesses, such as breast cancer and osteoporosis (American College of Sports Medicine, 2013). Not only are girls who are active and participate in sports healthier, but they are less likely to engage in unhealthy behaviors and lifestyles such as smoking, drinking, using drugs, and sexual activity that can result in unwanted pregnancies or exposure to sexually transmitted diseases (Jones-Palm and Palm, n.d.).

Participation in sports has also been identified as useful in alleviating many psychological issues girls face. Being active helps girls reduce stress, anxiety, and depression (Garcia, Archer, Moradi, and Andersson-Arntén, 2012). Anxiety and depression occur in boys and girls, but by mid-adolescence girls are more than twice as likely to be diagnosed with a mood disorder as boys (Steingard, 2014). Participating in sports combats many issues girls experience psychologically, such as a lack of self-esteem and confidence, and dissatisfaction with their bodies. Multiple studies have shown that playing a sport enhances a girl's self-esteem, improves confidence, and improves body image and self-worth (Hancock, Lyras, and Ha, 2013). Many psychological problems also create barriers to girls participating in sports, while sport participation helps eliminate those same barriers. There is, then, somewhat of a vicious cycle at work that needs to be broken if girls are to reap the psychological benefits that involvement in sport can confer on them.

Lack of access to sports has been linked to girls and women occupying a weaker position in society educationally, socially, politically, and economically (Hancock, Lyras, and Ha, 2013). By investing in sport programs for girls and women, sport can have a positive impact on society as a whole. Melinda Gates, an advocate for girls and women's rights, affirms, "If you invest in a girl or a woman, you are investing in everybody else" (Fortune, 2015, 1). Sport and recreational activities promote education, and reduce dropout rates, which can enhance female empowerment (Hancock, Lyras, and Ha, 2013). Girls who participate in sports are more likely to perform better in school and attain educational success, especially in areas dominated by men, such as the sciences. Sports foster the cultivation of attributes desirable in the workplace, such as the ability to be a team player, communicate, and compete. Increasing girls' access to sport allows them to develop these attributes, which in turn aids them in securing better jobs as adults. In this regard, more opportunities to play sports lead to greater female participation in many male-dominated occupations (Kotschwar, 2014).

Sports also provide girls opportunities to develop socially. Early in life girls spend a lot of time with their families. Sports open up another avenue of opportunity for peer-to-peer social interactions and friendships. Positive sport experiences thus contribute to girls experiencing social inclusion. Sports bring together individuals from a variety of social and economic backgrounds for a common and shared interest in activities. Being a part of a team, sporting community, program, or club can provide girls with a powerful sense of belonging. Sports help develop and extend social networks, as teams often consist of girls from different schools or towns. Players, coaches, and parents also note that sports can provide girls with opportunities to strengthen social skills such as working with others, resolving conflict, making friends, and developing leadership and negotiation skills (Hancock, Lyras, and Ha, 2013).

Role Models for Girls

Women are underrepresented in sport at all levels. Their absence can give girls a sense that they do not belong in sport. To ward off this perception, female role models are holding more and more key positions in sport organizations, including the National Basketball Association (NBA) and the National Football League (NFL). Becky Hammon, for example, was hired in 2014 by the San Antonio Spurs as the first female assistant coach in the NBA. Sarah Thomas was hired in 2015 as the first female official referee in the NFL. Jen Welter, also hired in 2015, was the first female coach in the NFL for the Arizona Cardinals. Welter stated, "I want little girls everywhere to grow up knowing they can do anything, even play football" (NBC News, 2015, 1). Women are thus slowly making their way into significant roles in a male-dominated sport industry. They serve as role models to look up to, and they are a source of inspiration for girls interested in sports.

Complicating the situation, however, is an imbalance in media coverage between women's and men's sports. This imbalance reduces girls' opportunities to see strong female athletes as role models. Approximately 4 percent of sports coverage in local and national media print is dedicated to women's sport, thereby conveying the message "that sports is still for, by, and about men" (Zirin, 2010, 1). The media play a central role in forming society's knowledge, opinions, and attitudes about women in sport, which influences girls' and women's participation levels. Left unchecked, a lack of coverage of women's sports leads to limited female role models available to cultivate the next generation of healthy, active women (Women's Sports Foundation, 2011b).

Effective role models do not need to be the most outstanding athletes. They may come from the home, school, or community (Bailey, Wellard, and Dismore, 2004). Dads also need to take a more active role in mentoring young girls in sports. One study found that only 28 percent of girls say their fathers taught them the most about sports, compared to 48 percent of boys. Dads tend to focus their mentoring on their sons instead of their daughters. Regardless of gender, dads should be providing mentorship to their children. Sport organizations and programs should also draw from local communities and schools to include women in key mentorship roles (Women's Sports Foundation, 2008).

Program Recommendations

Developmentally focused youth sports (DYS), which use sport as a medium to teach sport and life skills, have been proposed as a particularly promising program for girls. The program provides young girls with opportunities for physical, psychological, intellectual, and social growth. Sport programs provide a setting for life skills instruction, including "problem solving, goal setting, teamwork, communication, management of success and failure, and receiving and applying constructive feedback" (Debate, Gabriel, Zwald, Huberty, and Zhang, 2009). Sports help develop these life skills through demonstration, modeling, and practice. Girls acquiring sport and life skills may then sustain their interest in physical activity and their own social/psychological growth and development. Curricula in DYS address situations that are familiar to girls, including "peer pressure, gossiping, bullying, body image, healthy decision making, active listening, and getting along with peers" (Debate, Gabriel, Zwald, Huberty, and Zhang, 2009).

The World Health Organization also suggests a number of strategies that promote practices for positive sporting experiences for girls:

1. Girls do enjoy engaging in physical activities. Strategies should be implemented which build upon this enjoyment, and allow them to participate as fully as possible, in forms that offer them satisfaction and opportunities for achievement.
2. Practices should be established which recognise the importance of fun, health and social interaction in sports participation.
3. School physical education is a foundation of life-long physical activity. Fundamental movement skills need to be developed from an early age, *for all children*, with the emphasis on the individual body, rather than sporting outcomes.
4. Some girls regularly engage in sports and physical activities, as an integral part of their lifestyle. Any strategies concerned with raising participation among young people need to remember that neither girls nor boys are 'the problem'; rather, the difficulty lies with the ways in which physical activities are constructed and presented.
5. It is important to examine and highlight the practices inherent within sports which might deter children from participating. Sports provision may need to be adapted to encourage and accommodate all young people.
6. It is necessary to listen to voices from outside mainstream sports, for example, dance, mixed ability, non-competitive and co-operative activities.
7. Sports programmes should reflect local cultural needs if they are to engage and sustain girls' participation.

8. The organisation of sports groups and programs should include women in key roles, such as coaching and mentors, and role models drawn from within local communities and schools. These should reflect differences in perspectives and interests, and develop close links with schools and communities, to ensure continuity of engagement in sports and physical activities throughout life.
9. The more opportunities that are available for girls to be physically active, the more they are active. Strategies need to be put in place that ensures activities, settings and facilities are easily accessible and safe. (Bailey, Wellard, and Dismore, 2004)

Conclusion

Sports have the potential to serve important positive developmental functions for girls, but much work needs to be done in the personal, family, school, community, and social realms to level the playing field for girls and boys. The benefits of involvement in sports for girls are largely untapped because substantial barriers to girls' full participation in sports still exist. This is a social problem that can be solved if sport administrators, parents, physical education teachers, coaches, and other community sport leaders take an active approach at breaking down these barriers for girls and give them the resources and opportunities they deserve.

Cait Wilson

Further Reading

Allender, Steven, Gill Cowburn, and Charlie Foster. 2006. "Understanding Participation in Sport and Physical Activity among Children and Adults: A Review of Qualitative Studies." *Health Education Research*, *21*: 826–835.

American College of Sports Medicine. 2013. *ACSM's Guidelines for Exercise Testing and Prescription*. Philadelphia: Lippincott Williams and Wilkins.

Bailey, Richard, Ian Wellard, and H. Dismore. 2004, February 18. *Girls Participation in Physical Activities and Sports: Benefits, Patterns, Influences and Ways Forward*. Accessed July 25, 2015, at https://www.icsspe.org/sites/default/files/Girls.pdf.

Bustle. 2015, August 2. *6 Feminist Quotes from Ronda Rousey That Prove She's More Than Just a Trash Talker*. Accessed August 8, 2015, at www.bustle.com/articles/101566-6-feminist-quotes-from-ronda-rousey-that-prove-shes-more-than-just-a-trash-talker.

DeBate, Rita DiGioacchino, Kelley K. Pettee Gabriel, Marissa Zwald, Jennifer Huberty, and Yan Zhang. 2009. "Changes in Psychosocial Factors and Physical Activity Frequency

Among Third- to Eighth-Grade Girls Who Participated in a Developmentally Focused Youth Sport Program: A Preliminary Study." *Journal of School Health, 79*: 474–484.

Dilworth, Virginia. 2010. *Dimensions of Leisure in Your Life: Contemporary Leisure.* Champaign, IL: Human Kinetics.

Dusenbury, Maya, and Jaeah Lee. 2012. *Charts: The State of Women's Athletics, 40 Years after Title IX.* Accessed September 23, 2015, at http://www.motherjones.com/politics /2012/06/charts-womens-athletics-title-nine-ncaa.

Eime, Rochelle, Jack Harvey, Neroli Sawyer, Melinda Craike, Caroline Symons, Remco Polman, and Warren Payne. 2013. "Understanding the Contexts of Adolescent Female Participation in Sport and Physical Activity." *Research Quarterly for Exercise and Sport, 84*(2): 157–166.

Fortune. 2015, March 9. *Melinda Gates: Why Hiring Women Is Good for Business.* Accessed August 1, 2015, at www.fortune.com/2015/03/09/melinda-gates-why-hiring-women-is -good-for-business.

Garcia, Danilo, Trevor Archer, Saleh Moradi, and Ann-Christine Andersson-Arntén. 2012. "Exercise Frequency, High Activation Positive Affect, and Psychological Well-Being: Beyond Age, Gender, and Occupation." *Psychology, 3*(4): 328.

Hancock, Meg, Alexis Lyras, and J. P. Ha. 2013. "Sport for Development Programmes for Girls and Women: A Global Assessment." *Journal of Sport for Development, 1*: 15–24.

Jones-Palm, Diane H., and Jurgen Palm. n.d. *Physical Activity and Its Impact on Health Behavior among Youth.* Accessed September 27, 2015, at https://www.icsspe.org/sites /default/files/PhysicalActivity.pdf.

Kelley, Bruce, and Carl Carchia. 2013. *Hey Data Data—Swing!* Accessed September 23, 2015, at http://espn.go.com/espn/story/_/id/9469252/hidden-demographics-youth-sports -espn-magazine.

Kotschwar, Barbara. 2014, March 1. *Women, Sports, and Development: Does It Pay to Let Girls Play?* Accessed August 4, 2015, at https://www.piie.com/publications/pb/pb14-8 .pdf.

Myer, Gregory D., Avery D. Faigenbaum, Andrea Stracciolini, Timothy E. Hewett, Lyle J. Micheli, and Thomas M. Best. 2012. "Exercise Deficit Disorder in Youth: A Paradigm Shift toward Disease Prevention and Comprehensive Care." *Current Sports Medicine Reports, 12*: 248–255.

National Institute of Diabetes and Digestive and Kidney Diseases (NIDDK). 2012, October 2. *Overweight and Obesity Statistics.* Accessed July 30, 2015, at www.niddk.nih .gov/health-information/health-statistics/Pages/overweight-obesity-statistics.aspx.

NBC News. 2015. *Arizona Cardinals Hire First Female Coach in NFL History.* Accessed September 28, 2015, at http://www.nbcnews.com/news/sports/arizona-cardinals-hire -first-female-coach-nfl-history-n399386.

Sagas, Michael, and George B. Cunningham. 2014. *The Aspen Institutes PROJECT PLAY.* Accessed September 23, 2015, at http://www.aspeninstitute.org/sites/default/files/content /docs/education/Project_Play_Underserved_Populations_Roundtable_Research_Brief .PDF.

SHAPE America. 2014. *Title IX,* Accessed July 30, 2015, at http://www.shapeamerica.org
/advocacy/titleix.cfm.

Steingard, Ron J. 2014, August 25. *Mood Disorders and Teenage Girls.* Accessed August 1,
2015, at www.childmind.org/en/posts/articles/mood-disorders-teenage-girls-anxiety
-depression.

Title IX. 2015. *Athletics under Title IX.* Accessed July 23, 2015, at www.titleix.info/10-key
-areas-of-title-ix/athletics.aspx.

United Nations. n.d. *Sport and Gender: Empowering Girls and Women.* Accessed August 2,
2015, at www.un.org/wcm/webdav/site/sport/shared/sport/SDP%20IWG/Chapter4
_SportandGender.pdf.

U.S. Department of Education. 2015, April 22. *Title IX and Sex Discrimination.* Accessed
July 24, 2015, at www.ed.gov/category/keyword/title-ix.

Women's Sports Foundation. 2008, October 1. *Go Out and Play: Youth Sports in America.* Accessed July 23, 2015, at http://www.womenssportsfoundation.org/home/research
/articles-and-reports/mental-and-physical-health/~/media/PDFs/WSF%20
Research%20Reports/\go_Out_and_Play_Exec.ashx.

Women's Sports Foundation. 2011a. *Title IX Myths and Facts.* Accessed July 24, 2015, at
http://www.womenssportsfoundation.org/home/advocate/title-ix-and-issues/what-is
-title-ix/title-ix-myths-and-facts.

Women's Sports Foundation. 2011b. *Do You Know the Factors Influencing Girl's Participation in Sport?* Accessed July 31, 2015, at http://www.womenssportsfoundation.org
/home/support-us/do-you-know-the-factors-influencing-girls-participation-in-sports.

Woods, Ronald B. 2011. *Social Issues in Sport* (2nd ed.). Champaign, IL: Human Kinetics.

Zirin, Dave. 2010, July 6. "The Dramatic Drop in Women's Sports Coverage: An Interview with Mike Messner." *The Nation.* Accessed July 30, 2015, at www.thenation.com
/article/dramatic-drop-womens-sports-coverage-interview-mike-messner.

Goal Setting for Performance Enhancement

Michael Jordan, a Hall of Fame basketball player who many consider the greatest of all time, said, "I'm a firm believer in goal setting. Step by step. I can't see any other way of accomplishing anything." Similarly, Roy Williams, the head basketball coach at the University of North Carolina and a member of the Basketball Hall of Fame himself, once said that "without goals you are like a ship without a rudder—heading in no particular direction." Goal setting is one of many psychological strategies that can help athletes achieve peak performances. The process of setting goals not only influences athletes' performances, but it is linked to positive changes in a variety of psychological states, such as motivation and confidence. Additionally, goal setting is a tool that can be beneficial in all areas of life, including academics.

How effective is goal setting? In a classic book titled *A Theory of Goal Setting and Task Performance* (1990), Edwin Locke and Gary Latham reviewed 201 separate studies evaluating the effectiveness of systematic goal setting on performance and productivity improvement. There were 90 different tasks involved in these studies, including laboratory tasks, business and industrial productivity, academic improvement, sport performance and skill achievement, and social skills attainment. The subjects included college students, engineers, scientists, athletes, loggers, factory workers, and college professors. In most of the studies, goal-setting conditions were compared with control groups that did not set goals or were simply told to "do your best." Significant positive effects were found in 183 of the 201 studies—a 91 percent success rate. Moreover, increases of up to 60 percent in task performance were found, with a median level of improvement of around 16 percent. That level of improvement would increase a baseball or softball player's batting average from .250 to .290; a 70 percent free-throw shooter in basketball would improve to 81.2 percent.

In light of such study results, goal setting is frequently characterized as a highly effective performance enhancement strategy that works across a variety of tasks and settings. Done correctly, advocates say that it is one of the best performance enhancement techniques available in the behavioral sciences. Thus, correct goal setting constitutes a set of learnable skills that can then be used in virtually any area of life to improve performance.

With regard to youth sports, coaches and parents can teach goal-setting techniques to their young athletes. To be effective, however, the process must involve a collaborative effort. Why is this true? If coaches or parents set goals for kids, they become the adults' dreams, not the athletes' objectives.

Why Goal Setting Works

According to advocates of the practice, there are many reasons why goal setting improves performance:

1. **Goal setting focuses and directs one's activities:** Goals direct the athlete's attention and action to important aspects of the task. For example, basketball players who set a goal of increasing their free-throw shooting percentage to 80 percent will concentrate on shooting free throws during practice time rather than taking many different kinds of shots.
2. **Goals help athletes mobilize effort:** Returning to our basketball player example, by setting this specific goal, an individual will likely exhibit greater effort and commitment in attempting to achieve this objective.
3. **Goals not only increase immediate effort, but also increase persistence:** As a case in point, the boredom of a long season is offset and persistence is increased when a golfer sets a number of short-term goals throughout the year.
4. **Athletes often develop and use new strategies for improving performance:** For example, baseball players may change the mechanics of their swing in order to achieve a goal of hitting a certain percentage of line drives. Thus, setting and trying to attain specific goals may help to increase motivation, commitment, and performance.

Goal-Setting Procedures

Not all goal-setting procedures are created equal. Some approaches to goal setting are more effective than others, according to proponents. Research on the effectiveness of various types of goal-setting strategies suggests several practical guidelines:

1. **Set specific goals in terms that can be measured:** Specific goals are more effective in improving performance than are general "do your best" goals

or no goals at all. An effective goal clearly indicates what a person needs to do to accomplish it. This means that you must be able to measure the performance that relates to the specific goal. For example, it should be possible to measure how much an athlete has improved on a specific skill or task (e.g., percent of successfully completed free throws) or the frequency of desirable behaviors (e.g., the number of times the athlete praised teammates).

2. **Set difficult but realistic goals:** Difficult or challenging goals produce better performance than moderate or easy goals. The higher the goal, the higher the performance, as long as the goal does not exceed what the athlete is capable of doing. Goals should not be so difficult that the athlete will fail to take them seriously or will experience failure and frustration in meeting them. It is therefore important for an athlete to set goals in relation to his or her ability level. The goals should be set so that they are difficult enough to challenge athletes but realistic enough to achieve.

3. **Set short-range as well as long-range goals:** Breaking down any long-term goal into smaller more attainable goals helps to promote achievement and success. The motto here is, "Yard by yard it's awfully hard, but inch by inch it's a cinch!" Short-term goals are effective for two main reasons. First, they are more flexible and controllable. Thus, they can be more easily raised and lowered to keep them challenging but realistic. Second, goals provide more frequent evaluations of success. The object of each step is to give athletes a sense of accomplishment, which motivates them to eventually reach long-term objectives.

One way to understand the relationship between short- and long-range goals is in terms of a staircase. The top stair represents the athlete's long-range goal or objective, and the lowest stair is his or her present level of performance. The steps in between represent a progression of short-term goals of increasing difficulty that lead from the bottom to the top of the stairs. The short-term goals allow athletes to enjoy successes and accomplishments as they move toward the top of the stairs.

4. **Set performance goals as opposed to outcome goals:** American society places tremendous emphasis on the outcome of athletic events, and it is not surprising that many athletes of all ages are accustomed to setting only outcome goals. Outcome goals focus on the product of performance. Good examples include wanting to win a league championship or all-star recognition. Although outcome goals can provide a sense of direction and purpose, they do have built-in flaws. For instance, if your goal is to go undefeated all season and you lose your first game, "it's all over."

The more important and inherent problem with outcome goals, however, is that athletes have only partial control over them. An athlete may achieve the best performance of his or her life and yet fail to achieve the outcome goal of winning an event because someone performed even better. Youth advocates emphasize that it is far better to set goals in terms of personal performance standards, for then success is seen in terms of athletes exceeding their own goals rather than surpassing the performance of others. When winning (outcome) becomes secondary to achieving their own personal goals, athletes are much more motivated to practice. Practice gives athletes the opportunity to work toward their personal goals with assistance from the coach. Athletes do not judge themselves as having succeeded or failed purely on the basis of whether they have won or lost, but in terms of their achievement of the specific performance and behavioral goals they have set. Thus, the amount of personal satisfaction that athletes achieve from sport does not need to be tied to winning. Athletes at all levels of ability can enjoy success through attainment of their personal goals. Stating goals in such terms also helps athletes to learn the valuable lesson that winning has more to do with *doing their best* than *being the best.*

5. **Express goals in positive rather than negative terms:** Youth sports researchers urge athletes (and coaches) to set goals positively (e.g., number of passes made or shots-on-goal) rather than negatively (e.g., number of mistakes reduced). Positive goal-setting helps athletes focus on success instead of failure.

6. **Set goals for both practices and competition:** It is just as important, if not more so, to set goals for practice sessions as it is for competitive events. Practices are the times when athletes often make the greatest advancements in developing and honing their skills. When practice becomes meaningful as a result of being tied in with specific goals, athletes become more engaged. Moreover, setting specific goals related to practice and tracking progress toward them help reduce the drudgery of practice and makes it more meaningful for the athlete. During practice, athletes can work toward specific performance goals that are geared to their areas of strength and weakness. Thus, one football player's goals may be keyed to improving blocking, while another's may relate to tackling.

Since the presumed goal of every competitor is to win, it might seem meaningless to set additional goals during competition itself. However, such goals can be very useful in that they provide one means by which winning will be achieved. For example, a basketball team can set a team goal for a game, such as holding the opponent's best player to 15 points, out-rebounding the other team, or limiting turnovers to no more than 10. By focusing on the attainment of specific performance goals, coaches can create a "game within the game" in which athletes can be successful in some important respects, even if they are not victorious in terms of the final score. Many coaches have found that this technique helps prevent players from being discouraged if the team does not win and helps promote steady improvement in the team's play.

7. **Identify specific goal achievement strategies:** All too often, goals are not accomplished because athletes fail to identify and commit themselves to goal achievement strategies. Setting goals without identifying ways of achieving them is not very effective. Thus, hockey players who wants to improve their skating speed by 5 percent may choose an achievement strategy of doing an additional 10 sprints after practice each day.

8. **Record goals, achievement strategies, and target dates for attaining goals:** Once (a) specific goals have been set, (b) achievement strategies decided on by the athlete and coach, and (c) target dates for goal accomplishment have been established, these should be written down so that they can be referred to frequently. Some coaches and parents actually establish a formal contract with their young athletes to keep them focused on the activity and committed to it.

9. **Set up a performance feedback or goal evaluation system:** In the words of Don James, Hall of Fame college football coach, "The best way to build confidence in your players is to show improvement through statistics." In support of this, goal-setting research indicates that performance feedback is absolutely necessary if goals are to enhance performance. Therefore, athletes must receive feedback about how their present performance is related to both short- and long-range goals. Without such feedback, athletes cannot track their progress toward goals and may be unable to see improvement that is actually occurring.

Feedback can also correct misconceptions. Athletes, like other people, often have distorted perceptions of their own behavior. Objective evidence in the form of statistics or numbers can help correct such misconceptions and may help motivate corrective action. For example, it can be a sobering experience for basketball players who fancy themselves great ball handlers to find out that they have more turnovers than assists. But, after being provided this statistical feedback, basketball players can then use the information to make changes and set statistical goals for improvement.

Feedback also creates internal consequences by causing athletes to experience positive (or negative) feelings about themselves. Athletes who are dissatisfied with their level of performance will experience feelings of self-satisfaction when

subsequent feedback indicates improvement. This also functions as positive reinforcement. The feelings of pride and self-confidence that arise can be even more
important than external reinforcement from the coach in bringing out improved
performance. Promoting self-motivation in athletes also reduces the need for coaches
to reinforce or punish. When feedback is public, as in the posting of statistics, the
actual or anticipated reactions of others can serve as an additional motivator of
increased effort and performance.

10. **Goals should not be "set in stone":** Goals should be made to be revised,
    and they should be used as a guide. When athletes are helped to set realis-
    tic goals, they inevitably experience more success and feel more compe-
    tent. By becoming more competent, they gain in self-confidence and
    become less fearful of failure. Perhaps most important, they discover that
    commitment to goals helps lead to success.

11. **Goal-setting programs are most effective when they are supported by
    those individuals who are important in the athlete's life:** This typically
    includes the coach, teammates, and the athlete's family. Therefore, it is
    important that significant others promote the recognition, encouragement,
    and support of individual and team movement toward goals. Coaches and
    parents are central figures in providing such support.

Common Problems with Goal Setting

In addition to the goal-setting principles presented above, there are some pitfalls to
avoid. It is not particularly difficult to set up a goal-setting program. However, problems can arise when proper goal-setting procedures are not used. One such problem occurs when too many goals are set too soon, resulting in system overload. If
too many goals are set, athletes cannot properly monitor performance, or they find
it very difficult to do so. To avoid this, an appropriate approach is to prioritize goals
and focus attention on the one or two that are most important.

A second problem arises in setting goals that are too general. We have emphasized the importance of setting specific, measurable goals. The general principle
here is that if you can't measure the goal in terms of specific numbers, it is too vague
and general to be used effectively. And again, remember that *performance* goals
are preferable to *product* goals because athletes have greater control over them.

Finally, some athletes have negative attitudes about goal setting. In such cases,
it is best not to force their participation in a goal-setting program. Quite frequently,
they will see the benefits and enjoyment that other athletes are experiencing as a
result of goal setting and will come on board later on.

Establishing a Goal-Setting Program

To be successful in carrying out a goal-setting program, some sort of goal-setting system or procedure must be employed. The simplest and most effective system has three main phases: (1) the planning phase, (2) the meeting phase, and (3) the follow-up or evaluation phase. In this final section of this entry, we discuss each phase in terms of how coaches can initiate a goal-setting program in sport situations. Aspects of the approach also apply to parents' implementation of goal setting in a more general context.

The Planning Phase

Setting up a goal-setting program obviously requires a good deal of planning. First of all, individual and team needs must be identified. These may be in a variety of areas including performance, conditioning, sportsmanship, care of equipment, relations among teammates, and so forth. Once the most important of these are decided on, coaches must decide how they can help their athletes achieve these goals. In other words, coaches must engage in a goal-setting program with respect to identifying goals and specifying how they are going to help athletes attain them.

Meeting with Athletes

After goals have been decided on, it is important that the coach communicate these to the athletes and indicate why they are important. The amount of detail will of course depend on the level of maturity of the athletes. With older and more experienced athletes, it may be beneficial to meet with each one individually after the general meeting in order to mutually decide on goals and strategies. For younger athletes, team rather than individual goals may be more appropriate, but it is essential that these goals be very specific and measurable.

It may be necessary to involve athletes in the measurement of behaviors relating to specific goals. For example, an athlete who is not currently playing in a soccer match may keep track of the number of passes made before each shot, if one of the goals is to work the ball around the defense before shooting.

Follow-Up/Evaluation

In order to ensure that movement toward goals and possible revision of goals can occur, it is a good idea to set up several evaluation meetings with individuals, subgroups of athletes, or the entire team. A critical part of the entire process is the feedback procedure that coaches choose to employ. The procedure should allow coaches and athletes to clearly see where things stand in relation to the goals that have been set. If athletes are mature enough, coaches might require that they monitor their own target behaviors to supplement whatever statistics are used to chart progress toward goals.

Conclusion

When coaches and parents help athletes to set realistic goals and provide ways for them to attain those goals, youth sport athletes inevitably experience more success and feel more competent. By becoming more competent, they gain in self-confidence and become less fearful of failure. Perhaps most importantly, they discover that commitment to goals helps lead to success. They also learn, with help from coaches and parents, that failure indicates they should try harder, not that they are unworthy. Deemphasizing winning and emphasizing attainment of personal and team goals can greatly increase the positive impact that adults can have on the athlete's performance and enjoyment of the sport.

Frank L. Smoll and Ronald E. Smith

Further Reading

Gould, Daniel. 2015. Goal setting for peak performance. In Jean M. Williams and Vikki K. Krane (Eds.), *Applied Sport Psychology: Personal Growth to Peak Performance* (7th ed., pp. 188–206). New York: McGraw-Hill.

Locke, E. A., and Gary P. Latham. 1990. *A Theory of Goal Setting and Task Performance.* Englewood Cliffs, NJ: Prentice-Hall.

Smith, Ronald E., and Frank L. Smoll. 2012. *Sport Psychology for Youth Coaches: Developing Champions in Sports and Life.* Lanham, MD: Rowman & Littlefield.

Smoll, Frank L., and Ronald E. Smith. 2012. *Parenting Young Athletes: Developing Champions in Sports and Life.* Lanham, MD: Rowman & Littlefield.

Smoll, Frank L., and Ronald E. Smith. *Coaching and Parenting Young Athletes* [Blog]. Accessed at https://www.psychologytoday.com/blog/coaching-and-parenting-young-athletes.

Hazing

Although there are many positive outcomes and benefits from participating in youth sports (e.g., increased physical activity, socializing, teamwork), the experience for some young athletes is spoiled due to hazing. Hazing is commonly defined as any activity expected of someone joining a group that humiliates, degrades, abuses, or endangers, regardless of the person's willingness to participate. It has been documented in sports settings from middle school to professional leagues (e.g., NFL, NHL). In general, hazing occurs when veterans, or experienced members of a team, require new or prospective teammates to perform actions or activities beyond normally accepted athletic expectations. These actions or activities typically embarrass or humiliate the victim, and they can also be physically painful or otherwise detrimental to physical health and well-being. Experiencing hazing in youth sport, either as a participant or victim, can profoundly impact a child's future involvement in, and enjoyment of, sport. The current state of hazing in athletics requires coaches, administrators, parents, and student-athletes to scrutinize traditions on their teams and develop positive team-building initiations and activities inside the context of legal, ethical, and child development standards. Despite an enhanced awareness of the negative implications from hazing, and the multiple efforts on behalf of leagues and administration to thwart hazing activity, these negative "team-building" traditions, which in practice often amount to no more than bullying, continue to plague the various levels of sport.

Hazing Defined

In addition to the definition of hazing above, other characterizations have been developed by researchers, youth advocates, and other observers. Karen Savoy of Mothers Against School Hazing (MASH) advanced a more broad description, contending that hazing is any action or activity that does not contribute to the positive development of a person. Others have defined hazing based on the degree of severity or impact on victims. Hazing that does not result in emotional or physical harm is termed "lowercase h" hazing. Hazing that causes quantifiable physical or emotional harm is considered "Uppercase H" Hazing, which is often an outgrowth of unchecked "lowercase h" hazing.

Developing a strong, clear, and comprehensive definition of hazing that can be understood by young athletes is important, but arriving at such a definition can be problematic on three fronts. First, academicians and researchers, who in some cases can be detached from the realities faced by young people, have developed these definitions. Second, often these same researchers make the language in a hazing definition purposefully broad and vague to cover a wide variety of activities; listing every specific activity that falls under the wide-ranging definition of hazing would take reams of paper. In addition, when addressing young athletes, listing every insidious act that could constitute hazing is risky, as it may focus their attention on hazing endeavors they had never considered before and may ultimately try. The third reason that defining hazing can prove challenging is that 90 percent of hazing victims, based on the above definitions, do not consider themselves to have been subjected to hazing (Allan and Madden, 2008). This gap between what researchers, parents, coaches, administrators, police, and prosecutors consider hazing, and what young people consider hazing, is wide and appears to be widening. It is within this cavernous space where most hazing takes place.

Crow and MacIntosh (2009) proposed a new definition of hazing in athletics that recognizes that often coaches, not athletes, determine whether a player (hazed or not) remains on a team. They define hazing as:

> Any potentially humiliating, degrading, abusive, or dangerous activity expected of a junior-ranking athlete by a more senior teammate, which does not contribute to either athlete's positive development, but is required to be *accepted* as part of a team, regardless of the junior-ranking athlete's willingness to participate. This includes, but is not limited to, any activity, no matter how traditional or seemingly benign, that sets apart or alienates any teammate based on class, number of years on the team, or athletic ability.

Persistence of Hazing

That hazing exists and persists in sport is a function of three main concepts: (1) that it creates team cohesion and unity, (2) that it shows who on a team is dominant, and (3) that it proves commitment to the team (Cimino, 2011). Although on the surface, theories (1) and (2) seem to be in direct contrast to one another, this dichotomy is often cited by hazers who believe that new teammates should be subservient to veterans in order to improve or maintain team cohesion.

Indeed, one of the more insidious attributes of hazing is that it is often considered a tradition by its perpetrators, victims, and coaches in some cases and thus is acceptable because others have done it before them. The overwhelming majority of perpetrators were once themselves victims of hazing (whether or not they considered it to be hazing at that time). They in turn want to ensure that the following newcomers have to endure the same, and many times worse, hazing rituals than they did. This continual building of more egregious and potentially dangerous hazing then becomes mistaken for tradition, and is repeated with the arrival of every new cadre of rookie teammates looking to build rapport and be accepted. Veteran members, knowingly or unknowingly, use hazing rituals as an attempt to establish a hierarchical structure. Researchers have studied why current members of the group insist on accelerating the severity and intensity of initiation rites such that it crosses over into hazing. When current members were hazed as rookies, they had no power. Now, as veterans, they are in a position of power, and since they allowed themselves to be hazed, they expect to engage in such activities with those next in line. However, what is clear is that Uppercase H Hazing should never be considered traditional; athletic traditions should be centered around athletic achievement (e.g., league titles, championships), academic achievement (e.g., team grade point average, graduation rates), or both. These traditions can be celebrated through periodic rituals or ceremonies throughout the season.

In addition, hazing exploits the basic human desire to belong to a group. Newcomers regularly subject themselves to this behavior, often fully aware of the impending danger and risks. Perpetrators and victims alike can believe that surviving hazing ensures a bonding experience and strong team cohesion. This belief strengthens the subversive culture of hazing. In addition, each veteran involved in hazing feels empowered by a legion of colleagues who enthusiastically encourage the behavior. Countless young people have given in to peer pressure and allowed themselves to be hazed just to gain the empowerment that goes along with being part of a formidable and socially desirable group.

All told, however, experts emphasize that hazing is not team building. Team building is a purposeful effort where leaders (whether coaches or veteran athletes of the team) study and examine their own processes of working together, and as a result create a more positive culture that propagates values and contributes to enhancing a more collaborative and shared vision of success. Team building can also allow for more open and honest communication among members of the team, which helps to formulate a more cohesive unit.

Legal Issues

As of 2015, 44 states had antihazing laws in place. These statutes are generally classified as misdemeanors, with insignificant penalties and fines. However, even though a particular state may not have enacted a specific hazing statute, actions that constitute hazing often can be prosecuted under other criminal statutes, such as assault, kidnapping, providing alcohol to minors, or reckless endangerment. Historically, there have been very few successfully prosecuted cases involving hazing statutes. Perhaps this notable case of hazing, although not directly related to athletics, provides the best example of the potential outcomes and punishment that can occur when hazing turns deadly:

In the fall of 2011, Robert Champion, a drum major in the world famous Florida A&M University (FAMU) Marching Band, known as the FAMU Marching 100, died as a result of methodical and preplanned beating at the hands of fellow band members in a hazing tradition known as "crossing bus C." Hazing had a long history in the FAMU band, and in fact, the band director had suspended 26 members of the band barely one week before Champion's death (Montgomery, 2012).

In October 2014, a jury found Dante Martin, a fellow member of the marching band, guilty of manslaughter and other charges in the hazing of Champion and two other band members. He was sentenced to 77 months in prison. Most of the other 15 band members who were charged with felony hazing received probation, but no jail time. Martin, who had refused to speak with detectives investigating Champion's death and who did not testify at his trial, spoke publicly for the first time about the hazing. "Sometimes we just go with what is tradition," Martin said of hazing at FAMU. "We don't second-guess it, we don't doubt it" (Montgomery, 2012).

Hazing in Sport

In Canada, where hockey is by far the most popular youth sport, hazing is prevalent, particularly in the junior ranks. In 2011, 16 players and the coaching staff from the Neepawa Natives of the Manitoba Junior Hockey League were suspended for the hazing of 5 newcomers to the team. Most of this hazing took the form of sexual misconduct or assault and the underage consumption (often forced) of alcohol. Hockey Canada, the country's governing body at all levels of the sport, has recently strengthened its antihazing policies, and there are calls from hazing victims to have a dedicated antihazing officer in the organization. The Hockey Canada policy currently defines hazing as "an initiation practice that may humiliate, demean, degrade, or disgrace a person regardless of location or consent of the participant(s)." The full statement from Hockey Canada (2015) reads:

Hockey Canada developed the Speak Out program in 1997 in order to educate and prevent bullying, harassment and abuse in hockey across Canada. Since then, a comprehensive program of training, education and awareness of bullying, harassment and abuse has been accomplished through workshops, resource materials and branch and association initiatives. All of these factors have focused on coaches, managers, safety people, parents, players and administrators. Furthermore, it is the policy of Hockey Canada that there shall be no abuse and neglect, whether physical, emotional or sexual of any participant in any of its programs. Hockey Canada expects every parent, volunteer and staff member to take all reasonable steps to safeguard the welfare of its participants and protect them from any form of maltreatment.

Hazing, however, is not isolated in sport to Canada or hockey; it is pervasive in all sport systems.

In 2015, the men's and women's swimming and diving programs at the University of Western Kentucky, in Bowling Green, Kentucky, were suspended for five years, the coaching staff lost their jobs, and at least one member of the team faces criminal charges as a result of wide-ranging hazing allegations. The charges involve sexual assault, harassment, underage drinking, and numerous violations of the school's student code of conduct (Highland, 2015). In the same year, the women's softball program at St. Joseph's University in Philadelphia had the remainder of its season canceled amid hazing allegations that have thus far resulted in two lawsuits against the institution and the head coach (Snyder, 2015).

Role of Society

Hank Nuwer (2004), the foremost authority on hazing in the United States and abroad, suggests that the flippant manner by which members of local and national media cover hazing incidents that occur in professional North American sport may "ripple down" and lead to incidents of hazing in high school and college athletic settings. These same media members, who vilify and castigate student-athletes involved in hazing, conversely make light-hearted or humorous comments of professional athletes acting the same way. Media coverage of hazing has shown that young athletes can be impacted by observing the media coverage of ostensibly "harmless" activities, including challenges occurring on "reality" television and hazing in professional sports.

Many young athletes see initiation and hazing activities conducted by professional athletes on television, in print, and on social media. Often the media personnel that deliver the story make light of the initiations, and although some of the activities portrayed are fairly benign, make no mistake, they involve demeaning behaviors that are antithetical to good sportsmanship and foster a climate of class structure. For example, the consumption of alcohol might be perfectly fine for the majority of professional athletes, but consider the player whose family has a secret history of alcoholism and is hesitant to consume. Or, the rookie forced to sing the words to his college alma mater's fight song, but whose learning disability prohibits him from remembering the words. The scars from this type of humiliation are not visible, but may certainly be long lasting.

In the National Football League, hazing generally occurs during, and near the end of, training camp, which often takes place on a college campus. Several players have been injured so severely they were no longer able to participate in training camp activities, yet often sport media personnel covering the teams characterize these hazing rituals as pranks. Think for a moment what would happen in a youth sport setting if veteran, returning players on a team taped their brand-new teammates to a goalpost, covered him in shaving cream or analgesic cream, made a video of the activities, then shared them with the local news team. These young athletes would be punished, and rightfully so, but in the NFL it is considered a fun, humorous, tradition.

In the National Basketball Association, one of the most common rookie hazing activities, besides making rookies carry the veterans' luggage on road trips, is to wait until a rookie buys a new car, then fill it with loose popcorn or other food items. While seemingly harmless, many would argue there is no positive outcome from that behavior either. Examples of unrealistic behavior and challenges on TV shows like *Survivor* and *Fear Factor* also encourage impressionable kids and make it harder to distinguish what activities are hazing. In perhaps the most inharmonious example of sport media "approval" of hazing, Alyson Footer (2008) wrote an article for the Major League Baseball's official website, entitled "Rookies Face Hazy Days of Spring." Part of the story included guidelines for new professionals:

> Most young players know their roles during Spring Training. The rules are simple. Don't talk too much. Keep your head down. Work hard. And when your veteran teammates pick on you, you must take it. And for good measure, it doesn't hurt to pretend you're enjoying it (p. 1).

To perhaps acknowledge the disrespectful tone of the article, Major League Baseball placed a disclaimer at the bottom of the webpage stating the story was not subject to its approval (most likely to protect Major League Baseball or any of its clubs). This is one simple illustration of a larger and more complex problem in sport that seemingly propagates the notion that hazing is acceptable in some circumstances.

Impact on Young Athletes

Most coaches, parents, and young athletes agree that hazing does more harm than good to the members of any group. What should also be clear is that hazing in youth sport has the potential to exploit and damage the spirit and psyche of the young person. Historically, many sports for both genders have been rife with hazing incidents that have included abuse of alcohol, sexual exploits, bodily harm, public displays of embarrassment, and generally degrading activity. More and more parents, coaches, and athletic administrators have come to realize that initiation onto a team as a rookie should not take the form of something embarrassing, harmful, degrading, or negative in any way. Making and being a part of a team should be a positive experience. It is becoming more common for administrators to understand their responsibility to produce a positive environment for athletes, coaches, fans, and media alike, and part of this responsibility is educating and enforcing important policies to protect the rights of its stakeholders. Creating a positive culture starts with the leadership of the organization, the coaches and players of the team, and even the parents who can act by speaking out against hazing-related behavior before it goes too far. A collective effort is needed through education, activation, and positive examples of team building if hazing activities are to stop. The eradication of hazing is necessary to help clean up the sport system and allow young people to positively experience the attributes that sport should bring to the playing field.

R. Brian Crow and Eric W. MacIntosh

Further Reading

Allan, E., and Madden, M. 2008. *Hazing in View: College Students at Risk*. National Study of Student Hazing. Accessed June 15, 2015, at http://www.stophazing.org/wp-content /uploads/2014/06/hazing_in_view_web1.pdf.

Cimino, A. 2011. "The Evolution of Hazing: Motivational Mechanism and the Abuse of Newcomers." *Journal of Cognition and Culture, 11*: 241–267.

Crow, R. B., and MacIntosh, E. W. 2009. "Conceptualizing a Meaningful Definition of Hazing in Sport." *European Sport Management Quarterly, 9*(4): 433–451.

Footer, A. 2008. *Rookies Face Hazy Days of Spring Training*. Accessed June 15, 2015, at http://www.milb.com/gen/articles/printer_friendly/milb/y2008/m03/d03/c353782.jsp.

Highland, D. 2015, April 14. "WKU Swim Program Suspended for Five Years in Wake of Hazing Investigation." *Bowling Green Daily News*. Accessed June 15, 2015, at

http://www.bgdailynews.com/news/wku-swim-program-suspended-for-five-years-in
-wake-of/article_26df8e00-e2a7-11e4-8849-1f04b5a1dc98.html.

Hockey Canada. 2013, September 9. *Information Bulletin: Important Message Regarding Hazing.* Accessed June 15, 2015, at http://assets.ngin.com/attachments/document/0044 /9504/HazingAwareness2013.pdf.

Hockey Canada. 2015. *Speak Out Canada.* Accessed June 15, 2015, at http://www.hockey canada.ca/en-ca/Hockey-Programs/Safety/Speak-Out.aspx.

Lipkins, S. 2006. *Preventing Hazing: How Parents, Teachers, and Coaches Can Stop the Violence, Harassment, and Humiliation.* San Francisco: Jossey-Bass Publishers.

Montgomery, B. 2012. "Recounting the Deadly Hazing That Destroyed FAMU Band's Reputation." *Tampa Bay Times.* Accessed June 15, 2015, at http://www.tampabay.com/news /humaninterest/recounting-the-deadly-hazing-that-destroyed-famu-bands-reputation /1260765.

Nuwer, H. 2004. *The Hazing Reader.* Bloomington, IN: Indiana University Press.

Snyder, S. 2015, May 15. *Lawsuit: St. Joe's Softball Rookies Forced to Drink, Simulate Sex.* Accessed June 14, 2015, at http://www.philly.com/philly/blogs/campus_inq /Disturbing-allegations-in-St-Joes-hazing-lawsuit.html#iW7EY3IZxWqLqsiC.99.

Healthy Competition

In his controversial book *No Contest: The Case against Competition,* American author and lecturer of education, human behavior, and parenting Alfie Kohn asserted that the term *healthy competition* is a contradiction. Since the original publication of Kohn's book in 1986, some Americans have come to agree with Kohn's contention that cooperation and intrinsic motivation are more important cogs in striving for excellence and achievement than competition. In sports, workplaces, and schools—the three primary contexts addressed by Kohn—Americans have made some progress in terms of balancing their perspectives related to competition. Yet, to think that a day might arrive wherein competition is removed completely from these settings is unrealistic—and even undesirable according to many. Competition is simply and utterly too deeply ingrained in American society to be removed, and even the perception of doing so is anathema to most Americans. This entry will focus on one of the settings addressed by Kohn in exploring the current state of youth sports and break down why *healthy competition* has ironically become the preferred mode of delivery in that setting.

The Context and Commercialization of Sport

Sport as an industry has evolved into a multi-billion-dollar entertainment complex. The global sport behemoth keeps inundating American society with sports-related news and information 24 hours a day, seven days a week. Americans can choose to plug in or not, but to escape its grasp entirely would certainly be a monumental accomplishment. Whether sports-related content emerges at the proverbial water-cooler at work, plays on the television at the local restaurant, splashes across the front page of the newspaper, or is advertised on passing buses or the Internet, sport makes its way into daily life. Many Americans grew up on sport and competition, and without the ability to follow their favorite teams and/or sports, their lives would not be as meaningful. However, adults have long since learned to process what competition means to them, and ultimately the highly business-oriented enterprise associated with the professional model of sport is something that many adults have learned to digest without even giving it a second thought.

When examining the impact of commercialized professional sport on America's youth, it is certainly an ever-changing and nuanced landscape. Rising concurrently with mass media in the form of television and now online broadcasts, the last 50 years have seen an explosion in the average person's access to professional, intercollegiate, and even interscholastic sports. With this rise has come an enormous influx in the money associated with the professional model of sport. That commercialization has certainly filtered down to youth sports as well. In the last 25 years, for example, television coverage of Little League International has increased exponentially to the point that state and regional Little League competitions are broadcast on ESPN. Many observers have expressed concern about the possible negative impact of this commercialization on the nation's youth.

Many youth sport advocates, including Up2Us Sports, the National Alliance for Youth Sports, and John O'Sullivan and the Changing the Game Project, among others, take this concern very seriously. Youth sport advocates are all dedicated to helping parents, coaches, and administrators achieve a healthy balance in their perspectives toward sport and align themselves and their programs toward the goal of holding youth development above winning and losing. These reformers hasten to add that they recognize that there are values and lessons to be learned through competition. Most believe in the inherent values associated with competition, and that sport has the potential to impart fabulous life lessons children and adolescents need in the course of growing up to be contributing members of society. However, they emphasize that unchecked competitiveness and a win-at-all-costs attitude have a potentially far greater negative impact on our society. Some reformers even assert that some of the more notorious ills of American society, whether Wall Street malfeasance or gang violence, can be attributed at least in part to an ill-conceived notion or ill-developed concept of ruthless competition. According to their perspective, it is important to recognize that all people go through a process, starting at a very young age, whereby they process and develop varying levels of understanding related to competition. This is one of the keys in moving toward a conception of healthy competition.

The Developmental Process for Children

Some people, particularly parents, believe that competition is an innate characteristic. Why? Parents see their children want to always be first in line or fight, cheat, and even grow upset with games as they age. However, the truth is that it may never be known for sure whether or not competition in humans is innate. Scientists have targeted biological traits in other species that naturally point to competition being innate as a survival mechanism. However, in our more evolved state, the separation between competition as a learned or innate element is a more problematic determination. Ultimately, that distinction matters less for youth sports than the child development tendencies related to competition. The point then is not whether or not children are competitive; many children exhibit signs of competitiveness at very young ages. The point is that research in developmental psychology points to the notion that most children's conception of competition is not fully developed until after age 10.

One important item to note is that child development is not like a chemistry experiment. Scientists can isolate molecules in a lab, but child development theory is in many ways more complex due to the myriad of interpersonal and sociocultural mitigating factors. Researchers can develop a theory that generally applies, but it will never apply to all children. Children and their development are simply too dynamic. Therefore, parents with children ages 8–10 may differ when asked whether or not their child understands competition. Yet, the perception of the complexity of competition and its true meaning may in fact escape even adult parents. When most people are asked to define competition, the answer invariably gets boiled down to winning and losing. Yet, winning and losing (and tying) are simply game-level outcomes associated with competition. Competition, in actuality, is more complex than these game-level outcomes.

Competition is an advanced interplay between ability, effort, and luck that ultimately yields an outcome of winning, losing, or tying. So, in revisiting the typical age of understanding, little Pat prior to age 10 believes that trying hard alone will equate to success in athletic endeavors and may get incredibly frustrated when trying hard does not equal success. Little Jordan after age 10 begins to understand that one's ability level coupled with effort (with a little luck mixed in) is the driving force behind achievement in youth sport competition. This is why standards have been developed to assist youth sport professionals with structuring positive developmental settings for children.

Developmental Standards and Competition

The very labels that are utilized to describe youth sport environments for children ages 4–8 point to the prevailing orientation associated with these settings. Youth sport programs for children in these age groups are not structured or framed as "noncompetitive" but rather as *developmental* and *instructional* due to the associated child development. The following are the *National Standards for Youth Sports,* as developed by the National Alliance for Youth Sports (2017):

Developmental programs for children 6 years old and under:
- Informal teams
- Focus on motor skill development
- Scores and/or standings not emphasized
- Roster size, rules, equipment, and fields modified
- Limited uniforms
- Postseason tournament or all-star competition highly discouraged
- Encourage boys and girls to participate together whenever possible
- No travel
- Coaches permitted on playing surface

Instructional sports programs for 7- to 8-year-olds:
- Focus on skill development and rules of the game
- Scores and standings not emphasized
- Roster size, rules, equipment, and fields modified
- Limited uniforms
- Encourage a variety of positions and situational play
- Postseason tournament or all-star competition discouraged
- Encourage boys and girls to participate together whenever possible
- Travel discouraged
- Coaches permitted on playing surface

As children age, their collective and individual understanding of competition matures along with them. Therefore, the *National Standards for Youth Sports* (as developed by NAYS), reflects this aspect:

Organizational programs for 9- to 10-year-olds:
- Scores kept but standings deemphasized
- Roster sizes, rules, equipment, and fields modified when necessary
- Encourage a variety of positions and situational play
- Out-of-community postseason play only when necessary
- No national tournament participation

Skill enhancement and enrichment programs for 11-year-olds and above:
- Scores and standings deemphasized
- Proper grouping and selection procedures to ensure fair and equitable teams
- Encourage a variety of positions and situational play

Cynics and generational purists have a tendency to point toward the coddling of today's youth, and many times these developmental measures that have been implemented in youth sports environments are targeted as evidence of that notion. However, youth sports advocates assert that, ultimately the message from those who care about the health, well-being, and lifelong fitness for the next generation is that child development does matter. When the orientation of these settings is left to those without a grounding in child development, what inevitably ensues is overt and unchecked competition and adults living their lives vicariously through children—a dynamic that is not healthy for children or society.

The *Healthy* Promise of Competition

So, what constitutes and makes competition *healthy*? Let's start with the most complex setting for competition—that of life—and work from there. Does winning and losing manifest itself in "real" life? Some might argue that at the microlevel, in everyday endeavors that take place in work and social settings, winning and losing is absolutely manifested. Others might take a more bird's-eye approach in looking at one's life in totality and say that the many and varied aspects of our life combine to make declaring a *winner* or *loser* in life not only impossible but counter to the realities of our complex lives as human beings. Whether we answer affirmatively or negatively to the question of winners and losers in life, we can likely all agree that it is more complex than a simple winner or loser (as in sports).

Many Americans believe very strongly in the context of sports as a training ground where valuable lessons about life are learned. However, is it a naturally occurring phenomenon? Leonard Wankel and Bonnie Berger noted, "Sport, like most activities, is not *a priori* good nor bad but has the potential for producing both positive and negative outcomes" (Wankel and Berger, 1990, 167). The prevailing message among youth sport experts is to be explicit (i.e., targeted or intentional) in working to achieve our goals relative to youth development. Just as the program in which we participate matters, coach, peer, and parental role models matter greatly as well for a healthy competitive sports environment.

So, again, what constitutes and makes competition *healthy*? One word: *balance*. American society will never be able to completely remove the potentially negative and/or damaging elements associated with competition, as doing so would effectively necessitate removal of it entirely (as Alfie Kohn indicated). However, if those more negative perspectives and/or elements are balanced with positive notions and/or qualities, youth sport settings can be developed that are more effective in fostering healthy competition. The following *balanced* perspectives are the key to healthy competition:

- Balance the notion of one's competitor as an enemy or combatant with the view of a competitor as partner or collaborator.
- Balance aggression and hate toward one's competitor with a playful nature and a spirit of camaraderie.
- Balance an overtly ego orientation centered on beating or destroying others with a task orientation of mastering the task at hand or striving to be one's best.
- Balance extrinsic motivation focused on rewards, money, and fame with intrinsic motivation of playing for the love of the sport.
- Balance the overbearing messages to win-at-all-costs with messages centered on personal growth and achievement across domains.

If these perspectives are promoted and fostered in youth sports, or any achievement-oriented environment for that matter, healthy competition and its associated benefits will be manifested.

The starting point for balance is a fundamental understanding that competition, if left unchecked, can certainly devolve into what David Light Shields and Brenda Light Bredemeier (2009) labeled *decompetition* and described as a state that is ultimately anticompetition. Unfortunately, decompetition has been present in sporting culture throughout history in the form of cheating, scandal, violence, and hatred—all the negatively associated elements that ruin what so many hold dear about sport and competition. This notion of decompetition should be balanced by a wholly different perspective toward competition, one that is healthier and aligned with wellness gains across the physical, psychological, emotional, social, and intellectual domains for children and adults alike.

The metaphorical connection of sports to war runs deep in our evolution as human beings. Historians and anthropologists have documented that connection across many ancient cultures. Whether Roman gladiators fighting animals or each other or Aztec warriors playing the Ball Game in mortal combat, the foundations of sport are mostly violent with negative associated outcomes. In fact, it was not until the turn of the century in the United States, with the concurrent rise of the Muscular Christianity movement—a Christian life of brave and cheerful physical activity—with that of the playground and recreation movements, that we as a society began to embrace sport (albeit skeptically) as an environment where we might teach children lessons about life. In addition to the rich history of sport as a violent training ground for war, it was also associated with heavy drinking and gambling, and hence, there was considerable consternation and even outright opposition related to sport's place in the positive development of youth. However, thanks to noted leaders like Joseph Lee (playgrounds), Jane Addams (recreation), and Luther Gulick (Muscular Christianity), organizations such as the Young Men's Christian

Association (YMCA) eventually embraced youth sports as part of their core mission to positively impact the lives of youth. The community centers that gave rise to municipal parks and recreation departments followed suit, and youth sports have prevailed as integral programming in the United States ever since. Despite this evolution in public attitudes toward sports, however, war metaphors still run deep within the lexicon of sport.

An understanding of this underlying metaphor and its associated tendency to promote a combative and aggressive approach to sport settings is critical in working toward a more balanced and healthier conception of competition in our youth sport environments. Some may disagree as to the validity of catharsis theory as applied to adult sports. Catharsis theory posits that aggressive sports like boxing and American football provide an outlet to release aggressive emotions that might otherwise manifest in violent acts in life. The theory has long been debunked in psychological circles, but it is seemingly accepted by popular sentiment (due in part to a fundamental lack of understanding that theories may work in isolation but must be applied more broadly). Setting aside the viability of catharsis theory for adults, youth sports advocates agree that some balance to that warring aggressive perspective is warranted in youth sport environments. They point out that although the United States has certainly made strides in reducing youth violence since the height of the gang violence epidemic in the 1990s, in many communities the daily reality is one where rival colors still mean life or death. So, is it really healthy to promote a similar perspective on the playing surface? Likely not. Yet, sports environments are often shaped by youth, coaches, and volunteers who do not necessarily have a firm grasp on the metaphorical realities of an overly aggressive and combative competitive environment. In so doing, American society may be failing to provide the empowerment necessary to promote a more playful environment wherein one can still compete at a high-spirited level but with an orientation of camaraderie and respect rather than aggression and hate. This is a simple lesson that could go a long way toward manifesting a more positive developmental outcome in the lives of youth. Yet, it is not the only lesson in the path toward a healthier conception of competition.

Does the motivation to play sports matter? Research says it does. Those who are more oriented towards extrinsic motivation (i.e., external rewards like money, fame, and fortune) receive far fewer benefits than those who are more intrinsically motivated by a love for and/or enjoyment of the game. Why? Many believe the answer to be tied to our achievement orientation in competitive environments. Are we oriented toward achievement for the sake of ego or for the task at hand? Those involved in sport in any meaningful capacity have heard the saying "Check your ego at the door" in reference to the need in team sport environments in particular to be humble and a quality teammate. Many youth, however, are not taught this message. The label *prima donna* is often used to label young elite athletes who are consistently bombarded with praise and develop an inflated sense of self-worth or ego. In achievement domains like sport, an ego orientation is associated with a desire to beat others in order to earn or maintain a lofty status in one's own mind and among peers. An overdeveloped ego orientation in sport, particularly when not balanced by a task orientation wherein the athletes also are oriented toward mastery of the task at hand and striving for their personal best, has been shown in countless studies to be associated with variables that may lead to negative outcomes. For example, Greenwood and Kanters (2009) in a sample of adolescent males engaged in a summer football camp found that those with high ego orientation and low task orientation scored lower than their peers on self-reported measures of character. This finding is relatively consistent across many studies examining both achievement orientation (i.e., ego/task) in isolation and when combined with motivation (i.e., extrinsic/intrinsic).

Therefore, if proceeding from this basic level of understanding relative to achievement orientation and motivation, youth sports advocates call for fostering a culture wherein love of the game and mastery of the task at hand are held in higher esteem than defeating others. In so doing, a message is conveyed that personal growth and achievement across domains ultimately means more than winning in sports. Yet, while individual sports like cross-country, swimming and diving, and golf naturally foster that intrinsic task-oriented perspective, team sports are a different story. Team sports do not necessarily promote task orientation, and therefore the need for such an orientation to be taught and fostered is even greater in these environments. Unfortunately, providing a balanced perspective along those lines is easier said than done, given the omnipresent commercialized sport entertainment behemoth that exists in the United States.

Even youth sport programs with curriculum fully and completely centered on fostering healthy competition may struggle with balancing the underlying message that winning is held above all else. Legendary American football coach Vince Lombardi has infamously and erroneously been associated with the quote, "Winning isn't everything; it's the only thing!" The actual source of this quote was another coach of his decade, "Red" Sanders. Lombardi, instead, preferred the saying, "Winning is not a sometime thing, it is an all the time thing" (Maraniss, 1999, 500). The difference between these two quotes is subtle but all important to the quest for *healthy* competition. Winning as the "only thing" denotes a win-at-all-costs mentality, while winning as an "all the time" thing denotes that the path to success or achievement is constant and should never wane. In other words, people should strive for excellence in all of our life's endeavors. Rather than promote the corrupted "Winning is the only thing" quote, youth sport advocates believe that the real Lombardi message should be carried forward to the next generation.

Youth sports advocates assert that the underlying negative messages associated with reports of cheating, corruption, and scandal at all levels of sport can and must be addressed. If such efforts are successful, the impact on society could be extraordinary. Already, many international (e.g., Basketball Without Borders), national (e.g., America Scores), regional (e.g., Junior Giants) and local (e.g., Smart Fit Girls) sports-based youth development organizations are carrying out that positive and balanced perspective toward youth sports. Focus on being great at reading, learn how to treat others with respect, win humbly, care for your teammates *and* your opponents (as without both, we have no game). The messages that align with healthy competition are needed in all sport environments, and they do not have to compromise competition in order to be successful in navigating this more balanced perspective in youth sports.

P. Brian Greenwood

Further Reading

Dweck, Carol S. 2006. *Mindset: The New Psychology of Success.* New York: Ballantine Books.

Greenwood, P. Brian, and Michael A. Kanters. 2009. "Talented Male Athletes: Exemplary Character or Questionable Characters?" *Journal of Sport Behavior, 32*(3): 298–324.

Kohn, Alfie. 1986/1992. *No Contest: The Case against Competition.* New York: Houghton-Mifflin.

Kohn, Alfie. 2014. *The Myth of the Spoiled Child: Challenging the Conventional Wisdom about Children and Parenting.* Boston: Da Capo Books.

Maraniss, David. 1999. *When Pride Still Mattered: A Life of Vince Lombardi.* New York: Simon & Schuster.

McLean, Daniel, and Amy Hurd. 2015. *Kraus' Recreation and Leisure in Modern Society* (10th ed.). Burlington, MA: Jones & Bartlett Learning.

National Alliance for Youth Sports. 2017. *National Standards for Youth Sports.* Accessed January 6, 2016, at https://www.nays.org/resources/nays-documents/national-standards-for-youth-sports.

Powell, Robert Andrew. 2004. *We Own This Game: A Season in the Adult World of Youth Football.* New York: Grove Press.

Shields, David Light, and Brenda Light Bredemeier. 2009. *True Competition: A Guide to Pursuing Excellence in Sport and Society.* Champaign, IL: Human Kinetics.

Wankel, Leonard M., and Bonnie G. Berger. 1990. "The Psychological and Social Benefits of Sport and Physical Activity." *Journal of Leisure Research, 22*(2): 167–182.

Low-Income Minority Youth

Despite a growing body of evidence that touts the role of physical activity and sports in helping youth lead healthy lifestyles, be successful in school, and stay away from violent delinquent behaviors and unsafe sexual activity, there are fewer and fewer opportunities for young people to play due to rising financial costs of participation. This is especially true for the youth who may need these opportunities the most: kids from low-income and minority communities and girls.

Trends in Youth Sports Participation

Over the last few years, there has been growing attention paid to the fact that fewer youth are playing sports. Thousands are dropping out when they reach middle school (True Sport, 2015). Considerably more are focusing only on one sport at a time. And the number of youth who don't play any sports at all is increasing rapidly (King, 2015). This precipitous decline can be attributed to a whole host of causes: burnout or injury from having to focus too seriously on one sport at an early age; the allure of other activities, like video games that keep kids in front of their screens; and concerns that youth sports have become too many parts business and not enough parts fun. Although all of these factors certainly contribute to the decline, there is one factor that is disproportionately affecting kids from low-income households: the rising cost of opportunities to play, particularly in school-based sports.

Of greatest concern among the decreasing participation trends in sports is the fact that because of budget cuts, school sports are no longer available to all. A core aspiration of public education in this country is that it can serve as a vehicle for equity. We have, as a society, long believed that by making access to public education a right, not a privilege, we have created a pathway to success for any citizen. Until recently, the expectation of access to school sports has been part of that promise. But over the last 10 years, opportunities for youth to play sports are disappearing from schools (Up2Us Sports, 2012). And they are disappearing more quickly for populations that already had fewer chances to play.

Given what is known about the benefits of sports on health, education, and community cohesion, critics assert that marginalizing this vulnerable population from sports is counterintuitive. Instead, youth advocates and other reformers contend that the United States should be expanding sports opportunities for kids in low-income minority communities.

In the Aspen Institute's 2015 Project Play report, the Sports and Fitness Industry Association (SFIA) provided data that showed dramatic changes in youth sports participation in the five-year period between 2008 and 2013. They reported that only 40 percent of kids played sport on a regular basis in 2013, down from 44.5 percent in 2008. The percentage of youth who participated in sports even once during the year was also down, from 58.6 percent to 52.2 percent. In the five sports that can easily be considered the "big five" of American youth sports—basketball, soccer, track and field, football, and softball—there were 2.6 million fewer kids playing in 2013 than in 2008. Finally, in 2008, there had been approximately 9 million kids, between the ages from 6 to 12 that regularly engaged in high-calorie-burning or fitness activities. That number dropped almost 9 percent to 8.2 million in 2013.

The percentage of children who are not playing sports or engaging in physical activity at all is also growing. According to PHIT America's 2015 *Inactivity Pandemic* report, inactivity among children ages 6 to 17 is approaching 20 percent, which means that approximately 10 million children are totally inactive. Even among those youth who are active, two-thirds of them don't get the recommended amount of physical activity (PHIT America, 2015c).

The picture in school sports is also bleak. In the 2012 report *The Decade of Decline,* researchers Don Sabo and Philip Veliz report that in the decade between school years 1999–2000 and 2009–2010, the number of U.S. schools that offered no sports almost doubled, from 8.2 percent to 15.1 percent. During the same period, 9.6 percent of urban high schools, 5.8 percent of suburban schools, 6.6 percent of town schools, and 7.7 percent of rural schools dropped interscholastic sports.

During this time, participation in school sports, which had been growing rapidly in the preceding decades, slowed. Data from the National Federation of State High School Associations show that while interscholastic high school sports participation grew in the decade between school years 1999–2000 and 2009–2010, it increased at a slower rate than it had in the previous decade. Whereas participation grew by close to 1.3 million students between 1989–1990 and 1999–2000, it slowed to just more than 1 million students between 1999–2000 and 2009–2010. In the five years since 2009–2010, the rate has slowed even more, with participation numbers increasing by less than 200,000 during that period. That includes the first drop in participation by boys in almost 15 years: approximately 10,000 fewer boys in 2011–2012 (NFHS, 2015).

Opportunities to participate in intramural activities are also shrinking. In a 2011 report from the American Alliance for Health, Physical Education, Recreation and Dance (AAHPERD), now the Society of Health and Physical Educators (SHAPE America), researchers found that only about 50 percent of high schools have more than one-quarter of their student population participating in at least one physical activity club or intramural sports. That number drops to 40 percent of schools where at least one-quarter of the girls in the school are playing (NASPE, 2013). A national study of middle school sports programs revealed that only 58 percent of schools had intramural sports programs (McEwin and Swaim, 2009).

When considering the landscape of school sports opportunities, the rise of the charter school movement also has been cited as a significant factor. According to the National Alliance for Public Charter Schools, as of 2015, 25 states have no laws that govern charter school student eligibility or access to extracurricular or inter-scholastic activities, including sports. The impact of charter schools on participation rates is still unknown, but given a common ethos of achievement against standardized metrics, it is easy to imagine that extracurricular activities like sports are considered low priorities.

If the trends of the past decade continue, Sabo and Veliz predict that by 2020, 27 percent of U.S. public high schools—a total of 4,398 schools—will not offer school-based sports. This means that close to 3.5 million young Americans will be going to schools that don't provide them with opportunities to play (Sabo and Veliz, 2012).

The Impact on Marginalized Groups

Within the larger trends, there are certain populations who are disproportionately affected by the decline in opportunity to participate in sports. On the whole, when it comes to opportunities to participate, boys fare better than girls; white students have more chances to play than their minority counterparts; and kids who live in higher income communities are less likely to be left out than those in lower income communities.

A 2015 study by the National Women's Law Center (NWLC) found that heavily minority schools, defined as those where at least 90 percent of the student body is minority, offer far fewer opportunities to play sports than schools where at least 90 percent of the student body is white. On average, the NWLC found only 25 spots on sports teams for every 100 students at heavily minority schools. At heavily white schools, by contrast, the NLWC found 58 opportunities per 100 students. Heavily minority schools also have fewer opportunities for girls. Participation rates among youth from wealthier homes, where the income is $100,000 or more, are almost twice as high as that of youth living in households with the lowest incomes, $25,000 or less (Aspen Institute, 2015). According to the Robert Wood Johnson Foundation, only a quarter of the 8th to 12th graders enrolled in the poorest schools played school sports (Kelley and Carchia, 2013).

Given such research findings, it is not surprising that low-income minority girls have the fewest opportunities to play and are, as the NWLC puts it, "finishing last." In 2010, boys in higher income schools had the most chances to play: 65 for every 100 students. Girls who attended lower income schools had the fewest: 34 for every 100 students (Sabo and Veliz, 2012).

Budget Cuts and "Pay to Play"

Budget cuts are crippling schools. Since the depths of the recession in 2009, states have made steep cuts to education funding, and in many states those cuts continue. In 2013–2014, per-student funding was lower in 15 states than it had been in 2012–2013. In 35 states the 2013–2014 school year funding was below the 2007–2008 school year. Fourteen of these states cut per-student funding by more than 10 percent during that time period (Leachman and Mai, 2014). Urban districts, where the percentage of low-income and minority students is high, have been particularly hard hit by the cuts in federal education spending. Nearly 90 percent of big-city school districts spent less per student in 2012 than when the recession ended in 2009 (Casselman, 2014).

As school systems scramble to make do with less, sports and other extracurricular activities are often first on the chopping block. Up2Us Sports estimated that more than $2 billion was cut from school sports budgets during the 2009–2010 school year and an additional $1.5 billion in the 2010–2011 school year (Up2Us Sports, 2012).

In some schools, budget cuts have not necessarily meant the end to school sports. Booster clubs and local businesses have stepped up and brought new resources to the schools in some communities to keep sports opportunities from disappearing. In communities where there are lots of other opportunities to play sports, the blow of losing school sports opportunities has been minimized by community-based sports organizations picking up the slack and offering expanded opportunities for kids to play. But these solutions happen most often in communities with an abundance of financial and human resources.

In communities where resources are scarce, budget cuts have meant something far different. In many places, it's meant that the opportunities just disappear. In others, fees have been implemented in order to offset the cost of teams. And while this "pay to play" strategy was born out of a well-meaning desire not to eliminate school sports opportunities entirely, it has only served to widen the opportunity gap between kids who have resources and those who do not (Rowe, 2012).

According to Up2Us Sports, as of 2012, the practice of "pay to play" had been instituted in approximately 40 percent of school districts nationwide (Up2Us Sports, 2012). Fee amounts vary greatly, ranging anywhere from $50 to more than $1,000 and averaging around $126 per child. On top of the participation fee, researchers conducting a national poll on children's health found that parents reported an average of $275 in other sports-related costs like equipment, raising the total average out-of-pocket cost for a student to join a school team to more than $400 (C. S. Mott Children's Hospital, 2015). It's not hard to see that for many families, especially those in low-income communities, the cost of participating is prohibitive.

Some propose that the answer to this challenge is to offer fee waivers. But when virtually all members of the study body of a low-income school would need a waiver to overcome a $400 barrier to participation, it is not viable for these communities to rely on waivers. Further, as many coaches and athletic directors have noted, it can be very difficult for a student who wants to play to navigate the waiver process—either because the process is not clear or because the student or family is embarrassed to have to ask for help. As one high school coach said, "Most students will not ask for help, they just won't show up" (Cunningham, 2012).

Impact of the Decline in Youth Sports Participation

Whether they are eliminated completely or simply placed out of reach because of the cost of participation, the decline of school-based sports impacts communities differently. For kids who live in communities with an abundance of resources, the impact of the school cuts is not as severe. Such communities have the youth sports and physical activity infrastructure to pick up the slack. This "sports safety net" is comprised of a variety of community-based or privately run sports teams and leagues, family financial resources to travel outside of their community to find other sports teams or leagues, and parents and other adults who can either commit to running a sports team or league or advocate for the creation of one. Kids in resourced communities are also more likely to be able to take advantage of informal opportunities to participate in sports: access to safe facilities, parks, bike paths, playgrounds, etc., that encourage kids to be active and play even in the absence of structured sports opportunities.

In underserved urban communities, the impact of school sports cuts is felt more deeply. Most times, there are not community-sponsored teams or leagues for kids to join. When there are, they are usually nonprofit community-based organizations whose mission is to provide opportunities to kids who do not otherwise have them. And while these programs often serve as lifelines for the kids they reach, their reach is often small and almost always limited to one sport. Kids in communities without a lot of resources are subsequently forced to join the one program that is offered and do not have the opportunity to explore other sports that better fit their interests or aptitude.

The informal opportunities to play are also limited in such communities. According to Active Living Research, communities of color and/or lower income communities have significantly less access to safe places to play. Approximately 70 percent of African American communities and 81 percent of Hispanic communities lack recreational facilities. Although racial and ethnic minorities tend to live in more densely populated urban environments with walkable neighborhoods, the actual walkability quotient is lowered by a lack of clean and well-maintained sidewalks, lack of natural scenery or trees providing shade, and a feeling of safety (Taylor and Lou, 2011). Girls who live in low-income urban communities have less access to parks and facilities than those living in more affluent communities (Babey et al., 2013). Finally, low-income and minority populations are more likely to live in violent neighborhoods. Children whose parents considered their neighborhoods to be unsafe were less active than those living in safer neighborhoods (Datar et al., 2013).

When school sports disappear from low-income minority communities, kids who live there do not have access to the same kind of sports safety net that kids in higher income communities do. The sports safety net in underserved communities is small, full of holes, and only catches a small percentage of kids. Therefore, the impact of school sports cuts is, yet again, disproportionately felt by already marginalized populations.

Implications for Health

Childhood inactivity has been noted as one of the top concerns of parents, and obesity has become the United States' number one public health concern (Berggoetz, 2012). Minority and low-income youth disproportionately suffer from both. They are more likely to be inactive, and the percentage of minority and low-income youth who are classified as overweight or obese is higher than their higher income white counterparts (RWJF, 2015). If opportunities to be active and participate in sports continue to shrink, low-income minority populations who already have the least access to these opportunities will have even fewer. The impact on the health of already vulnerable populations stands to be severe. Youth who are overweight or obese are more likely to suffer from long-term health problems like type 2 diabetes, heart disease, hypertension, stroke, and cancer.

Once a child is overweight or obese, poor physical health makes him or her more vulnerable to other problems as well. Youth who are overweight or obese are less likely to attend school, more likely to perform poorly in school, and less likely to continue their education after high school. They are more likely to suffer from depression and anxiety, to have low self-esteem, and to be bullied or victimized by peers. Conversely, there is a growing body of evidence that supports the idea that physical activity can protect the brain from anxiety, toxic stress, and depression.

Implications for Education

Given that a significant number of schools do not provide opportunities for youth to be active through physical education and recess, school sports are one of the last places where students can be active. And that activity has an important effect on their performance in school. Harvard neuroscientist John Ratey found that physical activity impacts chemicals in the brain that improve thinking, memory, focus, concentration, and impulsivity (Ratey and Hagerman, 2008). Studies in multiple states have shown that compared to their inactive counterparts, active students (defined as those who exercised regularly) significantly improved their scores on intelligence tests and performed better in core school subjects (Tomporowski et al., 2008). A study of more than 3 million students in California and Texas found that higher test scores were strongly correlated with higher fitness levels (PHIT America, 2015c).

The physical activity that students get from sports is not the only factor contributing to school success. Athletes are more likely to report liking school and are more likely to believe that teachers and other adults care about them. When children enjoy school and believe that the people in charge care about them, they are more likely to show up. A study of students in Kansas in 2008–2009 found significant differences between athletes and nonathletes when it came to school attendance and graduation. They found that nonathletes were 15 times more likely to drop out of school than athletes; male nonathletes were 12 times more likely, and female nonathletes were 24 times more likely to drop out than athletes (Lumpkin and Favor, 2012).

Violence Prevention

Studies indicate that the hours of 3:00 p.m. to 7:00 p.m. are the hours in which youth are most vulnerable to participate in or be victims of crime (OJJDP, 2014). Out of school time activities like sports are, if nothing else, ways of protecting kids from these risks. In addition, sports can offer kids the opportunity to learn how to work with their peers and become a vehicle through which kids learn to make good decisions. Sports also can help kids form meaningful adult and peer relationships that help them to be resilient in the face of challenges.

When armed with these skills, negative behaviors in youth can actually change for the better. For example, one study of a sports-based mentoring program in Chicago showed that program participants—youth who had previously been or were at high risk to be involved in violence or other crime—showed a 44 percent decrease in violent crime arrests during the intervention (Crime Lab, 2012).

Economic Costs

Obesity, incarceration, and disengagement from the education system are social issues that have a big cost to society. As vehicles for positive outcomes in these areas, sport programs have the potential to save the country hundreds of millions of dollars every year. The World Health Organization estimates that every $1 invested in physical activity returns a $3.20 savings in medical costs (PHIT America, 2015a). Add the costs of dropout prevention and crime reduction and the savings per dollar spent on sports programs becomes substantial. In fact, a United Kingdom study found that society saved more than 4,000 pounds (equivalent of $6,000 at time of the study) for each disadvantaged youth that participated in a sport for development program (Sported, 2015). Up2Us Sports has made a preliminary estimate that through their Coach Across America program, they can yield up to a $29 return on investment for every dollar spent putting trained coaches into the lives of youth who do not otherwise have the opportunity to play sports.

Conclusion

Knowing the significant benefits of physical activity and participating in sports on health, education, and social outcomes, it is easy to argue that there should be more, not fewer, opportunities for youth to participate. Obesity rates are highest among youth who also tend to have the hardest time accessing sports opportunities. If the United States wants to overcome the dual threats of inactivity and obesity among those who are most afflicted, the tables need to be turned. Instead of the least amount of sports opportunities, communities should be providing low-income and minority boys and girls with the most opportunities to play.

Advocates of such campaigns assert that keeping kids in low-income minority communities safe and engaged in something that will give them tools to navigate the world is a no-brainer. But time and time again, lawmakers and officials fail to invest in these communities in a meaningful way. Sports are a cost-effective investment that are uniquely suited to engage youth from these communities. Kids want to play. Sports teams could be one of the only things appealing enough to motivate kids to show up. And once they show up, a coach who makes the activity fun, helps kids see their own successes, and uses sport as an opportunity to teach broader lessons about succeeding in life can help keep them from engaging in risky behaviors that threaten their futures.

Finally, youth sports advocates claim that it is paradoxical to eliminate sports opportunities in the name of improving student performance. In fact, quite the opposite seems to be true; schools need to be increasing opportunities for youth to be active. Further, if educators are truly interested in closing the achievement gap between low-income minority youth and white youth with more resources, they should examine the opportunity gap in opportunities for kids to play sports. Narrow that gap, say supporters of increased funding for youth sports, and schools and communities will see better attendance, better performance, and higher achievement among these marginalized populations.

Megan Bartlett

Further Reading

Aspen Institute's Project Play. 2015, January 26. *Sport for All Play for Life: A Playbook to Get Every Kid in the Game.* Accessed August 14, 2015, at http://youthreport.projectplay.us.

Babey, Susan H., Joelle Wolstein, Samuel Krumholz, Breece Robertson, and Allison L. Diamant. 2013. *Physical Activity, Park Access and Park Use among California Adolescents.* Accessed August 14, 2015, at http://healthpolicy.ucla.edu/publications/Documents /PDF/parkaccesspb-mar2013.pdf.

Berggoetz, Barb. 2012, August 22. "Poll: Kids' Lack of Activity Is Top Health Concern." *USA Today.* Accessed August 14, 2015, at http://usatoday30.usatoday.com/news/health /story/2012-08-22/child-health/57219420/1.

CDC. 2015. *Childhood Obesity Facts.* Accessed August 14, 2015, at http://www.cdc.gov /healthyyouth/obesity/facts.htm.

Casselman, Ben. 2014, June 10. "Public Schools Are Hurting More in the Recovery Than in the Recession." *FiveThirtyEight.* Accessed August 14, 2015, at http://fivethirtyeight .com/features/public-schools-are-hurting-more-in-the-recovery-than-in-the-recession.

Crime Lab. 2012. *BAM-Sports Edition.* Accessed https://crimelab.uchicago.edu/sites /crimelab.uchicago.edu/files/uploads/BAM_FINAL%20Research%20and%20 Policy%20Brief_20120711.pdf.

C. S. Mott Children's Hospital. 2015. *Pay-to-Play Sports Keeping Some Kids on the Sidelines.* Accessed August 14, 2015, at http://mottnpch.org/sites/default/files/documents /012014_paytoplay.pdf.

Cunningham, Pete. 2012, August 28. "Pay-to-Participate Fees for Athletes Eliminated at Chelsea Community Schools." *The Ann Arbor News.* Accessed August 14, 2015, at http://www.annarbor.com/sports/high-school/chelsea-high-school-pay-to-play-school-board-meeting.

Datalys Center. 2015. *Sports Promote Youth Academic Achievement.* Accessed August 14, 2015, at http://www.stopsportsinjuries.org/LinkClick.aspx?fileticket=tJJcjjGbsKM%3D&tabid=296.

Datar, Ashlesha, Nancy Nicosia, and Victoria Shier. 2013. "Parent Perceptions of Neighborhood Safety and Children's Physical Activity, Sedentary Behavior, and Obesity: Evidence from a National Longitudinal Study." *American Journal of Epidemiology, 177*(10): 1065–1073.

Gardner, Amanda. 2012, June 14. "Does Obesity Affect School Performance?" *CNN.* Accessed August 17, 2015, at http://www.cnn.com/2012/06/14/health/obesity-affect-school-performance.

Kelley, Bruce, and Carl Carchia. 2013, July 16. "Hey, Data Data—Swing!" *ESPN.* Accessed August 14, 2015, at http://espn.go.com/espn/story/_/id/9469252/hidden-demographics-youth-sports-espn-magazine.

King, Bill. 2015, August 10. "Are the Kids Alright?" *Sports Business Daily.* Accessed August 14, 2015, at http://www.sportsbusinessdaily.com/Journal/Issues/2015/08/10/In-Depth/Lead.aspx.

Leachman, Michael, and Chris Mai. 2014. *Most States Funding Schools Less Than before the Recession.* Accessed August 14, 2015, at http://www.cbpp.org/research/most-states-funding-schools-less-than-before-the-recession.

Lumpkin, Angela, and Judy Favor. 2012. "Comparing the Academic Performance of High School Athletes and Non-Athletes in Kansas in 2008–2009." *Journal of Sport Administration & Supervision, 4*(1): 41–62.

McEwin, C. Kenneth, and John Swaim. 2009. *Middle Level Interscholastic Sports Programs.* Accessed August 14, 2015, at http://www.amle.org/BrowsebyTopic/WhatsNew/WNDet/TabId/270/ArtMID/888/ArticleID/324/Research-Summary-Middle-Level-Interscholastic-Sports-Programs-.aspx.

National Alliance for Public Charter Schools. 2015. *Extracurricular and Interscholastic Activities Eligibility and Access.* Accessed August 14, 2015, at http://www.publiccharters.org/law-database/extra-curricular-interscholastic-activities-eligibility-access.

National Association for Sport and Physical Education. 2013. *Before- and After-School Physical Activity and Intramural Sport Programs [Position statement].* Reston, VA: Author.

National Federation of State High School Associations. 2015. *Participation Statistics.* Accessed August 14, 2015, at http://www.nfhs.org/ParticipationStatics/ParticipationStatics.aspx.

National Women's Law Center. 2015. *Finishing Last: Girls of Color and School Sports Opportunities.* Accessed August 14, 2015, at http://www.nwlc.org/sites/default/files/pdfs/final_nwlc_girlsfinishinglast_report.pdf.

OJJDP. 2014. *Juveniles as Offenders.* Accessed August 17, 2015, at http://www.ojjdp.gov /ojstatbb/offenders/qa03301.asp.

PHIT America. 2015a. *Inactivity Kills More Than Obesity.* Accessed August 14, 2015, at http://www.phitamerica.org/News_Archive/Lack_of_Exercise.htm.

PHIT America. 2015b. *Physical Education for Stronger Bodies & Minds.* Accessed August 14, 2015, at http://www.phitamerica.org/Benefits_of_P_E__in_School.htm.

PHIT America. 2015c. *The Inactivity Pandemic.* Accessed August 14, 2015, at http://www .phitamerica.org/Assets/PHIT+America+Digital+Assets/Obesity+Sedentary+Crisis/In activity+Pandemic+2015+Edition+Consumer.pdf.

PHIT America. 2015d. *The PHIT Act.* Accessed August 14, 2015, at http://www.phitamerica .org/PHIT_Act.htm.

Ratey, John J., and Eric Hagerman. 2008. *Spark: The Revolutionary New Science of Exercise and the Brain.* New York: Little, Brown.

Rowe, Claudia. 2012, January 7. "Higher Fees to Play Sports Leaves Kids on Sidelines." *The Seattle Times.* Accessed at http://www.seattletimes.com/seattle-news/higher-fees-to -play-sports-leaves-kids-on-sidelines.

RWJF. 2015. *Income Disparities in Obesity Trends among California Adolescents.* Accessed August 14, 2015, at http://www.rwjf.org/en/library/research/2010/11/income-disparities -in-obesity-trends-among-california-adolescent.html.

Sabo, Don, and Philip Veliz. 2012. *The Decade of Decline: Gender Equity in High School Sports.* Accessed August 14, 2015, at http://irwg.research.umich.edu/pdf/OCR.pdf.

Shore, Stuart, Michael Sachs, Jeffrey Lidicker, Stephanie Brett, Adam Wright, and Joseph Libonati. 2008. "Decreased Scholastic Achievement in Overweight Middle School Students." *Obesity, 16*(7): 1535–1538. doi:10.1038/oby.2008.254

Sported. 2015. *Sport Works Summary Report.* Accessed August 14, 2015, at http://134.0.17 .66/~sportedorg/wp-content/uploads/2014/12/Sportworks-Summary-low-res.pdf.

Storch, Eric, Vanessa Milsom, Ninoska DeBraganza, Adam Lewin, Gary Geffken, and Janet Silverstein. 2007. "Peer Victimization, Psychosocial Adjustment, and Physical Activity in Overweight and At-Risk-for-Overweight Youth." *Journal of Pediatric Psychology, 32*(1): 80–89. doi:10.1093/jpepsy/jsj113

Taylor, Wendell C., and Deborah Lou. 2011. *Do All Children Have Places to be Active?* Accessed August 14, 2015, at http://activelivingresearch.org/sites/default/files/Synthesis _Taylor-Lou_Disparities_Nov2011_0.pdf.

Tomporowski, Phillip D., Catherine L. Davis, Patricia H. Miller, and Jack A. Naglieri. 2008. "Exercise and Children's Intelligence, Cognition, and Academic Achievement." *Educational Psychology Review, 20*: 111–131. doi:10.1007/s10648-007-9057-0

True Sport. 2015. *Why We Play Sport and Why We Stop.* Accessed August 14, 2015, at http:// truesport.org/resources/publications/reports/why-we-play-sport-and-why-we-stop.

Up2Us Sports. 2012 *Going Going Gone: The Decline of Youth Sports.* Accessed August 14, 2015, at https://0ea29dd9a16d63dcc571-314f1dcf5bee97a05ffca38f060fb9e3.ssl.cf1 .rackcdn.com/uploads/center_resource/document/561/Decline_of_Youth_Sports.pdf.

Media Coverage and Representation

Sport and media have become increasingly intertwined in American culture over the last several decades. Traditionally, most media attention remained squarely focused on college and professional competition. With the growing presence of multiple sport media outlets requiring 24/7 programming, however—and growing interest in recruiting of high school athletes for Division I athletic programs—there has been a surge in the media coverage of youth sports. Coverage of youth sports has thus expanded beyond the Little League World Series (LLWS) to include high school football and basketball games. Moreover, the advent of social media, coupled with the growing appetite for recruiting coverage, has led to young athletes possessing sizable social media audiences. These trends have created a visible platform for youth sports, but this attention also brings with it questions and concerns. The simultaneous effects of exposure and pressure are an important area in need of attention for youth sports.

Youth Sport and Media

The LLWS is one of the preeminent national broadcasts of youth sport. Whereas the Little League Softball World Series (LLSWS) has traditionally been well received by audiences, 2014 saw remarkable results. ESPN, which holds the media rights to the LLWS, drew 5 million viewers for a contest between the Las Vegas and Philadelphia teams, broadcast on August 20. The following day, August 21, the game between the Chicago and Philadelphia teams garnered 3.8 million viewers (Paulsen Sports Media Watch, 2014). The 5 million viewers who tuned in for the Chicago-Philadelphia contest represented up until that time, the largest audience for *any* baseball game shown on ESPN since a 2007 Yankees–Red Sox matchup. Certainly, some of the viewers were tuning in to follow the saga of Philadelphia pitcher Mo'ne Davis, who garnered national media attention for both her pitching and hitting performances, leading the Philadelphia team to the semifinals of the U.S.

Championship (Schwartz, 2014). Even taking into account the general public's fascination with Davis, however, these impressive viewing numbers reflect how significantly the LLWS has evolved since its inception. Indeed, when perusing the Little League World Series website (llwbs.org), there is an entire section devoted to media resources, including the Little League organization's press guide requirements (at the time of this writing, this section also contains a picture of three Little League players and two coaches sitting at a table being interviewed, a similar format to what one might see in Major League Baseball).

The growing media attention and commodification of the LLWS has been critiqued for placing kids under unnecessary pressure, all for the sake of ratings, which can then be used to generate more lucrative sponsorship deals (which notably is another prominent section of the LLWS website) (Hyman, 2009). Indeed, journalist Mark Hyman has noted the resistance that occurred in the 1950s to problematic commercialization of the LLWS. Yet, since that time, the LLWS has become a 10-day media megaevent that brings teams from across the globe to Williamsport, Pennsylvania. For example, television coverage of the Little League World Series has expanded from the championship game alone to include regional playoffs, wherein teams battle to get to the Little League World Series. Additionally, Little League Baseball provides a hefty, professionally designed media guide, and each of the players on the competing teams is individually featured on the Little League website with profiles that provide their statistics, player evaluation competencies, and videos.

The LLWS arguably can claim the title of the "pinnacle" of youth sport broadcasts. However, much like the Olympics, the Super Bowl, and other sport "megaevents," the attention soon fades once the LLWS is completed and audiences move on to other sporting events.

In the past, audiences generally had a respite from youth sport media events until the next year's LLWS. However, there has been a steady rise in media coverage, most notably by ESPN, of high school football and basketball contests, a previously untapped market for ESPN programming. These contests typically involve highly ranked programs competing in interstate competition. For example, for the opening of the 2015 football season, top-ranked De La Salle High School from California traveled to Texas to play Euless Trinity High School. This game was part of ESPN's high school kickoff, sponsored by GEICO, which included 10 games between teams from 10 states. The impetus to broadcast high school sports dates as far back as 2002, when ESPN broadcast the high school basketball games of LeBron James. Since that time, programming has steadily increased, and in the summer of 2014, ESPNU broadcast 60 hours of high school summer sport showcase events (Halley, 2014). Branded as "The Summer of Next," this programming appears to be designed to target viewers interested in future college football and basketball programs. As Dan Margulis, senior director of programming and acquisitions at ESPN, stated, "There's a coherent logic to having it on ESPNU because these are the kids you might see as college players in the future" (Halley, 2014).

This branding of youth sports media coverage not only illustrates the commodification of youth sports, but also brings with it questions regarding exploitation and ethics. Should high school athletic events be nationally broadcast? What about the effects the broadcast schedule has on athletes in terms of their academic performance? After ESPN elected to show LeBron James's high school contest, ESPN college basketball analyst Jay Bilas suggested that the answer to the question of whether it was appropriate to televise high school basketball games depended on the circumstances. Bilas further opined that determining the circumstances was a decision to be made collaboratively by school administrators, teachers, and coaches (Bilas, 2002). Whereas Bilas suggested that exploitation depended on the circumstances, there is little question that youth sporting events have surged in broadcast appeal, and it seems likely we have reached a "point of no return." That is, barring an unexpected decline in ratings, it is unlikely that viewers will be given less coverage of high school sports, or that coverage of events such as the LLWS will diminish. Indeed, many youth sports and sports media experts anticipate that athletes at ever younger ages will receive increasing media exposure. This outcome is influenced by the cycle of media coverage of youth sport and viewer demand. One particular domain where this relationship is vividly illustrated is college football and basketball recruiting.

College Recruiting and Media Coverage

With the growth of the Internet, sport coverage has expanded significantly, and perhaps in no area is that more evident than in college football and basketball recruiting. Historically, the recruiting of football and basketball players was largely an internal process about which fans knew little. Today, however, an entire industry has been built around recruiting high school football and basketball players. For example, Rivals, arguably the leading scouting service focused on high school football and basketball recruiting, claimed to employ more than 300 writers, reporters, and scouts in early 2017. For Rivals and its competitors, National Signing Day (the first Wednesday in February, when high school seniors can sign letters of intent), has become a major event that is treated as a virtual holiday by die-hard college sport fans. Indeed, many media outlets will report when these letters are faxed in, so fans can be certain that an athlete is indeed coming to their school. One aspect of National Signing Day that has become commonplace is for ESPN to live broadcast the college decisions of some of the top-ranked football players. These events are often shrouded in dramatic theater, with the athletes generally having three or four hats on a table in front of them representing the final list of suitors. The athlete will then don the hat of the school he is going to sign with to signify his choice.

As coverage of college football and basketball signings have increased, so has the drama surrounding them. For example, on National Signing Day 2013, Florida football player Alex Collins was prepared to sign with the University of Arkansas. However, Collins's mother did not want him to play for Arkansas and instead preferred him to play for the University of Miami. In an effort to thwart Collins playing for Arkansas, she took his letter of intent (which has to be signed by a parent/guardian) and refused to give it back to him. Eventually Collins's father was able to sign his letter of intent, but this turn of events illustrates the dramatic turns that can sometimes play out with college recruiting (Elliott, 2013). In another case, in January 2012, during the Under Armour All-American Game, a showcase event for top-ranked football players across the country in which many players announce their college choice, safety Landon Collins announced that he was going to play for the University of Alabama. This announcement noticeably aggravated his mother, who wanted him to play for Louisiana State University, which made the announcement rather uncomfortable. Collins was drafted into the NFL in 2015 after three years with the Alabama program (Spain, 2015). Although these two cases are not representative, they do illustrate how family relationships can be negatively impacted by the growing media coverage of recruiting. One of the challenges with youth sport is that parents sometimes exhibit negative behaviors toward their children when they cannot harness their desire for their children to earn college scholarships and/or play professionally. It is likely that parents are captivated by the allure of the recruiting process and the "celebrity" that it creates for their child. Whereas parent and child may be in agreement about the college destination, this decision may be a source of conflict, which can deteriorate family relationships, which introduces the question of whether the recruiting process is worth the consequences it can bring? Certainly, many people will seek the acclaim and notoriety that it provides, yet this process is also fraught with intense media coverage and contact from writers seeking to be the first to uncover the latest indication of a recruit's college choice. This process can become quite intrusive (Yanity and Edmondson, 2011), and many coaches and parents, as well as student athletes, opine that the issue warrants more investigation and intervention than currently seems to be occurring.

As fans consume information about recruiting from websites such as Rivals, 247 Sports, and ESPN.com, they become more identified and attached to these players. Indeed, many fans come to expect that a certain recruit will attend a particular school and start to feel as though they know the recruit. Indeed, this seemingly insatiable appetite for recruiting information has taken what many observers consider to be a problematic turn. In 2015, Rivals announced that it was ranking two sixth-grade football players after their performance at an elite camp (Smith, 2015). Thus, in these two cases, fans can now follow a player for *six years* before he is even eligible to attend college. One of the players, Daron Bryden, immediately went to his Twitter account to announce that Rivals had made a recruiting profile for him (Smith, 2015). This example illustrates another growing media outlet for youth sport—social media.

Youth Sport and Social Media

Social media technologies have significantly influenced sport. One of the more profound ways in which they have done so is by giving athletes the ability to become active media producers who generate content and interact with fans. As these capabilities can be conducted through a mobile phone, it is very difficult for teams to control the messaging that athletes disseminate via social media. Thus, some athletes have created public relations problems for themselves and their school programs by posting controversial or even illegal content for the world to see. However, whereas professional athletes often have the resources to withstand the consequences of these missteps (e.g., paying fines), social media missteps can result in significant harm for young athletes. In another case from 2012, Yuri Wright, a highly recruited football player from Don Bosco Prep in New Jersey was expelled after sexually explicit tweets he sent became public. Interestingly, Wright was tweeting from a private account, yet there is no way to control what those who are given access to the tweets can do with the content, making it not altogether surprising that Wright's tweets became public (Hinton, 2012).

At the time, Wright was being recruited by the University of Michigan, which stopped recruiting him after the tweets were made public. Wright eventually landed at the University of Colorado, but even three years after this event, when searching for his name on Google, these tweets still dominate the first page of results. In addition to incurring legal issues, young athletes, especially those who are being recruited, often are subjected to unceasing messages from fans via platforms such as Twitter, encouraging the athlete to attend the fan's favorite school. Although very difficult to enforce, this behavior is actually a violation of National Collegiate Athletic Association (NCAA) rules and has been labeled as reflecting stalking (DeShazo, 2015). Nevertheless, it has become so intense that many athletic departments take to social media to remind fans that they are not recruiters, and to request that the recruiting be left to the coaches. Although fans' behavior during the recruiting process is often encouraging, when a player elects to attend another school, these same fans will then bombard the recruit's social media accounts with hostile and inflammatory comments.

The Future of Youth Sports and Media Coverage

The increasing coverage of youth sports offers a number of compelling questions for parents, coaches, practitioners, and researchers alike. For youth sport megaevents like the LLWS, it seems important to ask about the effects of this media spectacle. For example, are 12- and 13-year-old children equipped to handle the pressure of having their performance shown to a national or even global audience? Although it is certainly easy to see the prestige that comes with playing in the LLWS, what happens after? What are the effects? One might look at Mo'ne Davis, who during the 2014 LLWS received misogynistic messages on her Twitter account from people—mostly men—who were upset that she was succeeding in a "male" sport. ESPN broadcast Davis's and other players Twitter handles during the broadcast, which raises questions about the appropriateness of exposing these young athletes to what can be a hostile audience.

Although these are more individual effects, what about collective outcomes? For example, concerns exist about the growing professionalization of youth sports, and the time and financial demands expected of players and parents (Peters, 2015). How does the broadcasting of events like the LLWS influence the behavior of those who run elite youth sport organizations, coaches, and parents? Might the allure of playing on national television and the prestige that accompanies it prompt coaches to push players in unhealthy ways? Might parents be more supportive of problematic coaching practices in an effort to see their child on national television? Some of the examples provided in this entry illustrate how family relationships can be compromised through the media coverage of youth sports, and it seems that the desire to receive media coverage, may strain family relationships.

Although there are "dead" periods where coaches cannot officially contact recruits, this does not stop fans from doing so, as well as more "unofficial" contacts being directed at recruits. How do athletes and their families manage their privacy amid an insatiable audience waiting to consume any morsel about the recruit's college plans? The fan side of this issue is equally compelling. What makes a fan contact a recruit via social media? Does a fan really believe that the recruit will make a decision based on the fan's messaging? Finally, given Rival's profiling of sixth-grade prospects, it seems that there is a need to critically think about the ethics of this practice. Clearly this process is driven by commodification—as more sites like Rivals provide information, the more the demand grows, and thus the more Rivals can charge for its services and its sponsors.

James Sanderson

Further Reading

Bilas, Jay. 2002, December 17. "Did 'Lebron Mania' Go Too Far?" *ESPN.com*. Accessed at http://espn.go.com/columns/bilas_jay/1477784.html.

Brady, Erik. 2014, November 30. "Why Are High School Football Players Dying?" *USA Today*. Accessed athttp://www.usatoday.com/story/sports/high school/2014/11/30/high-school-football-deaths-damon-janes/19712169.

DeShazo, Kevin. 2015, February 3. "Hey, Super Fans, Careful What You Tweet at Athletes, Coaches." *Sporting News*. Accessed at http://www.sportingnews.com/ncaa-football/story/2015-02-02/fans-tweeting-at-recruits-national-signing-day-athletes-coaches-creepy-rude-social-media.

Elliott, Bud. 2013, February 6. "Alex Collins' Mom Runs Off with Letter of Intent, Refuses to Let Running Back Recruit Sign with Arkansas." *SBNation.com*. Accessed at http://www.sbnation.com/college-football-recruiting/2013/2/6/3959996/alex-collins-mom-recruit-letter-national-signing-day.

Halley, Jim. 2013, August 22. "Should High School Sports Be Televised?" *USA Today* (McLean, VA). Accessed at http://www.usatoday.com/story/sports/highschool/2013/08/21/high-school-football-espn-fox-sports-1/2683177.

Halley, Jim. 2014, June 30. "ESPN Will Broadcast 60 Hours of Summer High School Sports." *USA Today*. Accessed at http://usatodayhss.com/2014/espn-will-broadcast-60-hours-of-summer-high-school-sports.

Hardin, Marie, Susan Lynn, Kristie Walsdorf, and Brent Hardin. 2002. "The Framing of Sexual Difference in SI for Kids Editorial Photos." *Mass Communication and Society, 5*: 341–359.

Hinton, Matt. 2012, January 20. "Recruits Say the Dumbest Things: Yuri Wright's Prospects Derailed by Vulgar Tweets." *Yahoo!Sports.com*. Accessed at http://sports.yahoo.com/blogs/ncaaf-dr-saturday/recruits-dumbest-things-blue-chip-cornerback-prospects-derailed-145734774.html.

Hyman, Mark. 2009. *Until It Hurts: America's Obsession with Youth Sports and How It Harms Our Kids*. Boston: Beacon Press.

Hyman, Mark. 2012. *The Most Expensive Game in Town: The Rising Cost of Youth Sports and the Toll on Today's Families*. Boston: Beacon Press.

Kassing, Jeffrey W, and Jimmy Sanderson. 2015. "Playing in the New Media Game or Riding the Virtual Bench: Confirming and Disconfirming Membership in the Community of Sport." *Journal of Sport & Social Issues, 39*: 3–18.

Kilgore, Adam. 2015, February 18. "Profiling 12-Year-Old Football Prospects: How Low Will It Go?" *Washington Post*. Accessed at http://www.washingtonpost.com/news/sports/wp/2015/02/18/profiling-12-year-old-football-prospects-how-low-will-it-go.

Messner, Michael A., and Michela Musto. 2014. "Where Are the Kids?" *Sociology of Sport, 31*: 102–122.

Paulsen Sports Media Watch. 2014, August 24. "Little League World Series Nets Record TV Audience, Blows Away MLB." *Sporting News.* Accessed at http://www. sporting-news.com/mlb/story/2014-08-24/little-league-world-series-2014-tv-ratings-llws -viewership-audience.

Peters, Justin. 2015, May 26. "Good Riddance to Little League." *Slate.com.* Accessed at http://www.slate.com/articles/life/family/2015/05/little_league_warning_it_s_time_for _organized_youth_sports_to_die.html.

Sanderson, Jimmy, and Blair Browning. 2013. "Training versus Monitoring: A Qualitative Examination of Athletic Department Practices Regarding Student-Athletes and Twit-ter." *Qualitative Research Reports in Communication, 14*: 105–111.

Schwartz, Nick. 2014, August 20. "Mo'ne Davis Strikes Out Six Batters in Little League World Series Loss." *USA Today.* Accessed at http://ftw.usatoday.com/2014/08/mone -davis-strikes-out-six-batters-in-latest-little-league-world-series-start.

Smith, Cam. 2015, February 18. "What Do Rivals.com 6th Grade Profiles Mean for the Recruiting Industry?" *USA Today.* Accessed at http://usatodayhss.com/2015/rivals-com -is-now-officially-tracking-6th-grade-football-prospects.

Spain, Sarah. 2015, May 1. "Three Years Later, Landon Collins and Mom Still Aren't Quite on the Same Page." *ESPNW.com.* Accessed at http://espn.go.com/news-commentary /article/12796424/three-years-later-landon-collins-mom-quite-same-page.

Wenner, Lawrence A. 2013. "The Media Sport Interpellation: Gender, Fanship, and Con-sumer Culture." *Sociology of Sport, 30*: 83–103.

Yanity, Molly, and Aimee C. Edmondson. 2011. "The Ethics of Online Coverage of Recruiting High School Athletes." *International Journal of Sport Communication, 4*: 403–421.

Officiating Youth Sports

As the game of youth sport continues to evolve and grow, one group of participants that are often neglected in the game are those that ultimately are in charge of it: the referees, umpires, or officials. Whether it is the volunteer referee mom at the soccer game or the highly trained umpire at a senior state championship, the official overseeing the match is vital to the overall success of the program. This entry will seek to outline the important role that officials can play in the youth sport environment, the ability of the official to ensure program success, and the pathway that officials may take in order to advance in their career. Officiating for most sports now has a very clear path that mirrors the athlete path to success and advancement and professionalism.

Even in leagues featuring participants as young as 4 and 5 years old, referees are still needed to enforce the rules, get players checked in, and organize the game for the duration of the schedule. Kids, often not much older than 12 or 13 years, are put in charge of refereeing the little 5- or 6-year-olds in the game. This potentially causes problems when parents try to intervene or influence the young referees into making decisions or complain about calls. In some instances, teen officials find themselves in situations where they either have to confront a grown adult about his or her behavior or ignore the behavior and continue to be yelled at. With more and more volunteers involved in youth sporting events and administrators that are challenged to be present at every sporting event their league puts on, there is an overall shortage of referees in sport across the country. In most sports, there are reports of upward of 40–50 percent of first-year referees not registering for their second year due to lack of proper training, lack of proper support, or being exposed to intimidation and other negative experiences while officiating. Simply put, no agency can provide a quality product when nearly half of its employees do not return year after year. Similarly, when so few referees return for a second season, the opportunity for referees to practice their craft and gain sufficient knowledge to provide support to younger, less experienced referees is diminished. A number of sport agencies state that if referees can make it past their second season in a league, they are more likely to remain for an extended period of time, often five years or more. Clearly a referee who has been in the same league for greater than five years has the experience, knowledge, and confidence needed to perform at a much higher level than a rookie referee new to officiating and unfamiliar with the nuances of the job. For this reason alone, it should be acknowledged that referee development in youth sport is equally as important as player development in order for the games to function smoothly and as expected.

For the purposes of the description of referee development, the process of a soccer referee entering the system will be used; however, the reader should know that virtually the same process can and does happen for most of the mainstream sports in the United States, such as baseball, basketball, volleyball, hockey, and in some respects football.

The New Teen Referee

Youth officiating often begins with a parent suggesting the youth soccer player get a part-time job to make some additional money as he or she is getting older. In many states, a referee can get an entry level certification as young as age 14 with a 6-hour course, a 50-question test, and a registration fee. In less than a day, training is complete, the young 14-year-old is certified with a badge and can potentially receive an assignment the very next day. It is widely known in the referee world that the real "training" is on the job, and one can hope that this new referee gets paired up with a more experienced referee to at least get started. Although a brand-new referee will often only be an assistant referee, meaning he or she will be providing support to a supposedly more experienced referee who is in control of the game, this is not always the case, particularly in certain areas where the number of referees are limited. The greatest challenge for inexperienced young referees is not usually the regular season games that might give them two or three games on a weekend, because assignors often utilize young referees heavily during tournaments out of sheer necessity. These young referees could make $300 or more in a tournament weekend. This means they need to officiate four or five games per day, often with little to no rest—and for outdoor sports, officiate in the sun, heat, or rain. Although the financial incentive for a young teen to consent to such an officiating workload is considerable, the physical and mental toll presents challenges. As a new referee who is still learning the rules of the game and the culture of a particular sport begins to fatigue as the day gets long, he or she tends to make more mistakes and lose focus on the job at hand. This increases the likelihood of conflict with players, coaches, or parents that can ultimately lead them to reduce future involvement in officiating. Assignors must be aware that while physically, the young teen might be capable of being involved with three, four, or five games in one day, mentally this level of work presents a challenge.

The New Adult Referee

The new adult referee often gets into officiating for different reasons than teens. Often the new adult referee is looking to either give back to the game they have been involved with for so many years as a player, or they have children playing in the game, and officiating allows them to continue to be involved or support their children in the game. Some parents have also pursued certification after attending athletic events in which the assigned referee or official failed to appear. They want to be available to help out if a similar situation arose in the future. Some adult parents even see certification as an opportunity to provide support to children getting involved with officiating. Unfortunately, statistics indicate that new adult referees do not end up staying in the game much longer than new teen referees do. Although they are less intimidated with irate parents or coaches, they still tend to have to negotiate the pressures of referee performance and expectations. In cases in which parent and child get involved in officiating together, if their child is not enjoying officiating and wants to stop, the parent often stops as well. In addition, because they are "older" they often get assigned to games at a higher level than their younger counterparts. For example, an assignor would likely not put a new teen referee who is 15 years old in a game with participants older than 13 or 14. It is generally understood that the stakes in games featuring elementary-age children are lower. Parents tend to be more forgiving in lower-aged leagues simply because it is understood that they are developmental. However, a new adult referee could be placed in games that involve 16- or 17-year-olds—athletes who are potentially playing for college scholarships and even (in rare cases) professional futures in the sport. This creates additional pressure on the new adult referee that may be well beyond what they anticipated when they signed up. Again, assignors need to be aware of the skill sets of new referees and recognize that an older referee does not always equate to a more experienced referee.

Post-Two-Year Rule It is widely accepted that if referees continue past their second season in a sport, they are much more likely (estimates of between 30 and 80 percent) to continue to officiate for five or more years. This is largely because the challenges the new official experiences like lack of training and integrating into a new social circle (of fellow officials) are overcome with experience and exposure. An experienced official begins to develop the tools to negotiate the challenges that are presented in games. If a parent gets upset, a more experienced official has a line or a response to calm the mood. A strange play occurs, and a more experienced official has seen this before and handles it much more smoothly than a new referee might. Perhaps even more importantly, a referee who has been in a particular league for a number of years begins to establish a rapport with coaches and players and thus their tools and tactics are more understood.

To retain a more experienced official, leagues need to understand that lack of referee administration and politics or sport administration policies, which fail to control overactive parents on the sidelines or in the stands, are the reasons that most experienced referees tend to stop officiating. In essence, the elements of the game are no longer the challenge to enjoyment of the referee, but rather the administrative elements of the job tend to be the roadblock that prevents the official with five or six years under his or her belt from becoming the ten-plus-year official who also moves into volunteer administration or mentorship of the younger referees.

Referee Advancement

Although there certainly are referees who are quite happy doing two or three games a week in their local park for decades, there are growing opportunities for advancement in all sports as an official. Particularly as the financial gains of the NCAA and professional sport continue to expand, the referee side of those leagues also has the potential to provide financial gains as well. For example, in U.S. Soccer, a referee typically begins at what is called a grade 8. This is often a referee between the ages of 15 and 18 who is certified to officiate youth games, both recreational and competitive. For soccer at least, the numerical grades then actually get smaller as the referee becomes more advanced. Grade 7 referees are certified to officiate adult amateur matches, and depending on their level of experience and competence, it is possible they might be exposed to top amateur divisions in their region. To continue to advance, referees often need to continue to seek out additional training and instruction necessary to upgrade their certification levels. Depending on the league, referees in soccer and other sports that have significant physical demands such as lacrosse or rugby, will be required to take a fitness test to some degree as well. In order to advance to a grade 6 referee, soccer officials typically need to meet a specified game count, meaning they must have to demonstrate they have been involved in a certain number of games to be eligible for "upgrade." An eligible official will then declare his or her intent to upgrade and will arrange for an assessor, often a very experienced official who is moving into a referee coaching or mentoring role, who will watch that referee perform in a match and provide feedback. If the referee performed well, he or she will be permitted to advance. Each state is responsible for determining the number and quality of assessments needed to advance to a grade 6 level referee. In some states, for example, there may be 5,000 or more grade 7 and grade 8 referees but no more than 30 or 40 grade 6 advanced referees. This obviously creates a clear gap in the number and quality of referees who can officiate the most competitive games in the state. It also puts this small pool of referees in a precarious position to be doing a number of high level games in a very short period of time. Recovery, both mentally and physically for a soccer referee who might run 5–8 miles in a high level adult match, can be challenging in a short period of time. For a referee at this level to do three or four high level games a week is not uncommon, however. In light of how commonplace these situations are, it is clear there is a need to retain and train more referees for more experienced rolls to spread the high level of games around.

The High Level Referee

Only a very small few ever make it to elite levels of sport. A number of officials will have an opportunity to officiate lower level professional games, AAA baseball, Division 2 soccer, D league basketball, for example, but very few will ever make it to the highest level their sport can offer in the country. Nonetheless, much like the progression of an athlete to a high level of recruitment and playing, a young referee goes through virtually the same step-by-step process to achieve advanced certification status as well. In order to advance, the referees need to register or be involved in the higher traveling competitive leagues to gain the experience and knowledge needed. If they perform well in those leagues, they often arrange for an assessment in which referee coaches witness their performance and make recommendations regarding the referees' grade level and suitability for different levels of competition. Once a referee has been recognized locally in youth leagues, he or she might be invited to attend state-level or regional-level youth championships where they would again be subject to review from more experienced and higher level officials. A small number of referees would then be invited to various national-level tournaments, where more advanced referee scouts and coaches would assess the referees and determine their level of progress into elite ranks.

At these more advanced levels of officiating, parents, coaches, and spectators rarely realize the level of training, scrutiny, critical self-reflection, and analysis that high level referees put themselves through for the sake of improving their skills. At the highest levels of all sports in this country, referees analyze videos of game play, discuss scenarios to deal with, undergo physically demanding fitness testing, and take tests on the rules. Referees at the highest levels have worked 15 or 20 years as an official to get to the point where they are at the top of their game. In addition, many of these very high level officials still continue to work the Saturday community youth game and strangely enough tend to be criticized and scrutinized by parents and recreational coaches who may not know that the professional game they were watching on TV was officiated by the very same official they have on their under-12 boys game the next day.

Many young referees look up to these advanced referees and do see refereeing as a potential job opportunity for them to advance into. The salaries of professional referees often begin around $75,000 and can reach upward of $200,000 per year, not including performance incentives and additional income for officiating postseason events. Although the example of referee growth and development was given for a soccer referee, most of the other sports are not all that different to soccer officiating. USA Hockey, for example, begins at level 1 and progresses to level 4. There are criteria to allow for advancement such as skill level, availability, performance in evaluation, online test taking, and seminar attendance. Some sports will offer "schools" for training or advancement, and in some sports, you need to attend specialized clinics to be able to officiate within that certain conference or region. Much like sport for athletes is big business, officiating, assigning, and training officials for sport has also become big business.

Skye G. Arthur-Banning

Further Reading

FIBA Recruitment, Retention and Education of Referees. 2016. Accessed at https://fibaamericasreferee.files.wordpress.com/2016/01/fiba-recruitment-retention-and-education-of-referees.pdf.

Special Report from National Association of Sport Officials: How to Get and Keep Officials. 2001. Accessed at http://www.naso.org/Portals/0/downloads/reports/SpecRept Conf.pdf.

Parent Education

It's Saturday afternoon in Florida, a beautiful day for a pee-wee football game between two teams of 6-year-olds. By the end of the game, however, police are called to control unruly parents. In Texas, a parent at a pee-wee football game charges the field and tackles the 18-year-old referee; other parents jump in and a brawl ensues. On a Friday night in Massachusetts, an angry parent attacks his child's coach, biting off the coach's ear in the process. Unfortunately, these are just a few examples of parents behaving badly at youth sports events. But these types of behaviors do not have to be the norm. An increasing number of organizations are offering parent education programs and resources to encourage parents to remain positive forces in youth sports. According to Devin Rankin of Positive Coaching Alliance (PCA):

> At PCA we firmly believe that parents serve an important role in ensuring that life lessons learned during athletic competition translate to success in life outside of sport. Bouncing back from mistakes, winning with grace and working as a team are core principles that will help all children be successful in life. Our Second-Goal Parent Training seeks to provide parents with tools and tips to help them use sport to teach these life lessons. (Rankin, 2016)

This entry will provide an overview of parent education programs including some common themes and approaches across various programs. In addition, in order to provide context to youth sport programs, the entry will examine the role of parents in youth sport programs, the parent experience, parent behavior, and what youth want from their parents.

The Role of Parents in Youth Sport Programs

Parents play essential roles in both the production of youth sports and in shaping the quality of the experience. Let's look at the example of Mia. Mia is an 11-year-old girl who plays soccer with her friends but has never played in an organized league. Mia hears her friends talking about their soccer team and asks her parents if she can play, too. Her parents research the information, going online and also asking other parents about their experiences. Finally, they agree and register Mia online, including completing all the relevant paperwork and paying the (sometimes considerable) registration fee.

But this is just the beginning of the roles of Mia's parents in the soccer program. On the first day of practice they learn that a uniform, cleats, and fees for playing in outside tournaments are not included in the registration fee. Already Mia's parents are paying more than they had originally budgeted for. In fact, the cost to participate in youth sports continues to rise with expenses reaching up to 10 percent of some families' gross income (Dunn et al., 2016). Although Mia's parents want her to participate, these fees create financial strain on the family.

Once the season begins, the time commitment for Mia's parents only increases. Mia's team practices two days a week and plays at least one game on the weekends. Her parents must arrange for transportation to and from practices and games, and they try to attend most games to cheer for Mia. Further, Mia's younger brother has also decided he wanted to play in a league, so the parents are juggling multiple practices and games.

In addition to being financier, chauffer, and cheerleader, parents frequently perform functions that are crucial to the league programming (Fredricks and Eccles, 2004). In this example, Mia's team needed an assistant coach, and the head coach asked Mia's mother—a former high school player—if she would help coach the team. Indeed, parents coach a large percentage of youth sport teams. In addition, parents also often serve as league administrators, field maintenance personnel, snack providers, and fund-raisers. Many youth sport programs would likely not exist without the extraordinary number of volunteer hours that parents put in.

As one might expect, parents not only provide key logistical support, but their attitudes, behaviors, and interactions with their children, coaches, and other parents greatly influence the quality of the youth sport experience. In fact, youth participants generally perceive the influence of their parents to be even greater than parents realize (Kanters, Bocarro, and Casper, 2008). For example, parents' views strongly influence youth decisions on dropping out of sport or continuing to play (Fraser-Thomas, Côté, and Deakin, 2005. If Mia's parents had a negative view of the league, the coach, or the overall experience, it is likely that Mia would no longer want to participate. On the positive side, when parents provide encouragement and positive support such as cheering (and not yelling) for their children at games, youth are more likely to enjoy the experience (Dorsch, Smith, and Dotterer, 2016). Parents can have negative impacts as well, however. For example, youth players often mirror negative sportsmanship behaviors of their parents, and parental anger can cause additional stress on youth participants (Arthur-Banning, Wells, Baker, and Hegreness, 2009; Omli and LaVoi, 2011). In these ways and more, parents exert tremendous influence on youth sport programs and the experience of youth participants.

The Parent Experience

Youth sport programs exist "for the kids." But the reality is that parents are such a crucial part of the experience that they have their own experiences—both positive and negative. In order to understand the purposes of parent education programs it is important to first view the youth sport experience from a parent perspective.

Being a youth sport parent may be a positive experience. Youth sports provide parents with an opportunity to spend quality time with their children, socialize with other parents, and develop their own sense of community (Legg, Wells, and Barile, 2015). Parents of youth sport participants spend a substantial amount of time together, help each other out with transportation and other tasks, and bond around a shared experience. Thus, it is not surprising that they frequently develop positive social bonds with other parents.

In the example of Mia above, her parents are juggling two children in youth sports, so they often share transportation duties with another parent from Mia's team. They also sit with this parent at games, share stories of the challenges of raising an adolescent, and bond over the game. This relationship may then develop into a lifelong friendship. In addition, Mia's father discovers a new common interest to discuss with Mia. He often had difficulty getting Mia to talk about school or friends, but by starting the conversation with soccer, he is able to improve his bond with her and get her to open up about school and other aspects of her life. Thus, although enrolling Mia in the soccer league added some financial burden and time stress, Mia's parents are also gaining new friends and improving their relationship with their daughter.

Parents also face a number of challenges. On a practical level, the duties of getting youth to and from games and practices and paying team dues, transportation costs, and other associated expenses can be enormously stressful, particularly given the rising costs of youth sport programs. Although parents may develop social relationships with other youth sport parents, the time commitment also means less time for relationships outside of the sport experience or work duties. Further, watching one's own child play a sport—a situation where the child is being watched by others and judged—can cause stress or anger if the parent comes to feel that his or her child is not safe or is being treated unfairly (Omli and LaVoi, 2011). This anger may also be exacerbated if a parent feels that the success of his or her child reflects on him or her as a parent. Unfortunately, this type of anger can also reach a boiling point, which leads to the extreme examples of parents behaving badly.

But are the extreme stories of parents assaulting officials, coaches, and other parents the norm, or are they simply extreme exceptions that make for good media stories? Unfortunately, while these stories may not be the norm, research suggests an overall pattern of escalating negative parent behavior. In 2010, a Reuters News survey reported that 60 percent of American adults said they had witnessed parents "become verbally abusive towards coaches or officials." In another study, coaches and administrators reported observing more negative than positive behaviors and interactions with parents (Ross, Mallett, and Parkes, 2015). In yet another case, researchers observed parent behavior and recorded their observations. In this case, researchers observed that as many as one-third of parent behaviors were negative (Arthur-Banning, Wells, Baker, and Hegreness, 2009). So what do young athletes want from their parents? Do they want them to stand up for them by yelling at officials and coaches, or do they prefer quiet and positive support? Let's look at that question next.

What Do Kids Want?

Parents want the best for their kids. They want them to be successful, have great experiences, and develop as athletes. In some instances, though, this leads to parents becoming overly involved and critical, or to otherwise engage in stereotypical "helicopter" parenting. They may see the shortcoming of the league or team more than their kids do. However, youth sport players frequently express a more positive view of their experience. Youth generally perceive positive outcomes in skill development, teamwork, character development, sportsmanship, and fun more than their parents do (Schwab, Wells, and Arthur-Banning, 2010). Returning to the example of Mia, who had never played organized soccer before, she was thrilled that she scored a goal during the season and also felt like she had learned a lot about teamwork. Her parents, however, set such high goals for Mia's overall experience that they often expressed disappointment that Mia's coach did not play her more in an offensive role. Examples like this may lead to coach-parent conflict, or the parent influencing their child to not play on the team the next year. Given that parental views exert substantial influence on their child's perceptions of skill and enjoyment (Brustad and Partridge, 2002), Mia's initial positive appraisal of her experience may develop into a more negative view.

Parents often see sport as a means to an end rather than simply valuing the experience for its intrinsic value (Shannon, 2006). For instance, although the odds of playing professional sports are infinitesimally small, over one-quarter of parents of high school athletes hope that their child plays professional sports one day. These ideas may be a result of parents overidentifying with the win/loss success of the athlete, or simply a response to being a protective parent and wanting one's child to succeed (Ross, Mallett, and Parkes, 2015). Although Mia may want to play soccer for the sheer joy of playing, her parents may be seeing sport participation as a means to burnish a college application or even secure a college scholarship.

In general, youth prefer parents who are supportive and encouraging and focus on being a loving parent more than on winning and losing. Some motivation and discipline may be appropriate, but simply being a loving parent is most important. According to Olympic gymnastics gold medalist Shawn Johnson (2016), "The most important role that a sport parent can play is to be a parent . . . a big mistake parents make is they try to be a coach as well. Be parents and love your children and support them no matter what and push them along the way, but in a very loving way." Existing research supports this approach, with higher levels of parent warmth and focus on skill improvement instead of just winning associated with positive feelings of youth (Ross, Mallett, and Parkes, 2015).

Recognizing behaviors that constitute parental support and positive encouragement are especially important. Parents may sometimes believe that their expressions of support are positive and encouraging, but their children may perceive some of those same behaviors as negative pressure (Kanters, Bocarro, and Casper, 2008). For example, Mia's parents may think that constantly yelling at Mia to hustle or shoot is simply encouraging her, but Mia may perceive this as negative pressure. Positive parent support may also lead to increased enjoyment, enthusiasm, and positive perception of skill by their children (Gagne, Ryan, and Bargmann, 2003).

Parent Education Organizations

Numerous organizations are stepping into the gap to create parent education programs and materials to improve parent behavior and the overall youth sport culture. Although these programs may be delivered at a local level, larger national organizations create much of the content. In general, three types of organizations develop parent education material: (1) not-for-profit organizations whose sole focus is related to improving youth sports, (2) sport-specific organizations, and (3) local community and recreation organizations. This section will give an overview of these types of organizations along with some examples of each.

Positive Coaching Alliance (PCA) and the National Alliance for Youth Sports (NAYS) represent two of the largest non-sport-specific organizations devoted to improving youth sports. Positive Coaching Alliance seeks to change the culture of youth sports through training programs for coaches, parents, and athletes, as well as a wealth of resources designed for each of these groups. Similarly, NAYS provides organizations and individuals with training programs for coaches, parents, administrators, and officials as well as background checks, specific program resources, and annual conference, awards, and youth sports apparel. The Parents Association for Youth Sports (PAYS) is an arm of NAYS that focuses on parents, including training (online or in-person), membership, and ongoing resources.

Other nonsport specific organizations may not offer specific parent training but do provide resources and information either directly or indirectly related to youth sport parents. Changing the Game Project, for example, states that part of its mission is to provide parents and coaches with the information and resources they need to make sports a positive experience for the whole family. In addition to a Speakers Bureau, Changing the Game Project offers "one-stop shopping" to a wealth of resources for coaches and parents including youth and talent development.

In addition to these nonsport specific resources, a number of sport-specific organizations, primarily national governing bodies (NGOs), offer resources and training for parents. U.S. Soccer, for instance, offers several online courses, a DVD, a blog, and links to additional resources for parents. Online courses include courses devoted to learning the game of soccer, concussions, health and fitness, and positive parenting. International sports organizations are also addressing parenting in youth sports. For example, the Australian Football League (AFL) developed Kids First—We're Not Playing for Sheep Stations. This program includes marketing and educational materials designed to influence the behavior of parents. Kids First seeks to remind parents that sport can be a vital part of growing up, that children primarily want to have fun, that parents serve as important role models, that parents should be proud of their child regardless of win/loss, and that sports function as a key contributor of a child's self-esteem.

Local communities and recreation departments may also provide their own parent-related training and information. These types of programs vary in scope and approach, but often take the form of information provided at parent meetings, e-mail communications, and signage at games. Interestingly, programs that understand that the parent is an integral part of the youth sport environment are ultimately programs that take a more serious approach to educating and training their parents as well.

Finally, multiple resources including books and blogs that are not affiliated with specific organizations are available. A quick search of "youth sports parents" in books on Amazon.com yields more than 500 results. Although some of these books are affiliated with organizations (e.g., *Why Johnny Hates Sports* [NAYS] and *Changing the Game: The Parent's Guide to Raising Happy, High Performing Athletes, and Giving Youth Sports Back* [Changing the Game Project]), a number of others were written by journalists, professors, researchers, parents, and coaches. In addition, numerous articles and blogs can be found online. *The Huffington Post*, for instance, includes an entire section on youth sports with much of the information focusing on parenting advice.

Parent Education Program Formats

Although offered by different types of organizations, parent education programs exist in three, often overlapping formats. First, some programs offer specific parent education training courses. These may be either in-person or online. For example, PCA offers its Second Goal Parent: Developing Winners in Life through Sports course. Organizations that partner with PCA may offer this in-person training, or parents can take the online course through the PCA website.

Marketing campaigns function as a second form of parent education. These campaigns use print, broadcast, and social media as well as on-site banners, e-mail campaigns, and print newsletters to encourage positive parent behavior. For instance, a number of youth baseball programs have posted signs at their field that read: "Please remember: (1) These are kids. (2) This is a game. (3) The coaches volunteer. (4) The umpires are human. (5) You do not play for the Yankees." Signs such as these use humor as a means to improve parent behavior. On a national level, Fox Sports Supports designated PCA as one of its national partners for 2016–2017. As part of this partnership, Fox Sports will air 30- and 60-second public service announcements (PSAs) that also use humor to demonstrate how absurd parent behavior can be. The PSAs first show parents yelling at their kids to "get some confidence" during a sports game. The tables then turn as kids show up at their parents' work presentation to deliver the same message. These types of humorous messages that poke fun at parent behavior appear to be increasing as a means of educating youth sport parents.

A third approach to parent education is to provide links and resources related to parenting and youth sports. This approach appears to be most common at sport-specific organizations or smaller organizations. USA Football, for example, provides a designated landing page for parents. On this page are links to a player-safety checklist, information about concussions, equipment fitting, and health. Similarly, USA Hockey provides a designated page for parents that provide a downloadable parent handbook as well as links to articles about role models, leadership, and fair play.

Parent Education Program Themes

Unfortunately, a magic formula for how to best educate parents does not exist. A review of multiple parent education programs and resources, however, suggests several common themes including teaching life lessons, positive reinforcement, good sportsmanship, and safety. This section will discuss these themes.

Teaching Life Lessons

Using sport to teach life lessons appears as one of the most common themes of parent education programs. In other words, parents should be parents first and focus on using the sports experience to teach life lessons rather than focusing on winning and losing. For example, PCA teaches that the parent role is different than the coach role. Coaches strive to be double-goal coaches. That is, they focus on two equally important goals—winning and teaching life lessons. In contrast, parents only have one goal. Their only role is to help use sports to teach life lessons. In a typical PCA parent training, the PCA trainer asks parents to make a list of the things they want their children to learn from participating in youth sports and then to prioritize those choices by assigning them points. Overwhelmingly, parents tend to list life lessons such as teamwork, the value of hard work and commitment, and dealing with failure. Winning and skill development tend to fall lower on the list. PCA trainers use this exercise as a reminder to parents to keep these life lessons at the forefront and not to get caught up in winning and losing. Similarly, PAYS asks parents to identify the top three things they want their child to get out of sports, to have their child complete the same exercise, and then compare answers. From these discussions, parents may learn that their child places less importance on certain aspects (e.g., winning) than the parent does. The hope is that the parent will then adjust his or her behavior accordingly. The AFL Kids First program also reminds parents of the value of sports in youth development, with this program specifically emphasizing that sports can have a tremendous impact on a child's self-esteem. Thus, it is important that parents help build a child's self-esteem through positive encouragement.

One way that parents can focus on teaching life lessons is by emphasizing effort, learning, and skill development as primary goals. This is called a "mastery or task-involving climate." A mastery climate is an environment that emphasizes goals that are self-referenced (e.g., improving and trying hard) rather than other-referenced (beating someone else) goals. A large body of research links mastery climates to positive youth development outcomes (Roberts, 2012). Positive Coaching Alliance teaches this concept through the "ELM Tree of Mastery"—effort, learning, and mistakes are OK. This approach contrasts to a scoreboard focus on results and winning.

Let's return to Mia and her parents. Mia returns home after a soccer game that her parents were unable to attend. What questions do Mia's parents ask about the game? A gut reaction of many parents would be to immediately ask the obvious question—did you win? Parents who focus on a mastery climate, however, would ideally ask if Mia had fun, if she tried hard, and if she learned anything. What about if Mia made a mistake in a game and her parents were there to see it? What do they say to Mia? According to the PCA ELM Tree model, Mia's parents should point out that mistakes are OK and that mistakes present opportunities to grown and learn.

Positive Reinforcement

Another theme common to parent education programs is that parents should remain positive and ensure that their child is having fun. The Parent Association of Youth Sports calls this "monitoring the smile factor." In the PAYS online training, ESPN journalist Chris McHendry (2016) tells parents to "cheer for everyone, and criticize no one." She continues by pointing out the value of cheering for everyone: "Think about how good that child will feel to hear parents from the opposing team recognizing him or her—and think about the boost in confidence and self-esteem your child would enjoy hearing the same from opposing parents. Set a standard of behavior in the stands for all parents. It can be contagious and everyone benefits." Providing positive support and encouragement will help kids enjoy the sport and continue playing. As Jerry Manual (2015), former major league baseball player and manager stated, "continue to encourage your child . . . get them to love that sport and have passion for that sport."

Both PCA and Changing the Game project talk about positive support as filling your child's emotional tank. Changing the Game states that a parent should be their child's number 1 fan and should be regularly telling their child that they love watching them play. According to PCA the magic ratio of positive to negative comments is 5:1. In other words, every one negative comment to a child should be accompanied by at least five positive comments, and ideally the negative comment is sandwiched in between the positive comments. For example, after a game Mia's parent's words to her may sound something like this, "Mia, I really loved watching you play today. You are out there working hard and improving every day. One thing I'd like to see you do is encourage your teammates when they make a mistake instead of yelling at them. You have so much enthusiasm, and are a great listener when your coach gives you instructions." By filling Mia's emotional tank, her parents are helping Mia feel positive and enthusiastic about her sport participation. As such, Mia is more likely to continue playing.

Good Sportsmanship

Although parents undoubtedly have the best intentions, we know that parents do not always exhibit the best sportsmanship. Parent education programs address this by emphasizing the importance of being a positive role model and exhibiting only the best behavior. In the online PAYS training, Dr. Dan Wann states it simply, "I have three tips for parents as far as sportsmanship is concerned: That would be find a seat, sit down and shut up." Both PAYS and Changing the Game Project suggest that parents sign an agreement with their child that includes behavior stipulations such as not booing bad calls, and not screaming at referees, players, or coaches. This process will remind parents of the importance of good sportsmanship as role models to their children. Positive Coaching Alliance (PCA) suggests that teams appoint a "culture keeper" whose role is to encourage positive behavior from all parents on the team.

Part of displaying good sportsmanship is getting along with coaches. Sometimes in their zeal to look out for their child's interests, parents interject themselves into the child/coach relationship. This may mean criticizing the coach for not playing one's child enough, in the right position, or not developing their child's skills enough. Unfortunately, more often than not, these conflicts simply add to the stress of the child. Parent education programs generally recommend leaving the coaching up to the coach, remembering that most coaches are volunteers, and thanking them for their time and efforts. As Claude Julien (2016), former head coach of the NHL's Boston Bruins, states, "As parents we should be supporting those coaches. It doesn't mean you always have to agree with their decisions . . . But at the end of the day, you have to know they are there for the right reasons." This idea of leaving the coaching decisions up to the coach and parents focusing on teaching life lessons is a key component of good parent behavior.

Safety

It is difficult to watch a college or professional football game without some mention of concussions. Concussions have become such a safety concern that the recent movie *Concussion* told the story of the doctor who initially sounded the alarm regarding concussions in the NFL. Perhaps because of this attention or perhaps because of general safety concerns, more parent education programs now include information about safety. Training offered by PAYS devotes particular attention to safety, covering topics including concussions, nutrition and hydration, and child abuse prevention.

Not surprisingly, parent information for sports where concussions are more prevalent spend more time on safety information. USA Football includes a player safety checklist, several links related to concussions, and information on general injury prevention, hydration, heat preparedness, and conditioning. The parent handbook for USA Hockey includes information about preventing child abuse, nutrition, hydration, and sleep.

Conclusion

Parents play an essential role in both the production of youth sports and as influencers of the quality of the experiences of youth participants. As a result of this, organizations have created a number of parent education training programs and resources. Both sport-specific organizations and organizations devoted to changing the culture of all youth sports offer parent education. These programs are delivered through in-person and online training, marketing campaigns, and links to resources. Although each program has its own focus, common themes include using sport to teach life lessons, positive encouragement, good sportsmanship, and safety. Although the current research provides limited information about the effectiveness of these programs, given the continued popularity of youth sports and the crucial role of parents, it is almost certain that resources and education programs geared specifically to parents will continue to gain popularity.

Eric Legg

Further Reading

Arthur-Banning, S., M. Wells, B. L. Baker, and R. Hegreness. 2009. "Parents Behaving Badly? The Relationship between the Sportsmanship Behaviors of Adults and Athletes in Youth Basketball Games." *Journal of Sport Behavior, 32*(1): 3–18.

Brustad, R. J. 1996. "Attraction to Physical Activity in Urban Schoolchildren: Parental Socialization and Gender Influences." *Research Quarterly for Exercise and Sport, 67*(3): 316–323.

Brustad, R. J., and J. A. Partridge. 2002. "Parental and Peer Influence on Children's Psychosocial Development through Sport." In F. L. Smoll and R. E. Smith (Eds.), *Children and youth in sport: A biopsychosocial perspective* (2nd ed., pp. 187–210). Dubuque, IA: Kendall/Hunt.

Dorsch, T. E., A.L. Smith, and A. M. Dotterer. 2016. "Individual, Relationship, and Context Factors Associated with Parent Support and Pressure in Organized Youth Sport." *Psychology of Sport & Exercise, 23*: 132–141.

Dunn, R., T. E. Dorsch, M. Q. King, and K. J. Rothlisberger. 2016. "The Impact of Family Financial Investment on Perceived Parent Pressure and Child Enjoyment and Commitment in Organized Youth Sport." *Family Relations, 65*(2): 287–299.

Engh, F. 1999. *Why Johnny Hates Sports: Why Organized Youth Sports Are Failing Our Children and What We Can Do about It.* New York: Avery Publishing Group.

Farrey, T. 2008. *Game on: How the Pressure to Win at All Costs Endangers Youth Sports and What Parents Can Do about It.* New York: Random House.

Fraser-Thomas, J. L., J. Côté, and J. Deakin. 2005. "Youth Sport Programs: An Avenue to Foster Positive Youth Development." *Physical Education & Sport Pedagogy, 10*(1): 19–40.

Fredricks, J. A., and J. S. Eccles. 2004. "Parental Influences on Youth Involvement in Sports." In M. R. Weiss (Ed.), *Developmental Sport and Exercise Psychology: A Lifespan Perspective* (pp. 145–164). Morgantown, WV: Fitness Information Technology.

Gagné, M., R. M. Ryan, and K. Bargmann, K. 2003. "Autonomy Support and Need Satisfaction in the Motivation and Well-Being of Gymnasts." *Journal of Applied Sport Psychology, 15*: 372–390.

Harwood, C. G., and C. J. Knight. 2015. "Parenting in Youth Sport: A Position Paper on Parenting Expertise." *Psychology of Sport & Exercise, 16*: 24–35.

Holt, N. L., and C. J. Knight. 2014. *Parenting in Youth Sport: From Research to Practice.* London: Routledge Taylor & Francis Group.

Johnson, Shawn. 2016, February 12. *Shawn Johnson's Advice to Sports Parents* [Video file]. Accessed at http://devzone.positivecoach.org/resource/video/shawn-johnsons-advice -sports-parents.

Julien, C. 2016, January 12. *How Critical Parents Affect a Team* [Video file]. Accessed at http://devzone.positivecoach.org/resource/video/claude-julien-how-critical-parents -affect-team.

Kanters, M. A., J. Bocarro, and J. Casper. 2008. "Supported or Pressured? An Examination of Agreement among Parents and Children on Parent's Role in Youth Sports." *Journal of Sport Behavior, 31*(1): 64–80.

Legg, E., M. S. Wells, and J. P. Barile. 2015. "Factors Related to Sense of Community in Youth Sport Parents." *Journal of Park & Recreation Administration, 33*(2): 73–86.

Manuel, J. 2015, April 6. *Sports Parenting: Realistic Views of Your Child's Potential* [Video file]. Accessed at http://devzone.positivecoach.org/resource/video/sports-parenting -realistic-views-your-childs-potential.

McHendry, C. 2016. *National Alliance for Youth Sports Parent Training* [Video file]. Accessed at http://www.nays.org/parents/training.

Murphy, S. M. 1999. *The Cheers and the Tears: A Health Alternative to the Dark Side of Youth Sports Today.* San Francisco: Jossey-Bass Publishers.

O'Sullivan, J. 2014. *Changing the Game: The Parent's Guide to Raising Happy, High-Performing Athletes and Giving Youth Sports Back to Your Kids.* New York: Morgan James Publishing.

Omli, J., and N. M. LaVoi. 2011. "Emotional Experiences of Youth Sport Parents I: Anger." *Journal of Applied Sport Psychology, 24*(1): 10–25.

Rankin, D. 2016, May 17. Personal interview.

Roberts, G. 2012. "Motivation in Sport and Exercise from an Achievement Goal Theory Perspective: After 30 Years, Where Are We?" *Advances in Motivation in Sport and Exercise, 3*: 5–58.

Ross, A, J., C. J. Mallett, and J. F. Parkes. 2015. "The Influence of Parent Sport Behaviours on Children's Development: Youth Coach and Administrator Perspectives." *International Journal of Sports Science and Coaching, 10*(4): 605–621.

Schwab, K. A., M. S. Wells, and S. G. Arthur-Banning. 2010. "Experiences in Youth Sports: A Comparison between Players' and Parents' Perspectives." *Journal of Sport Administration & Supervision, 2*(1): 41–51.

Shannon, C. S. 2006. "Parents' Messages about the Role of Extracurricular and Unstructured Leisure Activities: Adolescents' Perceptions." *Journal of Leisure Research, 38*(3): 398.

Thompson, J. 2009. *Positive Sports Parenting: How "Second-Goal" Parents Raise Winners in Life through Sports.* Portola Valley, CA: Balance Sports Publishing.

Parental Pressure

As the pitcher stood on the mound, it seemed his entire world was crumbling. His catcher was frustrated. His teammates were shaking their heads. His manager was at wit's end. Everyone in the stands was stunned, and yelling louder at every bad pitch.

He could not throw a strike. Try as he may, he threw balls. He threw wild pitches, and he hit batters. When he was finally removed from the game, his stat line for the inning read four runs, four walks, and five wild pitches.

This was not some child pitcher in a local little league game. The pitcher's name was Rick Ankiel, and he was pitching for the St. Louis Cardinals in the 2000 National League playoffs against the Atlanta Braves. After that horrific outing, Ankiel had several similarly disappointing appearances in the 2000 playoffs. He simply lost his ability to throw strikes, and within the span of less than a year went from one of the top pitching prospects in Major League Baseball to switching positions to the outfield. How can a promising young pitcher who had thrown thousands of pitches in his life fall so far and so fast? Rick Ankiel succumbed to the pressure and lost confidence in his ability to throw strikes (O'Sullivan, 2014).

Pressure can crack even the most seasoned professional athletes. Imagine what it can do to a young child playing sports, especially when the pressure is coming from his or her own parents. Parental pressure in sports has become one of the biggest issues facing child athletes. From the gymnastics mom yelling at her prepubescent daughter as she fails to properly land a vault, to the angry dad watching his quarterback son throw interceptions in front of college scouts, there is an inordinate amount of pressure being placed on youth and high school athletes.

Many observers contend that this pressure to win and perform in every practice and every game is not making them better athletes; it is making them bitter athletes, and it is making them quit. While some leave to pursue other interests, or because they are not skilled enough to make a high school team, many other children—even top youth athletes—walk away because the pressure and spotlight become unbearable.

Children play sports for many reasons, but far and away the top reason is for the fun of it. They like to play with their friends, they like to learn new things, and they enjoy the excitement of competition. They quit when it is no longer fun, when they get yelled at and disrespected, and when they lose playing time to other, more advanced players due to coaches with a win-at-all-cost mentality. Winning is nice, but according to a 2014 study by George Washington University researcher Amanda Visek and colleagues, when asked to define "fun" in sports, children came up with 81 different characteristics. Winning came in at number 48 on the list (Visek et al., 2014).

The primary reason children are walking away from sports is the pressure and professionalization of youth sports. In this entry, the parental pressure in youth sports will be examined from two interrelated angles:

1. The pressure parents put on young athletes to succeed, which takes away enjoyment, ownership, and internal motivation from young athletes.
2. The pressure parents put on themselves, and each other, to be perfect parents, to keep up with the Jones's and become the next Earl Woods or Richard Williams, leading their child to athletic glory.

Parental Pressure on Young Athletes

When discussing pressure in youth sports, the most obvious thought that comes to mind is the pressure and expectations many parents place on their children to succeed at sports at a very early age. Many sporting associations in the United States have participated in, and contributed to, the downward creep in age when it comes to travel and select teams. Children as young as 6 years old are trying out for teams in hockey, soccer, baseball, and nearly every sport under the sun. Their parents are then shelling out thousands of dollars in coaching fees, uniforms, and travel expenses to keep little Johnny or little Jenny in the developmental pipeline.

This push to make an "elite" team at increasingly younger ages has led to a push toward early sport specialization that contradicts the best science, psychology, and sociology of child and athletic development. It has led to a win-at-all-costs mentality in elementary school-aged sports. It has turned youth sports into a path to a future scholarship and professional sports career, an investment strategy with financial returns instead of character development. Combine these elements, and the pressure on very young athletes to perform and get a return on that investment of time and money escalates quickly.

Scientific studies indicate, however, that the pathway of early specialization and win-at-all-costs is not the optimal player development path. Dr. James Andrews, the noted orthopedic surgeon and inventor of the famed "Tommy John" elbow surgery in baseball, sees the by-product of this alarming trend in his office every week. In a 2013 interview with *The Cleveland Plain Dealer*, Andrews stated, "I started seeing a sharp increase in youth sports injuries, particularly baseball, beginning around 2000. I started tracking and researching, and what we've seen is a five- to sevenfold increase in injury rates in youth sports across the board" (Manoloff, 2013, para. 9).

Andrews attributes this rapid rise in injuries to early specialization and the professionalism of youth sports. "Almost half of sports injuries in adolescents stem from overuse . . . Professionalism is taking these kids at a young age and trying to work them as if they are pro athletes, in terms of training and year-round activity. Some can do it, like Tiger Woods. He was treated like a professional golfer when he was 4, 5, 6 years old. But you've got to realize that Tiger Woods is a special case. A lot of these kids don't have the ability to withstand that type of training and that type of parental/coach pressure" (Andrews, 2013, para. 16–17). As alluded to by Andrews, physical injury is not the only potentially negative by-product of early specialization.

Early specialization has led to a rise of younger and younger so-called "elite" teams. How can a 6-year-old be elite? They are labeled as such due to parents and coaches striving to put these early specialists on the same teams and travel far and wide to compete against other early specialists. To be admitted to these "elite" events, teams must have a record of success, and critics assert that all too often, this leads to an emphasis on wins and losses at far too young an age. These critics contend that parents and coaches have turned their attention away from developing excellence in young athletes and now only focus on immediate success. As a result, teams often do the following:

1. Play too many games and do not practice enough.
2. Select "talent" for short-term gains instead of identifying and developing all athletes and focusing on long-term potential.
3. Make cuts and select all-star teams at younger and younger ages, making youth sports an elitist undertaking for early developers and those with the financial means to participate.
4. Require year-round participation to be a part of elementary school age youth teams, which goes against the advice of physicians, psychologists, and sociologists.
5. Teach and coach strategies that provide short-term results at the expense of long-term development.

Many observers believe that parents and coaches are thus short-changing children's athletic education by seeking success instead of excellence, and victories instead of development.

How Do Pressure and Professionalization Negatively Affect Sports?

Dr. Joe Baker, a sport scientist from York University in Canada, is one of the world's leading researchers on the subject of early sport specialization and elite athletic performance. He sees firsthand how thousands of hours of dedicated training can lead to elite performance on a world stage.

Baker also sees the physical, emotional, and social fallout for tens of thousands of children, caused by parents pursuing glory for their kids, and through their kids, but not in fulfillment of the dreams and ambitions *of their kids*. According to Dr. Baker, parents should instead ensure that their child's youth sports experience feature the following three characteristics:

- **Autonomy:** The experience must belong to the child. It must be in fulfillment of the child's goals and ambitions, not the parents. Parents must let their children own the experience.
- **Enjoyment:** Without enjoyment, play, and fun, talent matters very little. A child who does not enjoy a sport will rarely pursue it long enough to be good at it. Far too many parents focus on competence and practice, instead of love of the game, and as a result their kids walk away before they play long enough to have a chance to develop into good players.
- **Intrinsic motivation:** The athletes must be internally motivated to train and play; they must be the ones setting goals and challenging themselves. "Intrinsic motivation is the currency of athletic development," says Baker. "If they don't have it, it is very hard to give it to them" (interview with author).

These three characteristics are simple enough, yet for many parents they are incredibly difficult to follow and implement due to the pressure parents place on themselves.

Intense pressure and the *adultification* of youth sports—making it about the needs, values, and priorities of parents and coaches instead of the kids—destroys these essential ingredients for long-term success. Children lose ownership as parents and coaches tell them what to do, when to do it, and how often to do it, leaving no time for free play. They turn the focus off of short-term enjoyment and onto deliberate practice and long-term training, losing sight of why kids show up to play in the first place. And ultimately, the loss of ownership and enjoyment saps a child's motivation to show up, to practice and to play; and intrinsic motivation is lost.

Why Do Parents Ramp Up the Pressure?

Why do seemingly sensible parents suspend common sense when it comes to youth sports? They don't expect their third grader to master calculus or play Beethoven on the piano, but for some reason they get very upset when their child makes mistakes and does not display mastery of a complicated sport like hockey or soccer. Researchers cite several main or overarching reasons for the increased pressure parents place on their children.

No Patience for Development

Whether it stems from their investments in time or money, or the false promises of some coaches, far too many adults expect immediate results. They compare the adult version of games to the game their child is playing, and think, "What is wrong with my DNA out there?" The patience for development drops the more time and money parents invest, while their expectations for results increase. They soon reach a tipping point and start to lose a sense of reality.

Emotional Investment in Outcomes

According to Po Bronson and Ashley Merryman (2013) in their book *Top Dog: The Science of Winning and Losing*, there is a scientific explanation for why parents sometimes lose control and ramp up the pressure at games. Most parents who have attended sporting events will attest to the vast difference between casual viewing of a game and the much more intense viewing of one's own child participating in a competitive sport environment. Every perceived bad call from an official or coach, every aggressive foul from an opposing player, every intense situation is magnified. With the emotional investment of being personally involved through one's child, the stakes simply become much higher, and hence emotional reactions are intensified. Research has found similar results with heavily invested fans of professional sport teams.

As noted by Bronson and Merryman (2013), it is perfectly normal for parents to experience emotional reactions due to that intense emotional investment. Nearly every parent, player, and coach goes through these same emotions. Science tells us why: *mirror processing*. In the 1990s, Italian researchers stumbled on a class of neurons in the brain that fire not only when an individual performs an action, but when that individual witnesses another perform an action. Examples abound from everyday experience. If a person sees another yawn, he yawns; when an individual sees another stub her toe, there's a tendency to flinch. These reactions are governed by mirror neurons, which allow a person to not only simulate the actions of others but the emotions behind those actions. Researchers have used fMRI technology to test the effect of emotional attachment on brain function, and the results are extraordinary.

When coaching a youth sports game, watching a loved one participate in an athletic contest, or even viewing one's favorite football team on Saturdays or Sundays in the fall, a different region of the brain is being utilized than when in a neutral or nonemotional setting. In those emotionally charged settings, the neutral decision-making areas of the brain actually disengage, and the inferior parietal lobe (IPL) is utilized to judge a pass interference call or to assess whether offsides should have been called or not. The result: our brains react *as if we were* the ones performing the action. This is why there is a tendency for parents (and coaches) to act so irrationally during youth sports contests. Our brains react as if we were the one being fouled, or as if we were the one who *unjustly* had a goal called back.

The same mirror processing that governs this behavior is also why teams tend to feed off of each other's energy, often either peaking and dominating together, or sulking and giving up at the same time. Team emotions are contagious, both in a positive and negative way. Parents have a tendency to ramp up pressure on their children because, in a way, they are ramping up pressure on themselves to perform better.

Pressure to "Keep Up" with Peer Families

In speaking to tens of thousands of parents across the United States and the world about youth sports, coaching, and athlete development, many have confided that they are under intense pressure and feel frustration in trying to navigate the youth sports world. The pressure on parents to be perfect parents and to keep up with the proverbial Jones's has become astronomical. Questions from parents are plentiful: When should children be pushed to perform better, work harder, and dedicate themselves more to the sport? Is there a line of diminishing returns where parents push too much and their children respond negatively? Should parents expose children to as many opportunities as possible for athletic success? Or, should parents let their children choose which opportunities are pursued? These questions reflect the unease with which parents approach their children's youth sports experience.

Researchers have examined the dynamic of parents living vicariously through their children in youth sports, attempting to quantify the extent to which parents become emotionally invested in their children's sports performances as a way of fulfilling their own unrealized ambitions. They've found that the more that parents view a child as an extension of themselves, rather than as a separate individual with his or her own hopes and dreams, the more the parents live vicariously through their child's achievements. In other words, the more that children succeed in sports or school, the more validation parents living vicariously through them receive in their parental role. And, the more they are able to release their own regret and disappointment that they did not achieve those same accomplishments (Brummelman et al., 2013).

While parents who live vicariously through their children typically receive the most attention, it should also be noted that many parents do not live vicariously through their children. Yet, these parents feel the same pressure to keep up and be perfect parents. Ex-NFL punter turned Utah State professor Travis Dorsch has found that the more parents spend on their child's sports, the more they treat that spending as an investment, the more pressure their child feels to perform, and the less enjoyment their child may get from sports (Cook, 2014). "We have to change the conversation," Dorsch stated in an interview with the author, "from 'Did you win?' to 'Did you have fun, and what did you learn?'" It's a simple yet potentially very effective shift in the discourse surrounding youth sports.

Healthy Parental Attitudes about Youth Sports

The purpose of this entry is not to leave parents feeling hopeless, or more frustrated than when they started. The purpose is to shine a light on some of the main causes of pressure on children. That way, parents can do their best to avoid being a source of pressure themselves and can help their children navigate other sources of pressure. Researchers urge parents to do the following:

- Start by focusing on the three ingredients of long-term athletic participation: autonomy, enjoyment, and intrinsic motivation.
- Allow the sports experience to belong to the children.
- Have open lines of communication with sons and daughters. Learn why they play, what they enjoy most about sports, and what they most want to avoid.
- Surround them with great role models on and off the field, and help them understand that it takes a long time to become proficient at anything as complicated as sports.
- Focus on their effort and focus every time they take the field, instead of only on the outcome of each game.

Finally, parents should treat sports like any other family experience. As Dorsch explains, parents are better off making sports an experience instead of something that leads to a greater goal. "If you take your family to Disney World, you don't expect to take Mickey Mouse home with you. You go to have a great family experience, period. Youth sports should be the same thing, and that's a great way to start reducing the pressure" (interview with author).

John O'Sullivan

Further Reading

Andrews, James R. (with Don Yaeger). 2013. *Any Given Monday: Sports Injuries and How to Prevent Them, for Athletes, Parents and Coaches—Based on My Life in Sports Medicine.* New York: Scribner.

Bronson, Po, and Ashley Merryman. 2013. *Top Dog: The Science of Winning and Losing.* New York: Twelve Books.

Brummelman, Eddie, Sander Thomaes, Meike Slagt, Geertjan Overbeek, Bram Orobio de Castro, and Brad Bushman. 2013. "My Child Redeems My Broken Dreams: On Parents Transferring Their Unfulfilled Ambitions onto Their Child." *PLoS ONE, 8*(6). Accessed August 15, 2015, at http://journals.plos.org/plosone/article?id=10.1371/journal.pone.0065360.

Cook, Bob. 2014. *Punter Turned Prof: Kids Feel Pressure When Parents Spend a Lot on Sports.* Accessed August 15, 2015, at http://www.forbes.com/sites/bobcook/2014/04/11/punter-turned-prof-kids-feel-pressure-when-parents-spend-a-lot-on-sports.

Dweck, Carol S. 2006. *Mindset: The New Psychology of Success.* New York: Ballantine Books.

Hyman, Mark. 2012., *The Most Expensive Game in Town.* Boston: Beacon Press.

Manoloff, Dennis. 2013. *Noted Surgeon Dr. James Andrews Wants Your Young Athlete to Stay Healthy by Playing Less.* Accessed August 15, 2015, at http://www.cleveland.com/dman/index.ssf/2013/02/noted_surgeon_dr_james_andrews.html.

Matheny, Mike. 2015. *The Matheny Manifesto: A Young Manager's Old-School Views on Success in Sports and Life.* New York: Crown Archetype.

O'Sullivan, John. 2014. *Changing the Game: The Parent's Guide to Raising Happy, High-Performing Athletes and Giving Youth Sports Back to Our Kids.* New York: Morgan James Publishing.

O'Sullivan, John. 2015a. *Is it Wise to Specialize?* Accessed August 15, 2015, at http://changingthegameproject.com/is-it-wise-to-specialize.

O'Sullivan, John. 2015b. *Our Biggest Mistake: Talent Selection Instead of Talent Identification.* Accessed August 15, 2015, at http://changingthegameproject.com/our-biggest-mistake-talent-selection-instead-of-talent-identification.

O'Sullivan, John. 2015c. "Parental Athletic Dreams Can Become Youth Sports Nightmares." *Huffington Post.* Accessed August 15, 2015, at http://www.huffingtonpost.com/john-oasullivan/parental-athletic-dreams-_b_6850790.html?1426111942.

Pink, Daniel H. 2009. *Drive: The Surprising Truth about What Motivates Us.* New York: Riverhead Books.

Taylor, Jim. 2003. *Positive Pushing: How to Raise a Successful and Happy Child.* New York: Hachette Books.

Tough, Paul. 2012. *How Children Succeed: Grit, Curiosity, and the Hidden Power of Character.* New York: Houghton Mifflin Harcourt.

Visek, Amanda J., Sara M. Achrati, Heather Manning, Karen McDonnell, Brandonn S. Harris, and Loretta DiPietro. 2014. "Fun Integration Theory: Towards Sustaining Children and Adolescents Sport Participation." *Journal of Physical Activity & Health, 12*(3): 424–433.

Parents in Fan and Coaching Contexts

Many parents are productive contributors to youngsters' sport experiences. Unfortunately, however, the negative effects of a rather small minority of parents are all too obvious. The following are extreme examples of media reports concerning parents engaging in criminally violent actions toward coaches:

- In Massachusetts, a coach died after he was beaten unconscious following a hockey practice by a father who was upset about rough play in a scrimmage. The assailant was convicted of involuntary manslaughter.
- At a Philadelphia-area youth football game, a player's father brandished a .357 magnum during a dispute with a coach over his son's playing time.
- A Long Island, NY, soccer mom angered over being dropped from the team e-mail list for game-day directions was arrested after slamming a metal folding chair across the face of her daughter's coach. The woman was charged with second-degree reckless endangerment.

Fortunately, incidents such as these rarely occur. Yet, in their own dramatic fashion, they illustrate problems that have caused some programs to take steps to protect the welfare of youth sport coaches.

The importance of coach-parent relationships cannot be overemphasized. In forming a dynamic social system, coaches and parents interact in complex ways, and the nature of the interactions can have significant consequences for the psychosocial development of young athletes. Experts say, however, that there are a number of steps that can be taken to get coaches and parents "on the same page" and working cooperatively to create positive and harmonious sport environments. Although there are a myriad of issues associated with coach-parent relationships, positive relations are more likely when both parties work toward a mutual understanding of (1) developmental versus professional models of sport, (2) objectives of youth sports, (3) a healthy philosophy of winning, (4) parents' responsibilities and challenges, (5) parents' commitments and affirmations, (6) parental conduct at sport events, (7) responsibilities of coaching one's own child, (8) discussing disagreements about playing time, and (9) two-way communication between coaches and parents.

Developmental versus Professional Models of Sport

An important issue is the difference between youth and professional models of sport. Youth sports provide an educational medium for the development of desirable physical and psychosocial characteristics. The sport environment is viewed as a microcosm of society in which children and youth can learn to cope with realities they will face in later life. Thus, athletics provide a developmental setting within which an *educational process* can occur.

In contrast, professional sports are an explicitly commercial enterprise. Their goals, simply stated, are to entertain and, ultimately, to make money. Financial success is of primary importance and depends heavily on a *product orientation,* namely, winning. Is this wrong? Certainly not! Professional sports are part of the entertainment industry, and as such, they are enormously valued on a worldwide basis.

What, then, is the problem? Most of the negative consequences of youth sports occur when adults erroneously impose a professional model on what should be a recreational and educational experience for youngsters, the so-called "professionalization" of youth sports. When excessive emphasis is placed on winning, it is easy to lose sight of the needs and interests of the young athlete.

Objectives of Youth Sport

Youth sport programs provide miniature life situations in which children and adolescents can learn to relate more effectively to other people and to cope with realities they will face in later life. *Physically,* athletes can learn sport skills and increase their health and fitness. *Psychologically,* they can develop leadership skills, self-discipline, respect for authority, competitiveness, cooperativeness, sportsmanship, and self-confidence. Moreover, sports can be just plain *fun!* Youth sports are also an important *social* activity in which children can make new friends and acquaintances and become part of an ever-expanding social network. Furthermore, the involvement of parents in the athletic enterprise can serve to bring families closer together and strengthen family unity.

The basic right of the young athlete to have fun participating should be emphasized. One of the quickest ways to reduce fun is for adults to begin treating children as if they were professional athletes. Coaches and parents alike need to keep in mind that young athletes are not miniature adults. They are children, and they have the right to play as children. Youth sports are first and foremost a play activity, and youngsters deserve to enjoy sports in their own way. In essence, it is important that programs remain *child-centered* and do not become adult dominated.

A Healthy Philosophy of Winning

In terms of the educational benefits of sport, young athletes can learn from both winning and losing. But for this to occur, winning must be put in a *healthy* perspective. We have therefore developed a four-part philosophy of winning designed to maximize athletes' enjoyment of sports and their chances of receiving the positive outcomes of participation (Smith and Smoll, 2012, 27–28).

1. **Winning isn't everything, nor is it the only thing:** Young athletes can't possibly learn from winning and losing if they think the only objective is to beat their opponents. Although winning is an important goal, it is not the most important objective.
2. **Failure is not the same thing as losing:** It is important that athletes do not view losing as a sign of failure or as a threat to their personal value.
3. **Success is not equivalent to winning:** Neither success nor failure need depend on the outcome of a competition or on a won-lost record. Winning and losing apply to the outcome of a competition, whereas success and failure do not.
4. **Athletes should be taught that success is found in striving for victory (i.e., success is related to commitment and effort):** The only thing athletes can control is the amount of effort they give. They have incomplete control over the outcome that is achieved. Athletes at all levels of competition should be taught that they are never "losers" if they give maximum effort in striving for excellence. This philosophy of success is relevant to coaches as well as parents. In fact, it may be more important for parents to understand its meaning. They can apply it to many areas of their child's life in addition to athletics.

Parents' Responsibilities and Challenges

When a child enters a sport program, parents automatically take on some obligations. Some parents do not realize this at first and are surprised to find what is expected of them. Others never realize their responsibilities and miss opportunities to help their children grow through sports, or they may actually do things that interfere with their children's development.

To begin, parents must realize that children have a right to participate in sports. But this includes the right to choose *not* to participate. Although parents might wish to encourage participation, children should not be pressured, intimidated, or bribed into playing. Athletes who feel "entrapped" experience less enjoyment and lower intrinsic motivation, and they derive fewer benefits from being involved in sports. Consequently, they are more likely to drop out. In fulfilling their responsibility, parents should counsel their children, giving consideration to the sport selected and the level of competition at which the child wants to play. Parents should respect their children's decisions.

Parents can enjoy their children's participation more if they acquire an understanding and appreciation of the sport. This includes knowledge of basic rules, skills, and strategies. Coaches can serve as valuable resources by answering parents' questions and by referring parents to appropriate websites, community and school libraries, or bookstores for educational materials (e.g., videos, books, magazines). In addition, coaches should devote part of an early season practice to a lecture and/or demonstration of the fundamentals of the sport. Parents having little background in the sport should be encouraged to attend this session.

Some parents unknowingly become a source of stress to young athletes. One factor that might constitute the underlying basis of parent-induced stress is what we call the *reversed-dependency phenomenon*. All parents identify with their children to some extent and thus want them to do well. Unfortunately, in some cases, the degree of identification becomes excessive, and the child becomes an extension of the parents. When this happens, parents begin to define their own self-worth in terms of their son's or daughter's successes or failures. The parent who was a "frustrated jock" may seek to experience through his or her child the success they never knew as an athlete. Conversely, the parent who was a star may be resentful and rejecting if the child does not attain a similar level of achievement. Some parents thus become "winners" or "losers" through their child, and the pressure placed on the children to excel can be extreme. The child *must* succeed or the parent's self-image is threatened. Much more is at stake than a mere competition, and the child of such a parent carries a heavy burden. When parental love and approval depend on adequacy of performance, sports are bound to be stressful.

Coaches may be able to counteract this tendency by explaining the overidentification process to parents. They can tell parents that placing excessive pressure on children can decrease the potential of sports for enjoyment and personal growth. A key to reducing parent-produced stress is to impress on parents that youth sport programs are for young athletes and that children and youth are not adults. Parents must acknowledge the right of each child to develop athletic potential in an atmosphere that emphasizes participation, personal growth, and fun.

Parents' Commitments and Affirmations

To contribute to the success of a sport program, parents must be willing and able to commit themselves in many different ways. Six key questions serve as thought-provoking reminders of the scope of parents' responsibilities. Parents should be able to honestly answer "yes" to each question.

1. **Can the parents share their son or daughter?** This requires putting the child in the coach's charge and trusting him or her to guide the sport experience. It involves accepting the coach's authority and the fact that the coach may gain some of the admiration and affection the child once directed solely at the parent. This commitment does not mean that parents cannot have input, but the coach is the boss! If parents are going to undermine the coach's leadership, everyone concerned is going to have problems.

2. **Can the parents accept their child's triumphs?** Every child athlete experiences "the thrill of victory and the agony of defeat" as part of the competition process. Accepting a child's triumphs sounds easy, but it is not always so. Fathers, in particular, may be competitive with their sons. For example, if a boy does well in a competition, his father may point out minor mistakes, describe how others did even better, or remind his son of even more impressive sport achievements of his own.

3. **Can the parents accept their child's disappointments?** In addition to enjoying athletic accomplishments, parents are called on to support their children when they are disappointed and hurt. This may mean not being embarrassed, ashamed, or angry when their son or daughter cries after losing a competition. When an apparent disappointment occurs, parents should be able to help their child learn from the experience. By doing this without denying the validity of their feelings, parents can help their child see the positive side of the situation and thus change their child's disappointment into self-acceptance.

4. **Can the parents give their child some time?** Parents need to decide how much time can be devoted to their child's sport activities. Conflicts arise when they are very busy yet are also interested and want to encourage their child. To avoid this, the best thing to do is deal honestly with the time-commitment issue and not promise more time than can actually be delivered.

Parents should ask their child about their sport experiences and make every effort to watch some of their competitions.

5. **Can the parents let their child make his or her own decisions?** Accepting responsibility for one's own behavior and decisions is an essential part of growing up. Parents should offer suggestions and guidance about sports, but ultimately, within reasonable limits, they should let their children go their own way. All parents likely have ambitions for their child, but they must accept the fact that they cannot dominate the child's life. Sports can offer an introduction to the major parental challenge of letting go.

6. **Can the parents show their child self-control?** Parents should be reminded that they are important role models for their child's behavior. It is not surprising that parents who lose control of themselves often have children who are prone to emotional outbursts and poor self-discipline. Coaches can hardly be expected to teach sportsmanship and self-control to youngsters whose parents obviously lack these qualities.

Parental Conduct at Sport Events

The most noticeable parent problem is misbehavior at sport events. As part of their responsibilities, parents should watch their children compete in sports. But their behavior must meet acceptable standards. In addition to acknowledging some obviously inappropriate actions (using profanity, drinking alcohol, throwing objects, and so forth), six rules are recommended for parental behavior (Smoll and Smith, 2012).

1. **Do** remain in the spectator area during the event.
2. **Don't** interfere with the coach. Parents must be willing to give up the responsibility for their child to the coach for the duration of the practice or competition.
3. **Do** express interest, encouragement, and support to young athletes. Be sure to cheer good effort as well as good performance. Communicate repeatedly that giving total effort is all that is expected.
4. **Don't** shout instructions or criticisms to the children.
5. **Do** lend a hand when a coach or official asks for help.
6. **Don't** make abusive comments to athletes, parents, officials, or coaches of either team.

These rules make good sense. We also propose using a *video rule* that is easy to remember. Specifically, when parents attend practices and competitions, they should imagine they are being videotaped. The two-part rule is simple:

- **Don't** do anything that would embarrass yourself or your child.
- **Do** things that would make your son or daughter proud.

What about parents who violate the rules of conduct? When parents misbehave, it is the duty of program administrators, sport officials, and other parents to intervene. It is not the coach's *primary* job! Coaches have a huge responsibility in taking care of the team and cannot be expected to police the spectators as well. This perspective must be qualified for the sport of soccer. The rules of youth soccer specify that coaches are responsible for the behavior of parents. Because of this, the most effective approach is for coaches to enlist the assistance of parents. In other words, coaches should delegate authority to parents. They should be asked to step in and correct inappropriate behavior when they see or hear it.

Coaching One's Own Child

Many volunteer coaches find their way into youth sport programs because their son or daughter is participating. Therefore, the majority of coaches end up coaching their own child at one time or another. This can be a wonderful opportunity to spend quality time together, but it also presents some unique challenges for both the parent and the child.

The most difficult issue concerns confusion arising from the dual roles of coach and parent. To effectively deal with this, parents and children need to understand that coaching behavior and parenting behavior will be different. For example, a coach will not be able to give the immediate access or personal attention that a parent would give to a child at home. A coach must make time for all members of the team, not just one young athlete.

The four principles presented below explicitly target the coach-parent. The first two provide a basic parent-child foundation, which should be established in a preseason meeting. The last two principles can be implemented during practices and competitions.

1. **Ask your child how they feel about having you for a coach:** In other words, get your child's opinion prior to the season. If there are reservations, it is important to discuss them. Most children enjoy playing for their parent, but some would prefer another coach. Are some kids afraid to say they would rather play for someone else? Yes, because they might believe their mother or father will feel rejected. To counteract this, you must openly communicate with your children; hear your children; encourage them to express their true feelings.

2. **Discuss how your role will change when you are in the athletic environment, and why you need to treat your child like any other team member:** Does the youngster feel any undue pressure, such as perceived favoritism or excessive demands from you? Many coaches tend to be harder on their child, and they bend over backward not to show favoritism. Being fair does not mean being harder on your child. The challenge is to be impartial and treat your child no differently than anyone else on the team.

In addition to talking with your son or daughter, you should explain the situation to the whole team. This can be done at the first practice or team meeting. Some coaches tell their athletes that, even though their son or daughter is on the team, they consider every athlete as one of their children. Kids are able to understand the message.

3. **Be a parent at home and a coach in sports:** Make sure your separate roles are clear in your mind and in your child's mind. There are at least two ways to put this principle into operation:
   - Have your child refer to you as "Coach" when interacting in the sport environment. The labeling helps to solidify the separation of roles.
   - If you have an assistant coach, have that person work with your child in situations involving individual instruction. If the assistant also has a child on the team, use the *crisscross* technique of working with each other's children.
   - Don't overdo it! When driving home, you will likely talk about things that happened in the practice or competition. But set up a time interval, and don't go beyond it. Keep things in balance, and set some reasonable limits.
4. **Reaffirm your love, regardless of your child's level of performance:** Youngsters will go to extremes to please their parents, and too much emphasis on sports gets things out of kilter. Above all, demonstrate in words and actions that your love does not depend on athletic ability.

Avoiding Disputes about Playing Time

Perhaps the most common cause of coach-parent conflicts is a difference of opinions about the young athlete's abilities, which is the basis for determining playing time. To avoid disputes, it is critical for coaches to establish authority over playing time. This requires them to go beyond subjective evaluations of athletes' overall competence. Top-notch coaches usually develop and use a very basic performance evaluation system (PES) that can be easily understood by young athletes and their parents.

A PES is not the same as keeping game-related statistics. Rather, it provides an assessment of an athlete's abilities relative to the skills that are necessary to play the sport. For example, in baseball a PES would include evaluation of fielding, hitting, running, throwing, etc., and then specifics to playing the position. Other things like attitude, sportsmanship, and teamwork can also be included. In essence, the coach develops a fairly comprehensive sport grading system.

A PES can be used by coaches at any level of competition. Two major benefits can be derived. First, a PES is a valuable goal-setting/motivation tool for athletes because it provides them with objective feedback on their strengths and weaknesses. A coach can say, "Here are the areas that you've got to work on. When you see your grades go up in this area, you're going to see more playing time." Second, the carryover benefit with parents is that it takes the coach out of the position of being an arbitrary designator of playing time. A coach can say, "Here's the basis of my assessment, and here's where I'm coming from." In a very objective way, the coach can point out the strengths and weaknesses of the young athlete to the parent.

Promoting Two-Way Communication

Parents have both the right and the responsibility to inquire about *all* activities that their children are involved in, including sports. For this reason, coaches should be willing to answer questions and remain open to parents' input. The truism, *communication is a two-way street,* certainly applies here. If coaches keep the lines of communication open, they will be more likely to have constructive relations with parents.

Fostering two-way communication does not mean that parents are free to be disrespectful toward coaches in word or action. Rather, it is an open invitation for parents to express their genuine concerns with the assurance that they will be heard by the coach. There is, however, a proper time and place for parent-coach interaction. That time is not during practice or a contest, and it is never in the presence of the youngsters. Coaches should tell parents what times and places are best suited for discussions.

In some cases, it is desirable to have a program administrator serve as a mediator for a coach-parent consultation. The presence of a third person reduces the likelihood of conflict or hostility and can potentially contribute to the resolution process.

In establishing good relations with parents, coaches should be aware that most parents are really enthusiastic and have a true concern for their children. However, there are times when parents simply do not realize the trouble they are causing. Instead of being angry with them, coaches should recognize that they have a problem—one that the coaches can help solve. The task is to point out to these people, tactfully and diplomatically, the negative influences of their actions and get them to become more constructive and helpful.

Sometimes parents will disagree with what coaches are doing. The main thing is for coaches not to get defensive. They should listen to what the parents have to say. They might find some parents' suggestions helpful. However, even if they do not agree, coaches can at least *listen* and evaluate the message. They should realize that they have the final say and that no coach can please everyone. No one can ask any more than what coaches ask of their athletes, to do the very best job they can and to always look for ways to improve.

Frank L. Smoll and Ronald E. Smith

Further Reading

Smith, Ronald E., and Frank L. Smoll. 2012. *Sport Psychology for Youth Coaches: Developing Champions in Sports and Life.* Lanham, MD: Rowman & Littlefield.

Smoll, Frank L., and Ronald E. Smith. 2009a. *Mastery Approach to Coaching: A Self-Instruction Program for Youth Sport Coaches* [Video]. Accessed at http://www.y-e-sports.org.

Smoll, Frank L., and Ronald E. Smith. 2009b. *Mastery Approach to Parenting in Sports: A Self-Instruction Program for Youth Sport Parents* [Video]. Accessed at http://www.y-e-sports.org.

Smoll, Frank L., and Ronald E. Smith. 2012. *Parenting Young Athletes: Developing Champions in Sports and Life.* Lanham, MD: Rowman & Littlefield.

Smoll, Frank L., and Ronald E. Smith. *Coaching and Parenting Young Athletes* [Blog]. Accessed at https://www.psychologytoday.com/blog/coaching-and-parenting-young-athletes.

Pay-to-Play

Pay-to-play refers to an arrangement made between schools and activity participants in which a fee must be paid by the participants in order to represent their school in the sport. The term applies to more than sport, though, and can include any other activities deemed "extracurricular" or nonessential at the school. These are typically elective activities that are not required by the schools.

For those parents who have been paying for club or elite-level sports for their children, the concept is nothing new. Club sports have been using a pay-to-play model for decades. However, for many adults who grew up playing school-based or recreation sports, the cost to play was quite minimal. If there was a fee it may have only accounted for the equipment and some expenses. The rest of the cost to play school sports was mere sweat equity. Many people view the idea of paying an "entry fee" just to have a right to play the sport as a newer anomaly on the youth sports landscape, particularly for interscholastic sports participation (i.e., middle and high school).

As budgets tighten, funding diminishes, and schools seek to trim extraneous costs; however, the use of pay-to-play has become a far more common and accepted practice. That does not mean, however, that it does not arouse controversy. To the contrary, pay-to-play is fiercely debated in many communities. The issue has garnered an equal number of supporters and detractors. The subject is not only debated by parents, coaches, and athletes, but also by sport governing bodies, youth sport nonprofit organizations, research institutes, and even politicians.

Pay-to-play did not begin to emerge as a widespread strategy for funding middle school or high school sports programs until the 1990s. Prior to that time, most public school athletic programs were wholly funded by local property taxes, millages, and other government sources. But reductions in state and federal support for public education, economic downturns, Title IX mandates, and steady expansion in the ambition of high school sports programs all put increasing pressure on schools to find other revenue to pay for their sports offerings. By 2004, according to *USA*

Today, pay-to-play had become a relatively common practice in at least 34 states (Bradley and Glier, 2004a). The economic recession that gripped the United States toward the end of the first decade of the new millennium made pay-to-play even more attractive to school systems looking to offset the rising costs of extracurricular activities, failing levies, and dwindling funding. In July 2004, for example, the Fairfield School District in Ohio voted to institute a pay-to-play model when a levy it had been attempting to pass failed for the fourth time in three years. Parents, students, and community members, fearing major reductions in school sport offerings, agreed to work toward charging a fee for children to participate in extracurricular activities (Bradley and Glier, 2004b). Their goal was to use the fees to help cover the costs without further straining school budgets or losing sports programs.

Pay-to-play became more widely known in 2010, when groups like the American Civil Liberties Union (ACLU) shone a light on its use as a means of limiting access for certain groups. For example, the ACLU informed several public school districts in California that they might be violating the law established in 1879 to provide free public schools and by extension, free educational programs to include extracurricular activities, which includes participation in school sports (Sapp, 2010). This clash sparked increased scrutiny of the practice and heightened public debate about the financial pressures facing many American schools. Nonetheless, pay-to-play arrangements continued to proliferate. By 2011 more than 60 percent of public high schools across the United States were charging some kind of participation fee for varsity sports (Hill, 2014).

This trend is deeply alarming to many observers who assert that the ability to represent one's school in athletic competition should not be dependent on the financial security of one's family. Even so, pay-to-play is legal. As long as schools are *asking* participants to help offset extracurricular costs and not *requiring* participation in these activities, they are not in violation of any laws. Most state laws prohibit schools from requiring extracurricular participation but have no regulations regarding charging for participation. Private schools tend to be another matter altogether. They are not considered part of the public education paradigm and therefore do not have to follow the same guidelines and laws as public schools.

Though some pay-to-play costs can be as low as $50 per season, per sport, there are reports of schools charging an average of $1,124 (White, 2016) per season for a student athlete. If a family has multiple children, or a single child is a multisport athlete, the costs can become prohibitively high. Many school districts offer annual caps or multisibling discounts to partially offset the compounding fees, but critics contend that such provisions do not do enough for families with financial struggles.

Arguments in Support of Pay-to-Play

Some proponents argue there are advantages to the pay-to-play model that benefit children in the long run and outweigh the short-term issues. Those who argue in support of the model tend to present the following tenets:

Pay-to-Play Is Offsetting or Stabilizing School District Budgets

As tax levies fail, federal and state funding decreases, and schools struggle to keep afloat with increasing per-student educational costs, many districts seek to ease the budgetary pressure by cutting the peripheral or nonessential programs. This includes clubs, extracurriculars such as dances, and sports. Cutting these programs can reduce district costs by tens of thousands of dollars, and since schools are not required by law to provide sports and clubs, it is a very easy decision to cut them (particularly in areas lacking a strong tradition in a certain sport). Schools that do charge a pay-to-play fee can continue to offer these programs and offset the budgetary constraints. Supporters of the sports and the pay-to-play model point to the practice as a means to keep a school financially healthy without having to cut programs. Requesting that participants pay for the sport means the cost is not absorbed by the school and that only participating students bear any cost. For those willing and able to pay, this creates a win-win. The school stays in the black and the kids get to play.

Pay-to-Play Maintains a Vital Part of the Academic Experience

Many argue that school sports and extracurricular activities are part of the greater academic experience. Sports are considered arenas for learning and applying values; gaining important life skills; positively extending the classroom experience; developing better health, responsibility, and accountability; promoting school and community spirit; and creating lifelong friendships. Many parents are willing to pay these fees in order to provide those long-term benefits to their children. Without the fees, those benefits are lost when the schools cut the programs. Children do need a balanced activity diet that, similar to the nutritional full plate model, fills their various activity needs. Extracurricular activities like sports provide an outlet for fulfilling the balanced activity needs of youth. If these needs are met, intellectual, psychological, physical, social, and emotional benefits abound. Many argue that given today's financial constraints on school districts, pay-to-play is necessary to provide students with balanced activity diet resources.

Pay-to-Play Preserves Long-Standing School Traditions

Supporters also assert that playing school sports is an essential aspect of the community and family experience. Entire towns across the United States subscribe to the "Friday Night Lights" mystique of supporting and cheering for the local school teams. Some small towns virtually shut down for big sporting events and match-ups with neighboring rivals. Those events become points of pride of entire communities. Families center their social world around the school and the school sports experience. School sports defines many families, schools, and towns across the nation. It is part of the fabric of what and who many Americans are. Cutting school sports is, to many people, altering the very definition of what it means to grow up in the United States. Instituting a pay-to-play model may be the necessary element to maintain a community identity for many people. Pay-to-play is justified in the eyes of proponents and ultimately may be necessary to maintain social, familial, and community traditions through sport and other activities.

Pay-to-Play Provides a Valuable Outlet for Child Identity and a Resource to Combat Societal Pressure and Adolescent Issues

Many believe youth athletes identify with the sports they play, and having that foundational identity during the difficult teen years is key to keeping kids grounded and emotionally healthy. Engagement in school sports can also combat other teen issues like alcohol abuse, gang membership, drug use, and delinquency. The pay-to-play model helps maintain the activities that "keep kids out of trouble." Research does show that kids who play sports tend to be more attentive at school, miss less school, maintain better grades, and are more active with school participation. Without the model, supporters argue that more youth will drop out of school, engage less with school personnel, and find other outlets that may not be as healthy.

Pay-to-Play Assists with Funding and Resources for Other Programs

Defenders of pay-to-play contend that such programs help offset the costs of other extracurricular activities sponsored by schools, including programs that benefit non-athletes. If football, for instance, becomes more self-supporting, the resulting savings can be used to provide funding for after school clubs. As schools and communities look for solutions to keep children active, involved in school, and learning valuable skills outside of the classroom, a pay-to-play model that keeps sports intact and provides resources and funding to other activities is appealing. Ticket sales at a large, successful sport can help fund activities for a larger majority of students. Paying to keep those sports guarantees total extracurricular participation rates stay high. In many school districts 60 to 70 percent of students are engaged in extracurricular activities. If school sports are cut, those other activities that share resources and facilities are endangered as well, and the overall number of students engaged could dip significantly.

Pay-to-Play Provides Access to Quality Resources, Coaches, and Mentors

Most athletes do not play sports for college scholarships or to become professional athletes. At their best, however, youth sports can help participants learn the value of teamwork, hard work, and other life skills at the hands of coaches and other mentors. These experiences can influence young people long after their playing days are complete. Some advocates believe the pay-to-play model gives schools more money to attract qualified professionals as coaches and staff for their school sports. These professionals tend to have more experience working with children, backgrounds that lend to coaching sports, and other skills that help them better serve the athletes than a volunteer coach. If the athletes are provided with the best resources, safe equipment, quality facilities, and exemplary people to serve as role models and mentors, some argue that the pay-to-play model is wholly worth the cost. Coaches can sometimes have a greater impact on children than any other person in their lives, and parents fear missing out on the known benefits of youth sport such as enhanced leadership and positive self-perceptions (Neely and Holt, 2014). Rather than face the thought of their children missing out on positive role models or other social benefits, parents are willing to pay to keep those people and experiences in their children's lives.

Fear of Missing Out

A final factor contributing to the growth of the pay-to-play model is that many parents reluctantly participate because of anxiety that refusing to do so will result in their child "missing out" on important school experiences. The focus and goal of youth sports over the last decade or more have shifted dramatically toward a belief that sports are a vehicle to the next level. Many would argue that sports are opportunities for college scholarships, thereby offsetting the rising costs of college, or an avenue to professional career opportunities even though NCAA and many other sources will cite that less than 1% of high school athletes will get a college scholarship and less than 1% of college athletes will turn professional. In order to keep up with other athletes playing year-round, specializing in one sport, and hiring specialty coaches, many parents are willing to endure the pay-to-play model in order to allow their child to play year-round in school one season and in club sport the remaining year or in some cases, both in the same season. The belief is the more the child plays, the better the child will be, and the more opportunities at exposure to scouts and external entities the child will have. People are willing to pay to ensure their child has the best opportunity to leverage sports for the next level.

Arguments against Pay-to-Play

Most arguments against pay-to-play tend to center around the inequalities believed to be inherent within the model. These include the following:

Pay-to-Play Prices Out Certain Members of a School Population

One of the biggest arguments against the pay-to-play model for schools sports is that the rising costs may be pricing students from low-income families out of sports completely. As costs to participate continue to increase, inflation pinches, and the income gap widens, many fear the lower middle-class and low-income families are the groups who will suffer most from pay-to-play arrangements. Low-income families tend to reside in school districts that may not have the money to maintain athletic programming, and pay-to-play is not a viable option to keep them. Sport has long been viewed as a positive influence in the lives of children of all income levels, but research shows participation rates are already decreasing in low-income families (Pew Social Trends, 2015). As costs to participate rise, and entire programs are cut in less affluent districts, the low-income children, many believe, would be the ones hit hardest. Districts that have more than 60 percent of families on free and reduced lunches, or annual household incomes of less than $25,000, face the hard truth that families who cannot afford lunch certainly cannot afford sports. The pay-to-play model could potentially remove what many consider to be one of the most positive influences in the lives of underserved populations.

Meanwhile, more affluent school districts that see pay-to-play as a viable path still include lower income families that find such outlays to be a financial hardship. In 2015, for example, the University of Michigan's Mott's Children's Hospital released the results of a poll of families with middle or high school–aged children. The poll found that whereas 51 percent of families making more than $60,000 annually had a child playing school sports, only 30 percent of families making less than $60,000 had a child participating in school athletics. The study found that 14 percent of the parents of children not playing school sports cited cost as the primary reason for nonparticipation. "The average cost for sports participation was $400 for child," explained one of the poll's directors. "For many families, that cost is out of reach. Many schools base participation fee waivers on eligibility for income-based programs like Medicaid or free and reduced lunch. That could exclude working families who earn too much for a waiver but may not be able to afford the additional cost of sports fees" (*Pay-to-Play Keeping Kids on the Sidelines,* 2015).

Pay-to-Play Causes a General Reduction in Sports Participation

With an overall reduction in youth sport participation already and nearly 70 percent of youth athletes dropping at least one sport by the age of 13 (Aspen Institute Project Play, 2016), opponents of the pay-to-play model believe the participation rates will continue to decline at a faster rate with the higher cost to participate. Families can spend as high as 10 percent of their household income for youth sports when factoring the costs to play club sports, travel, equipment, off-season training, coaching fees, and more. As families feel the pinch of the sport participation costs, they begin to make choices between activities, opt for school teams over club teams, move to districts where participation is free, or quit the sport altogether. For families in low-income households, or families without the means to move to other districts, the choice is easier: quit sports. This is further compounded by the continued increase in club sport costs. Depending on the sport, families can pay as high as $10,000 per season for their child to participate in elite-level clubs. If the elite-level clubs are promising quality coaches, better facilities, top of the line equipment, access to college scouts, and potential avenues to Olympic and professional play, this makes the choice for many families a difficult one.

Pay-to-Play Changes the Emphasis of the Youth Sports Experience

As the pay-to-play model spreads across school districts and the price to play rises, opponents warn it could change the emphasis of the youth sports experience. The more it costs to play, the more the emphasis is on outcomes rather than on the process of learning, the acquisition of skills, the psychosocial benefits, and the values learned. Greater emphasis is put on results to justify the costs. A district that is charging upward of $250 per sport for the children to play should have some concrete data to show the sport is worth the cost. These data typically come in the form of wins. The more wins, the more justified a school is in charging money. If a school cannot show wins, or increased ticket sales and sponsorship dollars as a result of the sport, that is when parents, district officials, and community members begin to question the viability of the sport. Or, at the very least, they may question the cost to play. As everyone struggles to justify the cost, the emphasis continues to be more about outcomes. This increased focus on outcomes could potentially have an impact on the experience of the athletes. Youth and adolescents may find themselves in settings where the values, lessons, education, skills, or overall enjoyment are not the primary emphasis; instead, they are expected to play sports solely to win. Worse, they may not be playing for themselves, but rather, playing for those trying to justify the cost. Many believe this threatens the very nature and core mission of youth sports.

Pay-to-Play Causes Drastic Shift in Youth Sport Dynamics

Many parents and school districts feel the pay-to-play model creates a commodity dynamic in school sports. With parents as customers, schools and coaches are the service providers, and with this mindset comes the belief that customers have a greater say in the design, production, and delivery of the product. The more a parent pays for the child to play, the more the parent feels entitled to be a part of the process. Traditionally, school sports were run by the coaches and schools, and parents merely showed up to watch the games. Many argue that parents are more likely to attend practices, coach from the sidelines at games, and badger coaches and school officials with phone calls and e-mails when they feel their money has bought them a right to argue playing time, tactical formations, coaching philosophies, and the like. The dynamic, according to pay-to-play opponents, is now one of "I pay you a lot of money so I have a say in how things are done."

Pay-to-Play Causes Inequities for "Minor" Sports

Many believe the pay-to-play model is detrimental to the smaller, less popular sports such as tennis or golf because it deters people from participating. In some models, fees across sports such as soccer and baseball can be the same or very close in amount, so choosing one from the other is an option. However, participants not used to paying individual instruction in tennis, for example or believing it is too expensive may opt out of the sport altogether. In addition, the larger, more popular sports such as football or soccer can be perceived as being more worth the investment than a smaller sport, and therefore garner more participants largely because they receive more exposure, have more participants, and the perception is that more scholarships are available.

Pay-to-Play Creates an "Investment Mentality" in Adults toward Their Children

In addition to a commodity mindset evolving from the pay-to-play model, some argue that the model also creates an "investment mentality" among parents. School sports may no longer be seen as a rite of passage, a family or community tradition, or an extension of the academic experience; but, rather, it may be seen by parents as an investment in their children's future. The emphasis on the cost, and subsequent outcomes, opponents argue, also creates a belief in parents that they are investing in some long-term benefit for their child. The more a parent pays for the child to play, the more the parent believes there is a need for a return on this investment via financially beneficial outcomes such as athletic scholarships or professional contracts. Concerns have been expressed that some parents get so caught up in the investment mentality that they lose sight of the long-term benefits of youth sport participation.

Pay-to-Play Results in an Adultification of Youth Sports

There are also opponents to this model who argue that the focus on money, on outcomes, and on return on investment makes the youth sports experience less about the kids and more about the adults. With the focus on adults and their investment, topics and agendas surrounding youth and school sports tend to shift from a child-centered to an adult-centered mentality. The fear is that this will fully shift the emphasis away from youth development and the associated benefits.

Dealing with Pay-to-Play

Whatever the merits and drawbacks of pay-to-play, all sides agree that the practice is likely to be a staple of public school sports funding for the foreseeable future. As with other youth sports issues such as long-term athletic development models, early specialization, or athlete burnout, each individual child and each family has to evaluate their own position when weighing whether to meet pay-to-play fees.

There are some guidelines that athletes, parents, and families can use to help assist in their decisions regarding pay-to-play:

1. **Start with the end in mind (realistically):** There are two things that parents should remember and focus on when considering youth and school sports and pay-for-play. First, the percentages of athletes who earn college scholarships or become professional athletes is miniscule. Therefore, the focus should be on child development. Whether children are 5, 10, or 18 years old, sport can be a valuable tool to assist them in learning lessons that will stick with them through adulthood. Recognize this aspect, and start from this base of understanding in evaluating youth and school sport decisions.

2. **Include the athlete in the decision:** The ultimate winner or loser in the issue is the child. Paying money for a child and setting performance expectations based on that cost can be damaging to the child, especially if he or she is not that enthused about participating. On the flip side, if the child really wants to participate but has no say, it can undermine relationships down the road. Parents should have frank discussion with their children to discover their needs, wants, expectations, and dreams. Work together to ensure, at the very least, that the child is involved in the final decision.

3. **Seek out alternatives and compare:** If money is an issue, but parents want their child to participate, review all the options available and compare the benefits of each. Does the school approve waivers of fees for families that meet economic hardship criteria? Would another activity at a lower cost make more sense? In this process consider the intangible needs. If it is about certain values, skills, and relationships that can be found in a less expensive alternative, that choice may be a better option. Many sports-based youth development organizations, such as The First Tee, Girls on the Run, and RBI Baseball programs, provide free or low-cost options for children that provide fabulous environments promoting development of healthy choices, self-esteem, and empowerment.

4. **Do not look at it as an investment for some future return:** It is difficult to take this mindset when the check clears, but this is about what is best for children in the long run. Parents should view pay-to-play as providing opportunity rather than an investment for a future return.

Reed Maltbie

Further Reading

Aspen Institute Project Play. 2016. *Youth Report.* Accessed May 10, 2017, at http://www.youthreport.projectplay.us.

Bradley, Erik, and Ray Glier. 2004a, July 29. *To Play Sports, Many U.S. Students Must Pay.* Accessed May 30, 2017, at https://usatoday30.usatoday.com/sports/preps/2004-07-29-pay-to-play_x.htm.

Bradley, Erik, and Ray Glier. 2004b, July 29. *In a Lot of Cases They Have No Other Choice.* Accessed May 8, 2017, at http://usatoday30.usatoday.com/sports/preps/2004-07-29-pay-for-play-choice_x.htm.

Changing the Game Project [Blog]. Accessed May 30, 2017, at http://changingthegameproject.com.

Hill, Darryl. 2014, January 31. "Fighting against 'Pay-to-Play' Sports." *Atlantic.* Accessed September 13, 2017, at https://www.theatlantic.com/politics/archive/2014/01/fighting-against-pay-to-play-sports/430575.

Neely, K. C., and Nicholas L. Holt. 2014. "Parents' Perspectives on the Benefits of Sport Participation for Young Children." *The Sport Psychologist, 28*(3): 255–268.

Pay-to-Play Keeping Kids on the Sidelines. 2015, January 20. University of Michigan Institute for Healthcare Policy and Innovation. Accessed September 13, 2017, at http://ihpi .umich.edu/news/pay-play-keeping-kids-sidelines.

Pew Social Trends. 2015. *Pew Research Center: Parents.* Accessed May 31, 2017, at http:// www.pewsocialtrends.org/2015/12/17/5-childrens-extracurricular-activities.

Popke, Michael. 2007, November. *With Budgets Tightening, Schools Struggle to Keep Sports Affordable.* Accessed May 8, 2017, at http://www.athleticbusiness.com/budgeting/with -budgets-tightening-schools-struggle-to-keep-sports-affordable.html.

Sapp, David. 2010, September 15. *ACLU Sues California over Public School Fees for Students* [ACLU blog]. Accessed May 8, 2017, at https://www.aclu.org/blog/speakeasy /aclu-sues-california-over-public-school-fees-students.

Up2Us Sports. 2012. *Going, Going, Gone: The Decline of Youth Sports.* Accessed May 30, 2017, at https://s3-us-west-2.amazonaws.com/up2us/uploads/center_resource/document /561/GoingGoingGone_Up2UsReport.pdf.

White, M. C. 2016. *Here's the Insane Amount the Average Parent Will Pay for After-School Activities.* Accessed September 12, 2017, at http://time.com/money/4425114/parents -rising-costs-after-school-activities.

Performance-Enhancing Drugs

Involvement in athletics can have many positive benefits for individual participants. In most cases, these positive benefits far outweigh the negative aspects of participation in sports, often caused by expectations, pressure, and physical stress. However, at times, these negative pressures can lead to the use of performance-enhancing substances by athletes. The use of performance-enhancing substances such as anabolic steroids, hormones, and organic supplements to enhance physical performance and appearance is prevalent in many societies today. Ethical, physical, and psychological concerns surround the use of such substances in all populations, particularly youth. Since the early 2000s, several studies have expressed concerns with the use of these substances in younger populations and the fact that very little is known about their safety, use, and efficacy among adolescents (e.g., Barkoukis, Lazuras, Tsorbatzoudis, and Rodafinos, 2013; Castillo and Comstock, 2007; Yesalis and Bahrke, 2000). This entry addresses the current state of performance-enhancing substance use in youth sports and strategies for dealing with improper use.

Approximately 2 million high school athletic injuries occur annually within the United States, and roughly one-quarter of all emergency department visits among adolescents are the result of sport-related injuries. Research studies indicate that controlled medications prescribed to adolescents during emergency room and hospital-based outpatient clinic visits have continued to grow at an alarming rate (Fortuna, Robbins, Caiola, Joynt, and Halterman, 2010). Commonly prescribed to alleviate pain, medications are often reported as being misused by athletes as young as 9 years of age (Bahrke, Yesalis, Kopstein, and Stephens, 2000). In addition, studies have shown that many supplements recommended to youth athletes dealing with injuries do not pass tests for safety, purity, and ingredient quality, are imported from foreign countries, or are taken in incorrect doses for safe consumption (Fox, 2010; Green, Catlin, and Starcevic, 2001). Whether intentional or not, the misuse of prescription medications in youth can have detrimental effects on the health and well-being of adolescent athletes.

According to the American Academy of Pediatrics (AAP), any substances taken in nonpharmacologic doses specifically for the purposes of improving sport performance are considered performance-enhancing substances. These substances include pharmacologic agents (prescription or nonprescription), agents used for weight control, physiologic agents used to enhance oxygen-carrying capacity, substances used for unintended reasons such as weight loss, or supplements taken at higher doses than required to replace deficits created by a disease state. Addressing and understanding misuse of performance-enhancing substances among adolescents begins with an examination of the means through which the adolescents obtain these substances. To explore this issue, Laure and Binsinger (2005) conducted a study of 6,402 adolescent athletes to determine the methods and means by which performance-enhancing substances were obtained. The study found that many adolescents had multiple avenues through which to obtain the substances and most commonly received these substances from friends and parents. The multiple points of access to performance-enhancing substances among adolescents only adds to the challenges associated with understanding the controversial and crucial issue.

In addition to prescription drugs, nutritional supplements are generally available without a prescription and may be used by adolescent athletes in an attempt to optimize, or alter, performance in some way. One example of a supplement popular among athletes of all ages is Creatine. As of 2016, Creatine is the most popular nutritional supplement in the United States, with over $400 million in annual sales. Creatine is classified as a nutritional dietary supplement under the category of an ergogenic aid. Ergogenic aids are substances chemically designed to advance athletic performance. Some ergogenic aids, including growth hormones, anabolic steroids, and erythropoietin, have been banned by major sports organizations such as the International Olympic Committee, International Softball Federation, World Taekwondo Federation, International Volleyball Federation, and International Federation of Sport Climbing, among many others. These substances also have been linked to increased vulnerability to life-threatening health risks. They are also associated with poor sportsmanship, as their use is regarded as cheating. However, nutritional supplements such as Creatine that are largely made up of naturally occurring compounds have been marketed as safe and legal performance-enhancing alternatives to banned agents. Alarmingly, many of these substances can be purchased over the counter by individuals of any age.

Other examples of legal performance-enhancing substances include glucosamine, calcium, and beta-hydroxy-beta-methylbutyrate (HMB). HMB is a nutritional supplement that is used to assist in strength gains and lean body mass in athletes. It is advertised as assisting in protein breakdown and minimizing damage to cells that may occur with intense exercise. Proponents of these nutritional supplements draw attention to the point that Creatine, HMB, and others are found in many foods and do not need to meet any of the FDA drug requirements. However, research on the use and safety of these supplements is preliminary and has not produced reliable or consistent outcomes. Researchers question the safety of these supplements due to the lack of data documenting the effects of their use for adolescent athletes. At this point, long-term effects have not yet been determined.

Since the late 1990s the use of performance-enhancing substances in athletics has sparked a heated discussion among researchers, health care professionals, parents, athletes, and coaches. Although many may believe that the use of performance-enhancing substances is most commonly associated with sports emphasizing strength, one study found that adolescent athletes ages 10 to 18 participating in both strength and nonstrength sports such as wrestling, weight lifting, tennis, cheerleading, and field hockey reported taking performance-enhancing substances (Metzl, Small, Levine, and Gershel, 2001). Studies have also found that white males are the most identified group among adolescent athletes to use performance-enhancing supplements (Dodge and Jaccard, 2006; Evans, Ndetan, Perko, Williams, and Walker, 2012). The potential negative health effects (both physical and psychological), as well as the ethical implications of the use of such substances, have been central to both discussions and research focuses.

Health risks associated with adolescent use of performance-enhancing substances are plentiful and include "death and a wide variety of cardiovascular, psychiatric, metabolic, endocrine, neurologic, infectious, hepatic, renal, and musculoskeletal disorders" (Pope et al., 2013, 341). Although of concern for any age group, these types of serious health matters can be detrimental to growth and development for adolescents and have lasting impacts well beyond the competitive sport participation time span. In adolescents, a range of negative physical implications have been associated with the use of performance-enhancing substances, including impotence, loss of hair, stunted growth, worsening acne causing scarring or "pitting," heart and liver damage, and increased risk of blood clots. Due to the alarming number of identified health risks, doctors and researchers alike encourage parents of youth athletes to explain the consequences of use prior to engaging in any substance consumption routine.

In addition to physical health concerns, psychological concerns associated with performance-enhancing substance use are critically important for adolescent athletes. Adolescent years are commonly associated with increased concerns about peer acceptance, body image, and athletic prowess. Research has shown that adolescent's use of performance-enhancing substances is closely associated with the athlete's expectations of success in sports. However, many psychological costs have been associated with substance use including aggressive behaviors, mood swings, hallucinations, delusions, and addiction. Furthermore, many symptoms become prevalent when users withdraw from use. These effects include depression, anxiety, insomnia, anorexia, headaches, and muscle and joint pains, among others.

Many psychological causes have been identified as to why athletes pursue the use of performance-enhancing substances. These causes include a societal fixation on winning and physical appearance (Yealis and Bahrke, 2000), championship status, popularity, and financial compensation (Stewart and Smith, 2008). Other factors that have been identified as contributing to an adolescent's use of substances include a desire to gain muscle mass or strength, a negative body image, and pressure from parents or peers regarding weight or muscle. In hopes of protecting the health of athletes and maintaining the virtues of fair competition, the U.S. National Federation of State High School Associations, along with most overseeing athletic organizations, oppose the use of performance-enhancing drugs. However, research studies have indicated that the use of performance-enhancing substances remains an issue in both collegiate and high school athletics. An athlete's belief of improved opportunity for success in sports is one attributed reason for the use of performance-enhancing substances. Athletes that believe success is a result of personal agency and the advancement of skills are prone to "develop adaptive motivational and behavioral styles and achieve their performance goals, as compared to athletes using external attribution" (Barkoukis, Lazuras, Tsorbatzoudis, and Rodafinos, 2013, 213). Social conceptions of substance use in sports are commonly associated with deception and cheating, and the penalties for use include fines, loss of eligibility, suspensions, and a ban from participation.

Lastly, in addition to physical and psychological health concerns, ethical considerations are also central to understanding the use of performance-enhancing substances. Although many of those who oppose the use of performance-enhancing substances in sports state that it is considered cheating and unfair, this is not the only form of opposition toward athletes using or abusing these substances. Opponents of performance-enhancing substances state that drugs are against the "spirit" of sport (Hemphill, 2009). The argument is that using these substances places the emphasis of sport primarily on winning and dismisses the value of hard work, safe training practices, and team ownership.

Making the case that youth should not use performance-enhancing drugs is made more difficult by the fact that many professional-level athletes have been associated with using performance-enhancing substances. Users have been identified in a wide range of professional level sports including competitive road bicycling, baseball, wrestling, and football, among others. Although some of these elite-level athletes may be properly using substances, opponents of performance-enhancing substances state that allowing these substances in amateur athletics, without proper advice and monitoring, poses a greater danger and should be prevented.

Current strategies for dealing with performance-enhancing substance use by adolescents primarily involve education and prevention strategies as well as interdiction and drug-testing programs. The U.S. Supreme Court has ruled that random drug testing in school districts is constitutional under the Fourth Amendment. These tests can identify if an individual has used the anabolic-androgenic form of steroids. However, research has indicated that these methods of detecting use are flawed due to the fact that many athletes will discontinue their use in anticipation of being tested (Kammerer, 2000). In addition, testing is sometimes performed by individuals with very little training in maintaining test purity and security. Additionally, alternative means of dosing are available that allow athletes to adjust their dose as to remain below the maximum allowed level. These mediums include skin gels containing testosterone and transdermal patches, among other means. Lastly, the cost of testing is expensive at approximately $120 per test and thus is unaffordable for many high school and amateur sports programs. Research has called for the development of new approaches aimed at arresting the increasing rate of doping in adolescent athletes (Dodge and Hoagland, 2011; Harmer, 2010). These recommended approaches continue to emphasize the importance of social environments during adolescence on future health behaviors, as well as coach training to recognize the signs and symptoms of athletes using such substances.

Research published in 2007 in the *Journal of Sports Science and Medicine* indicated that the effects of supplement use in adolescents remained unclear and thus should be discouraged (McDowall, 2007). However, parents and coaches need to know what signs to look for in identifying inappropriate use in adolescents. Although health and illness prevention are found to be the main reasons for taking supplements, adolescent female use is most frequently associated with health, recovery, and inadequate dieting, whereas adolescent male use is more frequently linked to enhanced performance goals. Red flags that parents and coaches should be aware of include increased aggressiveness, dramatic changes in body build, increased acne, unusual marks in the thighs or buttocks, and unusual changes in hair growth. Emphasizing healthy alternatives to achieving the same goals is encouraged and, when appropriate, appointments should be made for youth to see his or her doctor for a medical evaluation and counseling.

In her book *Eat Like a Champion,* Jill Castile addresses the need to discourage young athletes from supplement use by providing natural food swaps for supplements. Castile states that catfish and citrus fruits, such as orange and grapefruits, can provide the same nutrients that supplements, such as HMB, claim to provide. This is just one example of educational initiatives aimed at discouraging performance-enhancing substance use in youth athletics. The American Academy of Pediatrics (AAP) strongly condemns the use of performance-enhancing substances during adolescent years and endorses efforts to eliminate misuse in youth athletics. Conveying factual information about the proven benefits and medical risks of substance use is one recommended strategy. Scare tactics, as a means to discourage use, are not recommended due to the fact that many adolescents engage in risk-taking behaviors and experimentation while coping with developmental tasks such as defining their sexual identity, achieving self-efficacy, and seeking a peer group they can identify with. Instead, coaches and parents who identify adolescents that are using performance-enhancing substances are encouraged to explore the athlete's motivation for using the substances, evaluate other associated high-risk behaviors, and provide guidance on safer, more appropriate alternative methods such as weight training and proper diet for meeting the individual's performance goals.

The American Academy of Pediatrics has recommended that parents take a strong stand in opposition of the use of performance-enhancing substances and demand that coaches be educated about the physical, psychological, and ethical concerns of use. The detrimental impacts of performance-enhancing substance abuse by adolescents are alarming and cause for immediate and focused efforts to address this issue. Through education initiatives and open conversations by all parties involved, the issue of performance-enhancing substance use in youth sports can be better understood and addressed.

W. Hunter Holland

Further Reading

American Academy of Pediatrics Committee on Sports Medicine and Fitness. 2005. "Use of Performance-Enhancing Substances." *Pediatrics, 115*: 1103–1106.

Bahrke, M. S., C. E. Yesalis, A. N. Kopstein, and J. A. Stephens. 2000. "Risk Factors Associated with Anabolic-Androgenic Steroid Use among Adolescents." *Sports Medicine, 29*(6): 397–405.

Barkoukis, V., L. Lazuras, H. Tsorbatzoudis, and A. Rodafinos. 2013. "Motivational and Sportspersonship Profiles of Elite Athletes in Relation to Doping Behavior." *Psychology of Sport and Exercise, 12*(3): 205–212.

Castillo, E. M., and R. D. Comstock. 2007. "Prevalence of Use of Performance-Enhancing Substances among United States Adolescents." *Pediatric Clinics of North America, 54*(4): 663–675.

Castle, J. 2015. *Eat Like a Champion: Performance Nutrition for Your Young Athlete.* New York: AMACOM Division of American Management Association.

Dodge, T., and M. F. Hoagland. 2011. "The Use of Anabolic and Rogenic Steroids and Polypharmacy: A Review of the Literature." *Drug and Alcohol Dependence, 114*: 100–109.

Dodge, T. L., and J. J. Jaccard. 2006. "The Effect of High School Sports Participation on the Use of Performance-Enhancing Substances in Young Adulthood." *Journal of Adolescent Health, 39*(3): 367–373.

Evans, M. W., Jr., H. Ndetan, M. Perko, R. Williams, and C. Walker. 2012. "Dietary Supplement Use by Children and Adolescents in the United States to Enhance Sport Performance: Results of the National Health Interview Survey." *The Journal of Primary Prevention, 33*(1): 3–12.

Fortuna, R. J., B. W. Robbins, E. Caiola, M. Joynt, and J. S. Halterman. 2010. "Prescribing of Controlled Medications to Adolescents and Young Adults in the United States." *Pediatrics, 126*(6): 1108–1116.

Fox, M. 2010. "U.S. Dietary Supplements Often Contaminated: Report." *Reuters.* Accessed January 1, 2017, at https://www.reuters.com/article/us-usa-supplements/u-s-dietary-supplements-often-contaminated-report-idUSTRE6721F520100803.

Green, G. A., D. H. Catlin, and B. Starcevic. 2001. "Analysis of Over-the-Counter Dietary Supplements." *Clinical Journal of Sports Medicine, 11*: 254–259.

Harmer, P. A. 2010. "Anabolic-Androgenic Steroid Use among Young Male and Female Athletes: Is the Game to Blame?" *British Journal of Sports Medicine, 44*: 26–31.

Hemphill, D. 2009. "Performance Enhancement and Drug Control in Sport: Ethical Considerations." *Sport in Society, 12*(3): 313–326.

Kammerer, R. C. 2000. "Drug Testing and Anabolic Steroids." *Anabolic Steroids in Sport and Exercise*, 415–459.

Laure, P., and C. Binsinger. 2005. "Adolescent Athletes and the Demand and Supply of Drugs to Improve Their Performance." *Journal of Sports Science and Medicine, 4*(3): 272–277.

McDowall, J. A. 2007. "Supplement Use by Young Athletes." *Journal of Sports Science and Medicine, 6*(3): 337–342.

Metzl, J. D. 1999. "Strength Training and Nutritional Supplement Use in Adolescents." *Current Opinion in Pediatrics, 11*(4): 292–296.

Metzl, J. D., E. Small, S. R. Levine, and J. C. Gershel. 2001. "Creatine Use among Young Athletes." *Pediatrics, 108*(2): 421–425.

Pope, H. G., Jr., R. I. Wood, A. Rogol, F. Nyberg, L. Bowers, and S. Bhasin. 2013. "Adverse Health Consequences of Performance-Enhancing Drugs: An Endocrine Society Scientific Statement." *Endocrine Reviews, 35*(3): 341–375.

Stewart, B., and A. C. T. Smith. 2008. "Drug Use in Sport: Implications for Public Policy." *Journal of Sport and Social Issues, 32*: 278–298.

Strulik, H. 2012. "Riding High: Success in Sports and the Rise of Doping Cultures." *The Scandinavian Journal of Economics, 114*(2): 539–574.

Yesalis, C. E., and M. S. Bahrke. 2000. "Doping among Adolescent Athletes." *Best Practice & Research Clinical Endocrinology & Metabolism, 14*(1): 25–35.

Personal Trainers and Other Consultants

Youth sports have changed over the past few decades, from a world characterized primarily by unorganized play to one dominated by organized competitive sporting events that place an emphasis on winning rather than on fun and physical activity. The typical household with a child playing on a competitive travel team spends on average $2,266 on participation fees per year, according to the University of Florida Sport Policy and Research Collaborative & Aspen Project Play, 2014 Sport Participation Survey. The same survey indicates that at the elite level, the expense rises up to $20,000 annually, depending on the sport and the organization.

The growing prominence of competitive youth sports has led to emerging career fields designed to serve the demand from parents for premier training for their youth athletes. In this entry, individuals in these emerging career fields will be referred to as consultants since they are providing professional advice or training to their clients. The remaining sections of this entry will focus on the young athlete's physical development and physiology, as well as discussions of consultants of youth sports such as personal coaches, personal trainers, sport psychologists, and nutritionists.

Are Youth Ready for Intense Training?

Parents often ask, "When is it OK for me to hire a strength trainer, or when should my child start doing weight or cardiovascular training and not have it influence her growth or get her injured?" This line of questioning has intensified in many youth sports, as the pressure to be bigger, stronger, and faster mounts.

The youth athlete was previously restricted from participation in strength training due to fears surrounding growth plate damage. The position of the American College of Sports Medicine as of 2017 is that if young people are ready to participate in organized sport or activities they are able to enhance their musculoskeletal strength through strength training (Faigenbaum et al., 2009; Sugimoto et al., 2017). The youth may appear to be physically ready for strength training but must be monitored due to the emotional immaturity of youth. The use of strength-training programs that are utilized with adults is not recommended for youth athletes because they differ in physical anatomy, physiology, and psychology, which potentially makes the case for a trainer who is able to modify to a youth level.

Physical Anatomy

The physical anatomy differences present in youth include differences in physical stature; youth athletes are shorter, which results in a misalignment of their positioning on strength-training machines commonly found in fitness centers. Parents of youth athletes are accustomed to training with strength-training machines and will introduce their youth athlete to strength-training machines rather than free weights for a perceived safety advantage. However, due to the shorter stature of the youth athlete, better options are activities such as push-ups, pull-ups, and other body weight exercises.

The shorter stature does not inhibit the ability to develop motor skills and does not have to be an inhibiting factor in strength training. Physical exercise and strength training are both beneficial by increasing tendon, ligament, and bone strength and thus potentially decreasing some sports injuries. The incorporation of strength training for youth athletes may enhance their athletic experience and overall enjoyment because they may experience a competitive advantage over their peers. The research indicates that the earlier children begin strength training, the more likely they are to be physically active and participate in sports throughout their lives. In addition, as youth athletes are moving toward a more specialized model and overuse injuries are common, some elements of "monitored" strength training can act as a preventive measure against overuse injuries (Sugimoto et al., 2017).

Physiology

The physiological adaptations that occur during adolescence are the linchpin to the muscular development for the older child. Once a child hits puberty, hormonal adaptations occur in the youth athlete. A male experiences an increase in testosterone, allowing for muscle development resulting in increased strength. But the boy must also be aware of overtraining, which can lead to decreased muscular performance and diminishment of gains experienced. A female experiences an increase in estrogen, which launches the menstrual cycle. Training postpubescent youth athletes is something that must be done with caution, especially female athletes. The growth of competitive youth sports for girls, particularly the early developing sports such as gymnastics and swimming, has raised concerns about increases in the prevalence of the female athlete triad, a condition that can lead to early onset osteoporosis and loss of the menstrual cycle if not monitored by trained professionals.

The hormonal changes that are brought about due to puberty are the driving force in the physiological changes in youth. Girls and boys are fairly equal physiologically until they reach puberty; girls typically reach puberty earlier followed by boys. Girls do not lose their natural testosterone, but the increase in estrogen overpowers testosterone, leading to the decreased ability to build muscle mass to the same extent as their male counterparts.

Psychology

Although "kids will be kids" can be a common approach to raising a child, in a sport-training setting an absence of proper supervision and coaching can result in both physical injuries and emotional harm. Risk taking is a natural aspect of life but is seen in higher occurrence in youth due to the lack of a fully developed prefrontal cortex in the brain; the child is not able to fully judge the risk associated with an activity until the prefrontal cortex is fully developed by around age 25 (Boyer, 2006; Steinberg, 2005; Steinberg, 2008). The lack of a fully developed prefrontal cortex helps to explain the need for an understanding of the youth athlete's psychological profile before beginning a serious physical training regimen. Youth frequently feel that they have no choice but to follow instructions and guidance of older authority figures, so it is essential for those authority figures to be responsible in their development of training programs for youth athletes. Training programs should reflect an awareness of the youth athlete's psychological profile and their level of psychological maturity.

As youth sport continues to grow in its level of competition and as the expense of participation escalates, parents are increasingly seeking outside support to provide their children with a competitive edge. The people who serve in supplemental roles to coaches in youth sport are referred to as consultants because they are hired by the youth athlete's parents to aid in the athletic development of their child. These consultants can range from personal coaches and personal trainers to sport psychologists and nutritionists. Whereas the coach's focus is the team, the consultant's focus is the athlete for whom the consultant is employed. The consultant is running a business and offers services to those who can pay. Often the parents will seek these services when they feel their child athlete has the potential to earn a college scholarship or embark on a professional athletic career, some with children as young as 6 or 7. Parents typically perceive the increased expenditure as an investment in their child's future by increasing the likelihood that their child achieves his or her full athletic potential.

Parents draw cues from the United States' sports-saturated cultural environment as to which consultants may be beneficial for enhanced athletic success for their child. The allure of specialized training through consultants is readily visible through the consumption of sports media, especially ESPN that features shows utilizing personal coaches, personal trainers, sport psychologists, and nutritionists.

Personal Coaches

The number of personal coaches associated with youth sports has blossomed in the 21st century, growing to match the increasing demand from parents. Perhaps most importantly, these coaches are often utilized outside of the scope of the "team practice" and involve extra training sessions or activities. In the past, personal coaches were often seen in baseball, such as a personal hitting coach. The hitting coach was commonly a previous player or coach who saw an opportunity to generate revenue from helping youth baseball players become better hitters. The focus in such training efforts typically focused on improving swing mechanics in order to improve overall batting performance.

Personal coaches have long been a fixture in sports such as tennis and golf as they lend themselves to such training as a more individualized type of activity. A youth athlete may participate in golf or tennis at his or her school with an assigned school team coach. It is not uncommon, though, for the parents of these athletes to supplement the instruction of their sons and daughters through personal coaches. It would not be uncommon for a parent to spend $100+ per hour of additional personal coach instruction and have these lessons 3–5 hours per week. As such, personal coaches provide a unique consulting service to their clients but are typically available only to families that can afford their services. The role of the team coach is altered but is still pivotal in the student athlete's progress and performance. This is becoming a serious downfall of youth sports in the United States, that top level sport is largely designed for those that can afford it rather than the historical context of sport being played in the backyard leading to the growth of skill development.

Personal coaches have assumed increased prominence in other sports as well. Often these consultants have avenues to showcase the athlete's skills in off-season events. Many parents feel this will increase their student athlete's chances for consideration for a college scholarship even though what they often spend on the consultants could have easily paid for tuition in the first place.

Personal coaches can come from any background, but they typically are former players of the sport they are coaching. An example of this would be college students who are majoring in sport coaching, exercise science, or any related major. who feel that they could coach a specific sport to youth. The individuals may look to volunteer their time at a local youth sporting organization, seeking clients and hoping to prove to parents their knowledge of the sport and their capacity to provide helpful instruction. As most people perceive a direct correlation between price and quality, the better personal coaches can often charge the most for their services, further widening the gap between the more wealthy families that can afford the best consultants and those that can only afford the local coach, for example. Personal coaches are good for youth sport because coaches who understand proper technique and skill for a certain position or skill in a sport are able to teach the youth athlete proper technique. A youth athlete who is able to understand and implement proper technique may be able to steer off injury caused from poor technique (DiFiori, 1999; Micheli, Glassman, and Klein, 2000). The incorporation of a personal coach has its advantages to the youth athlete in teaching proper form and the development of skills that will enhance the overall mastery and enjoyment of the sport.

When parents are considering a personal coach for their child, a careful examination of the coach's background and expertise should be considered. The irony is that parents will spend more time shopping for a car than they will for a youth sport coach, and yet their child might spend 5, 10, or 20 hours a week with that person. As long as the parents can achieve goals of performance for their child, little thought is put into the values, beliefs, or personal background of the coach. Parents should do their homework by speaking to parents of other youth athletes who the personal coach has previously worked with. The personal coach must not only have an expertise over a particular skill set, but also must create an environment that is conducive for the psychological development of the youth athlete. Personal coaches must be fully vetted by the parent to ensure that proper instruction is being given, but also that the coach is instilling good morals and values to fully ensure that the parent is receiving the largest return on investment for his or her youth athlete.

Personal Trainers

Unlike personal coaches, who tend to be very sport specific skill development specialists, a quarterback coach in football or a hitting coach in baseball, a personal trainer is often someone who can help an athlete build strength, speed, endurance, or power that will benefit the youth athlete in a number of different sport activities. Personal trainers offer their services in a variety of locations and under various titles. Personal trainers are often visible in fitness centers around the United

States, offering their services for a fee to enhance the performance goals of their clients. According to the United States Bureau of Labor Statistics, personal trainers are expected to see a steady growth of 10% between 2016 and 2026. Most clients of personal trainers are adults with disposable income, but there are indications that affluent parents increasingly view personal trainers as a potential resource to help their children better their athletic performance as well. This increase in personal training services for young athletes has led to adjustments in certification and training, although not all consultants calling themselves "trainers" have any level of certification at all. As a result, the various certification bodies have adjusted to the market by offering youth training certifications for professionals in the industry. Personal training certification for youth athletes is fairly easy to obtain and often only requires paying a fee of approximately $400–$500 for a training course. Upon completion of the course and passage of a certification exam, the personal trainer may be certified for working with youth. However, not all certification can be obtained so simply. For example, the American College of Sports Medicine and the National Strength and Conditioning Association require the completion of a college degree for one to be eligible for a certification exam, with an additional exam required for certification in training youth.

The cutting edge of personal training, though, is in the development of private performance centers aimed at youth sport athletes. The personal trainers at these facilities have rebranded themselves as performance specialists and market their services directly to youth sport athletes.

When seeking a personal trainer, it is imperative that the parent understands the personal trainer's background, education, and experience working with youth athletes. In addition, the goals of the personal training relationship need to be communicated to make sure that the youth client is best served in the relationship. As with the personal coach, the relationship between personal trainer and youth athlete is a critical component to the success of the partnership; the personal trainer must be able to develop a positive psychological relationship with the youth athlete.

As such, a detailed plan should be constructed between the personal trainer, youth athlete, and parents, and coaches from the sport should also be included so as to bring a more holistic understanding to the athlete's training regimen. Often youth athletes will not tell their sport coach that they are also seeing a personal trainer for fear of implying that the training they are receiving from their coach is not adequate. However, if the sport coach does not know a player is undergoing additional training "on the side," the young athlete may be at greater risk of suffering an overuse injury.

Depending on the age of the athlete when a personal trainer is utilized, a general strength and conditioning development plan should be instituted to increase overall strength, flexibility, and cardiovascular fitness Working with a personal trainer often teaches the foundations of training that will benefit the youth athlete later on in adulthood.

Sport Psychologist

Sport psychology is a budding area for youth sport athletes because of the demands that competitive sport, whether in club/travel or school settings, can place on the emotions and mental capacities of participants. Advocates of sports psychology say that it can help expedite the psychological maturity needed for an advanced level of competition and give young athletes, male or female, the tools to thrive in pressure-packed environments. With the thousands of dollars spent on youth sport, and many family budgets stretched thin simply to allow the child to participate at the highest levels, this brings with it an added stress that the youth athlete often feels the financial burden of the family is on the athlete's shoulders. So even beyond the pressures of the sport setting, the other elements of being involved in sport, particularly at a high level, are evident to the young athlete.

Although some universities offer specialized training in sport psychology, a majority of sport psychologists are trained in psychology and expand their practice to match market demands. Sport psychologists serve their clients by teaching them techniques to focus their minds in the correct state to maximize their competitive abilities and keep sport-related pressures from becoming overwhelming. However, often the pressures of adult or early adult athletes are radically different than those of a young 12-year-old athlete, and therefore a sport psychologist who deals particularly with youth is very important. Ideally, they can instruct the youth athletes in developing various coping techniques that will enable them to continue to enjoy sports, whatever the level of competition, and then to also continue to enjoy the sport beyond childhood.

Nutritionists

Nutritionists are also more likely to find themselves with young athletes as clients than ever before. They often provide services supplementary to those of personal trainers or coaches, who may be fairly well-versed on issues of nutrition but still typically do not possess the expertise of a trained nutritionist. The nutritionist can educate the youth athlete and her or his family on proper diet and food preparation practices that are conducive to high athletic performance. A nutritionist should be selected carefully, and an examination of background, education, and certification should be done to ensure that the nutritionist is knowledgeable in the field. The ideal situation for working with a nutritionist would be one that involves the whole family in an effort to improve the overall diet of parents and children alike. If the expense of a nutritionist is too much for the family, a family could seek prepared foods that are cooked by a nutritionist for the youth athlete to consume as a substitute for fast food meals that often prove convenient for families and athletes shuttling back and forth from home to school to practice and back.

Nicholas Schlereth

Further Reading

Boyer, Ty W. 2006. "The Development of Risk-Taking: A Multi-Perspective Review." *Developmental Review, 26*(3): 291–345.

DiFiori, John P. 1999. "Overuse Injuries in Children and Adolescents." *Physician and Sportsmedicine, 27*(1): 75–90.

Faigenbaum, Avery D., and Gregory D. Myer. 2010. "Resistance Training among Young Athletes: Safety, Efficacy and Injury Prevention Effects." *British Journal of Sports Medicine, 44*(1): 56–63.

Faigenbaum, Avery D., William J. Kraemer, Cameron J. R. Blimkie, Ian Jeffreys, Lyle J. Micheli, Mike Nitka, and Thomas W. Rowland. 2009. "Youth Resistance Training: Updated Position Statement Paper from the National Strength and Conditioning Association." *The Journal of Strength & Conditioning Research, 23*: S60–S79.

Micheli, Lyle J., Rita Glassman, and Michelle Klein. 2000. "The Prevention of Sports Injuries in Children." *Clinics in Sports Medicine, 19*(4): 821–834.

Steinberg, Laurence. 2005. "Cognitive and Affective Development in Adolescence." *Trends in Cognitive Sciences, 9*(2): 69–74. doi:10.1016/j.tics.2004.12.005

Steinberg, Laurence. 2008. "A Social Neuroscience Perspective on Adolescent Risk-Taking." *Developmental Review, 28*(1): 78–106.

Sugimoto, Dai, Andrea Stracciolini, Corey I. Dawkins, William P. Meehan III, , and Lyle J. Micheli. 2017. "Implications for Training in Youth: Is Specialization Benefiting Kids?" *Strength & Conditioning Journal, 39*(2): 77–81.

Role Models

A role model is defined by *Webster's Online Dictionary* (2015) as "a person whose behavior in a particular role is imitated by others." A role model can be a great teacher of values, skills, and knowledge—especially to youth (Cruess, Cruess, and Steinert, 2008). Most people who reflect back on their lives can remember someone who significantly impacted them, positively or negatively. Perhaps that person was a parent who took the child to all of her soccer games and cheered her on in positive ways. Maybe it was a peer on a tee-ball team who showed great leadership. Or a coach who was a reliable source of encouragement throughout the trials and tribulations of athletic performance. On the other hand, parents can shatter a young person's confidence by yelling about making mistakes during a game. Similarly, teammates can destroy confidence and enjoyment by belittling fellow players for underperforming, and coaches can make young players question their ability by depriving them of playing time. Such negative influences can lead young players to drop out of a sport altogether. Young players who recall these people, their actions, and how they made them feel know well that such individuals can have a powerful influence as role models, for better or worse.

Sport, in particular, is a context within which role models can have an influential impact on youth. It is the display of leadership from role models within sport that greatly affects the quality of youth experiences (Cuskelly, Hoye, and Auld, 2006). The benefits that flow from modeling positive behaviors are far-reaching, including enhanced self-concept, social competence, moral development, and regular physical activity (Malina and Cumming, 2003). At the same time, role models who display unwelcome behaviors such as poor sportsmanship or an overemphasis on winning can contribute to unwarranted stress, poor self-esteem, and a lack of respect for others (McCallister, Blinde, and Kolenbrander, 2000). Role models, in sum, have a responsibility to make their behavior worthy of imitation by the youth they serve. To that end, this entry focuses on individuals commonly considered to be role models in youth sports, discusses the impacts of their behaviors on youth, and concludes with recommendations for educating and employing role models to promote positive youth development.

Role Models at Different Stages of Life

Many people serve as role models in youth sport settings, including parents, peers, coaches, and professional athletes. Youth often identify with role models who share their own background, age, ability, and gender. Youngsters who identify with a role model experience increased self-efficacy and believe they can succeed like their role model. Once they see individuals as role models, youngsters begin to emulate them. For example, during early years of development, youngsters often look up to their parents as role models. When they enter school, peers and teachers play an increasingly important role. Moving into adolescence, youngsters often begin to aspire to be like their coaches and professional athletes. Although there are often differences between boys and girls in this shift from parents to peers and teachers to coaches and professional athletes, the centrality of role models in youth development continues (Bailey, Wellard, and Dismore, 2004). It is important, therefore, to examine parents, peers, and coaches, in particular, as role models in youth sports as well as acknowledging the special role professional athletes can play.

Parents

Parents can and should play an important supportive role in youth sports. They can be cheerleaders, offering words of encouragement, and can applaud effort regardless of outcome. Research suggests that youth experiencing positive parental reinforcement challenge themselves more, feel less pressured to play, and are intrinsically motivated to participate (Smith and Smoll, 2011). Alternatively, when a young person makes a mistake in the course of play, a parent's reaction can also lead to negative reinforcement. By yelling at a child, a parent can promote negative feelings. In such instances, shouts directed at referees, coaches, or other parents set the wrong example. Unfortunately, this is an all too common occurrence. An increasing number of parents have become disruptive while watching their children play in youth sport leagues. In a Survey USA poll (Bach, 2006), 74 percent of parents surveyed in Indianapolis reported witnessing other parents yelling at their children and referees, 55 percent reported witnessing others involved in verbal disputes, and 22 percent reported witnessing physical altercations.

A primary reason why parents exhibit bad behavior is that they forget youth sports exist to promote physical and psychosocial growth and development for their children (Smith and Smoll, 2011). Increasingly, sport administrators have embraced a professional sports model in their youth sports programs, where the emphasis is placed on winning-at-all-costs (Smith and Smoll, 2011). In such a competitive atmosphere, parents are prone to be highly critical and sometimes develop unrealistic expectations for their youngster's performance (Bach, 2006). Research has shown, however, that early specialization negatively affects youth sport experiences and does not prepare youth for being successful athletes later in life (Malina, 2010). Therefore, training sessions have been recommended for some parents to help them shift their mindset from treating youngsters like professional athletes to treating them like the highly impressionable young people they are.

Many parents are unaware of how their behaviors impact their youngsters in sport settings. To rectify this situation, as an example, the Parents Association for Youth Sports (PAYS) program conducts training sessions for youth sport parents that are intended to minimize bad parental behavior and provide resources to help parents exhibit positive behavior for youngsters to imitate. The PAYS training consists of a 40-minute session that can be carried out online or during a live meeting at a community sports organization's office. The training video features Chris McKendry, an ESPN Sports Center anchor, and covers topics such as safety, injury prevention, and modeling sportsmanship. The session educates parents regarding their roles and responsibilities, as well as what they can do to make their youngsters' sport experiences positive. Evaluations of the PAYS training program attest to its effectiveness. Indeed, many parents think the training should be mandatory. Most importantly, parents feel the program contributes to improving their behavior as well as that of other spectators (Bach, 2006).

Peers

Role models can also be peers such as a teammate, friend, or classmate. Peers can have a powerful positive or negative impact on a young person's effort, aggression, conflict resolution, sociability, and moral development (Smith, 2003). When peers in a sport setting demonstrate good behavior, youth benefit greatly. For example, a teammate may exhibit sportsmanship that another player emulates. Or a player may offer words of encouragement to a teammate who needs a confidence boost. A team that promotes player self-improvement, supports all teammates, and uses teammates' mistakes as learning experiences, creates a positive sport culture (Miulli and Nordin-Bates, 2011). This supportive culture increases youngsters' intrinsic motivation and persistence in sport (Joesaar, Hein, and Hagger, 2011).

A peer can also have a negative impact on a youngster's life. Undesirable behaviors among peers such as unsportsmanlike conduct, hazing, foul play, and brawling have been witnessed all too often in youth sports. There have been instances when teammates haze new players by making them perform embarrassing or humiliating team traditions to gain team membership. Unfortunately, research suggests that a young person is more likely to exhibit bad behavior when peers are doing the same (Fredricks and Eccles, 2005). Teammates who are deviant or distressed model their unwelcome behavior to other players (Fredricks and Eccles, 2005). A team that tolerates such negative behavior can exacerbate the behavior. Such negative behavior must be counteracted by players serving as good role models. Fortunately, encouraging peers to be good role models in sport can be fostered through moral and character development training sessions.

Character development education is readily available to youth sport teams. A good example is *Winning in Life: A Team Life Skills Program* (Stoll and Herman, 2002). In this program athletes examine moral and social issues in sport through reading, writing, discussion, and reflection. Athletes are challenged to discuss issues concerning honesty, fair play, responsibility, and decency toward others (Stoll and Beller, 2000). The goal is for players to develop a positive set of moral principles to live by in sport and life. This program is run by skilled and well-educated moral development specialists and has been highly effective in helping improve athletes' ethical behavior (Stoll and Beller, 2000).

Less time-intensive programs involve education through training videos. The *Fair Play Everyday* video was developed at the Center for Ethics at the University of Idaho. The video shows coaches and athletes in three common sport scenarios. Athletes and coaches are then asked if the scenarios seem honest, fair, and promote cooperation (Stoll and Beller, 2000). Studies assessing moral education strategies have shown them to improve athletes' moral conduct and reasoning (Beller, 2002). A U.S.-based organization called Stop Hazing also assists teams having difficulties with players subjecting their teammates to hazing practices. Stop Hazing aims to "promote safe school, campus and organizational climates through research, information sharing and the development of data-driven strategies for hazing prevention" (Stop Hazing, 2015).

Coaches

Coaches are also very important role models in sport settings. Youngsters look up to their coaches as "experts" for guidance and leadership, and their feedback and behavior are taken seriously. The responsibilities of a coach vary from providing direction during practices and games, to developing practice drills, to overseeing equipment, assigning team roles, contacting parents, as well as many other tasks. Many coaches volunteer their time and perform their duties without compensation. Indeed, youth sport leagues often allow anyone interested in coaching to do so. Frequently, however, coaches' backgrounds do not equip them with the skills needed to be effective role models who promote positive youth development (Wiersma and

Sherman, 2005). There are few guidelines on how volunteers should coach, leaving youth sport coaches largely on their own to develop their coaching philosophy, objectives for the season, and performance outcomes for youth (Gilbert and Trudel, 2004).

Coaching philosophies thus run the gamut. Coaches can be very positive and supportive, placing much emphasis on skill development and mastery. This type of philosophy is more apt to encourage and motivate youth to continue their involvement in sport, because they have more positive experiences with accomplishments/achievements, teamwork, fitness, energy release, skill development, friendship, and fun (Gilbert and Trudel, 2004). On the other hand, some coaches have a win-at-all-costs mentality, which puts youth at risk for harmful developmental effects. These coaches typically are less encouraging and supportive, and more controlling of their athletes. Coaches who place a heavy emphasis on winning have frequently been cited as a common contributor to youth dropping out of sports. Players feel there is too much pressure, time commitment, and lack of fun (Gilbert and Trudel, 2004). Most of these coaches have good intentions, but they are too often unaware that their coaching priorities can have far-reaching negative impacts on youth. Fortunately, educational resources are also readily available to help them recognize the effect their coaching behavior can have on a young player's development.

Youth sports advocates believe that coaches should be offered training sessions to ensure they possess the necessary skills to create a positive atmosphere conducive to youth development through sport. In other kinds of sport organizations, when a new hire or volunteer begins working, it is common for them to undergo training sessions to equip them with the requisite skills to be successful in their duties. Youth sport organizations, on the other hand, do not generally follow this approach. Many states, school districts, and sport organizations in the United States do not require coaching credentials or certifications. However, there are many formal coach training programs and curricula available, which can significantly improve the quality of sport programs offered. These training sessions provide high-quality resources, tools, and education to coaches. Examples include Coach Effectiveness Training (CET), American Coach/Sport Education Program (ACEP/ASEP), National Youth Sport Coaches Association (NYSCA), and Positive Coaching Alliance (PCA). Once coaches have completed such training, many programs confer a coaching certificate.

Coach Effectiveness Training (CET), developed by Ronald E. Smith and Frank L. Smoll, is good example of such a training program. It is a 2-hour program that teaches coaches how to develop programs that emphasize skill development, provide encouragement for players, and avoid negative behavior such as yelling and punishment. Coaches monitor their own progress by using a form they complete after each practice and game. The form allows coaches to reflect on the percentage of interactions in which they provide positive reinforcement, encouragement, and skill development instruction. The training also teaches coaches a technique called "the positive sandwich." When a player makes a mistake during practice or a game, the coach finds something positive that occurred during play, gives skill development instruction on how to resolve the mistake made, and then offers words of encouragement at the end. During the training sessions emphasis is placed on winning as a fundamental aspect of sports, but highlights that sport should be predominantly focused on fun, reducing anxiety, and improving individual performance as the best way to foster youth development (Munsey, 2010). Coach Effectiveness Training has evaluations to support its effectiveness as well. Coaches trained through the Coach Effectiveness Training program create an atmosphere that athletes perceive as more fun, resulting in increased team unity when compared to untrained coaches. Trained coaches heighten participation levels, increase athletes' self-esteem, and decrease anxiety. Moreover, fewer youth drop out of sports under their tutelage (Smoll and Smith, 2006).

Professional Athletes

Youth participating in sports also tend to admire elite athletes. Indeed, the media often lionize elite athletes. Consequently, people often expect elite athletes to be positive role models. Bill Bradley, American Hall of Fame Basketball player, reinforces this sentiment: "Sport is a metaphor for overcoming obstacles and achieving against great odds. Athletes, in times of difficulty can be important role models" (New University, 2012). Other athletes do not think they have an obligation to be a role model to youth. Charles Barkley, a retired professional basketball player, famously summarized this perspective in 1993 when he stated, "I'm not a role model, parents should be role models. Just because I dunk a basketball doesn't mean I should raise your kids" (St. Helena Star, 2014). There is an obvious difference of opinion about whether or not athletes should take on the responsibility of being a good role model to youth. Therefore, youth sport practitioners cannot endorse that professional athletes should undergo role model training. Still, professional athletes play a special role in influencing young athletes, and they can promote youth sport programs and model positive qualities for youth by acting as "champions" for youth sports leagues.

"Champions" are spokespersons for organizations and their programs. They communicate the organization's goals and objectives by "attending events, reaching out to media, and attracting a wider audience" (O'Reilly and Burnette, 2013). Many community sports programs, recognizing youngsters' attraction to famous personalities, make use of athletes who demonstrate positive behavior and consider themselves a role model to promote certain desirable qualities in sport and in life through discussions and other interactions with youth (Bricheno and Thornton, 2007). A champion is very effective in building awareness, expanding organizational networks, and broadcasting the credibility of the organization. When choosing an individual to champion a youth sports program, the athlete's success needs to seem attainable so he or she can encourage and inspire youth. Youngsters can be discouraged if elite athletes seem different from them and if their kind of success appears beyond reach (Vescio, Wilde, and Crosswhite, 2005). Therefore, when picking an athlete to champion an organization, one should consider the athlete's lifestyle and behavior. An athlete should be chosen whose lifestyle, habits, behavior, and values reflect those of the organization and youth being served (O'Reilly and Burnette, 2013).

Amy Purdy, a 2014 Paralympic Bronze Medalist in snowboarding, champions an organization called the Challenged Athletes Foundation. The foundation's mission is "to recognize the athletic greatness inherent in all people with physical challenges and support their athletic endeavors by providing unparalleled sports opportunities that lead to success in sports—and in life" (Challenged Athletes Foundation, 2015). Purdy has a similar background to many of the youth being served by the Challenged Athletes Foundation. She uses prosthetics that allow her to snowboard. Her success as a Paralympic snowboarder comes across as attainable to youth with disabilities, especially given the resources and equipment the foundation provides to support their athletic aspirations. Still other elite athletes champion their own organizations. NBA player Lebron James, for example, started the Lebron James Family Foundation, whose mission is "to positively affect the lives of children and young adults through education and co-curricular educational initiatives. We believe," James continues, "that an education and living an active, healthy lifestyle is pivotal to the development of children and young adults" (The Lebron James Family Foundation, 2013). These examples demonstrate that an elite athlete can be a positive role model for youth by being a "champion" of youth sport organizations and programs.

Conclusion

In sum, sport can be a powerful medium for turning young people into accomplished, responsible adults. Youngsters need positive role models, however, to demonstrate the best of behavior as they hone their life skills through youth sport. Sports administrators have a variety of resources at their disposal to help parents, peers, coaches, and elite athletes learn how their behavior impacts others, how they can improve their behavior, and how their improved behavior can enhance the lives of the youth they serve through sport.

Cait Wilson

Further Reading

Bach, Greg. 2006, August 1. *The Parents Association for Youth Sports: A Proactive Method to Spectator Behavior Management.* Accessed August 5, 2015, at http://www.tandfon line.com/doi/abs/10.1080/07303084.2006.10597888.

Bailey, Richard, Ian Wellard, and H. Dismore. 2004, February 18. *Girls Participation in Physical Activities and Sports: Benefits, Patterns, Influences and Ways Forward.* Accessed July 25, 2015, at https://www.icsspe.org/sites/default/files/Girls.pdf.

Beller, Jennifer Marie. 2002. *Positive Character Development in School Sport Programs.* Washington, D.C.: ERIC Clearinghouse on Teaching and Teacher Education.

Bricheno, Patricia, and Mary Thornton. 2007. "Role Model, Hero or Champion? Children's Views Concerning Role Models." *Educational Research, 49*: 1–22.

Challenged Athletes Foundation. 2015. *What We Do Overview.* Accessed August 3, 2015, at www.challengedathletes.org/site/c.4nJHJQPqEiKUE/b.6449069/k.F6A2/What_We _Do_Overview.htm.

Coakley, Jay. 2011. "Youth Sports: What Counts as 'Positive Development'?" *Journal of Sport & Social Issues, 35*: 306–324.

Cruess, Sylvia R., Richard L. Cruess, and Yvonne Steinert. 2008. "Role Modelling— Making the Most of a Powerful Teaching Strategy." *BMJ, 336*: 718–721.

Cuskelly, Graham, Russell Hoye, and Chris Auld. 2006. *Working with Volunteers in Sport: Theory and Practice.* New York: Routledge.

Fraser-Thomas, Jessica, Jean Côté, and Janice Deakin. 2005. "Youth Sport Programs: An Avenue to Foster Positive Youth Development." *Physical Education & Sport Pedagogy, 10*: 19–40.

Fredricks, Jennifer A., and Jacquelynne S. Eccles. 2005. "Developmental Benefits of Extra-curricular Involvement: Do Peer Characteristics Mediate the Link between Activities and Youth Outcomes?" *Journal of Youth and Adolescence, 34*: 507–520.

Gilbert, Wade. D., and Pierre Trudel. 2004. "Role of the Coach: How Model Youth Team Sport Coaches Frame Their Roles." *Sport Psychologist, 18*: 21–43.

Joesaar, Helen, Vello Hein, and Martin S. Hagger. 2011. "Peer Influence on Young Athletes' Need Satisfaction, Intrinsic Motivation and Persistence in Sport: A 12-month Perspective." *Psychology of Sport and Exercise, 12*: 500–508.

The Lebron James Family Foundation. 2013. *Mission.* Accessed August 1, 2015, at http://lebronjamesfamilyfoundation.org.

Malina, Robert M. 2010. "Early Sport Specialization: Roots, Effectiveness, Risks." *Current Sports Medicine Reports, 9(6)*: 364–371. doi:10.1249/JSR.0b013e3181fe3166

Malina, Robert, and Sean P. Cumming. 2003. *Youth Sports: Perspectives for a New Century.* Monterey, CA: Coaches Choice.

McCallister, Sara, Elaine Blinde, and Bill Kolenbrander. 2000. "Problematic Aspects of the Role of Youth Sport Coach." *International Sports Journal, 4*: 9–26.

Miulli, Michelle, and Sanna M. Nordin-Bates. 2011. "Motivational Climates: What They Are, and Why They Matter." *International Association for Dance Medicine & Science, 3*: 5–6.

Munsey, Christopher. 2010. "Coaching the Coaches." *Monitor Staff, 41*: 58.

New University. 2012. *Role Models: Athletes Hold the Responsibility to be Good Examples.* Accessed September 5, 2015, at www.newuniversity.org/2012/04/sports/role-models -athletes-hold-the-responsibility-to-be-good-examples.

O'Reilly, Norm, and Michelle Burnette. 2013. *Public-Private Partnerships in Physical Activity and Sport.* Champaign, IL: Human Kinetics.

Smith, Alan L. 2003. "Peer Relationships in Physical Activity Contexts: A Road Less Traveled in Youth Sport and Exercise Psychology Research." *Psychology of Sport and Exercise, 4*: 25–39.

Smith, Ronald E., and Frank L. Smoll. 2011. "Cognitive-Behavioral Coach Training: A Translational Approach to Theory, Research, and Intervention." In J. Luiselli and D. Reed (Eds.), *Behavioral Sport Psychology* (pp. 227–248). New York: Springer.

Smoll, Frank L., and Ronald E. Smith. 2006. "Enhancing Coach-Athlete Relationships: Cognitive-Behavioral Principles and Procedures." In J. Dosil (Ed.), *The Sport Psychologist's Handbook* (pp. 19–37). Chichester, England: John Wiley & Sons.

St. Helena Star. 2014. *Remembering Charles Barkley's Role Model Theory.* Accessed September 7, 2015, at napavalleyregister.com/star/sports/remembering-charles-barkley-s -role-model-theory/article_e8855e8f-ba4e-5b95-a899-1a084a8b06ca.html.

Stoll, Sharon K., and Jennifer M. Beller. 2000. "Do Sports Build Character?" In J. R. Gerdy (Ed.), *Sports in School: The Future of an Institution* (pp. 18–30.). New York: Teachers College Press.

Stoll, S. K., and C. R. Herman. 2002. *Winning in Life: A Team Life Skills Program.* Center for Ethics, University of Idaho, Moscow, ID.

Stop Hazing. 2015. *About Us.* Accessed September 14, 2015, at http://www.stophazing.org/about.

Taylor, Jim, and Gregory Scott White. 2005. *Applying Sport Psychology: Four Perspectives.* Champaign, IL: Human Kinetics.

Vescio, Johanna, Kerrie Wilde, and Janice J. Crosswhite. 2005. "Profiling Sport Role Models to Enhance Initiatives for Adolescent Girls in Physical Education and Sport." *European Physical Education Review, 11*: 153–170.

Webster's Online Dictionary. 2015. *Role Model.* Accessed July 30, 2015, at www.merriam -webster.com/dictionary/role%20model.

Wiersma, Lenny D., and Clay P. Sherman. 2005. "'Volunteer Youth Sport Coaches' Perspectives of Coaching Education/Certification and Parental Codes of Conduct." *Research Quarterly for Exercise and Sport, 76*: 324–338.

Role of Play in Sports-Based Youth Development

Children love to play. Play is a foundational experience that allows children to explore their world, express themselves, enjoy the company of others, and practice a wide range of skills. With characteristics like challenge, novelty, learning, and time (Jensen, 2001), play represents the full integration of body and mind (Hannaford, 2005). As one of the four core pathways of human experience, play (along with work, ritual, and civic celebration), represents a primary pathway for human expression (*American Journal of Play,* 2015). For many youth, play and sport go hand in hand, but the relationship between sports and play has evolved over time. What children once experienced as free time "pickup sports" has quickly become structured, adult-directed activities. As Dr. Peter Gray, a Boston College developmental psychologist and an expert on the evolution of childhood play notes, "over the decades, [there] has been a continuous and ultimately dramatic decline in children's opportunities to play and explore in their own chosen ways" (Gray, 2013, 2). With these changes in mind, this entry explores the notion of play within the context of sport, examining not only how play may contribute to youth development through sport, but also how play experiences may be dwindling. Through this examination of youth play and sport, we will explore the current state of play and consider what the future of play may hold.

The term *play* can be applied to a wide range of activities and behaviors that are freely chosen, enjoyable, and creatively engaging (Stegelin, Fite, and Wisneski, 2015). Children play on their own, and they play with others (Stegelin, Fite, and Wisneski, 2015). Play can be quiet and thoughtful or energetic and engaging. It can take many forms, including free or unstructured play, indoor and outdoor games, and even participation in a play-based curriculum. Due in part to the diverse ways that play can be expressed, play experiences can make a rich contribution to a child's growth and development. For example, research suggests linkages between play and memory, language, social development, and school success (National Association for the Education of Young Children, 2009).

Declines in Youth Play

In *Children at Play: An American History* (2007), Howard Chudacoff described the first half of the 20th century as the golden age of children's free play. Because the need for child labor declined around 1900, children had much more discretionary time. However, by the late 1950s, adults began to greatly shape children's free time, increasing the amount of time spent on schoolwork and reducing their freedom to play on their own (Gray, 2013).

Contemporary contexts for youth play are diverse, from in-school recess and physical education to after-school free and adult-directed play. Recess, which has long been a critical time for youth play during the school day, is shrinking. Since the early 1990s, there has been a broad trend toward reduction of recess in some schools and outright elimination of recess in others (Jarrett, 2013). Studies conducted in 2006 and 2011 suggest a decline from 57 percent to 40 percent in schools that require regularly scheduled recess. There is also inequity in terms of the children who are receiving access to recess, with white students being more likely to have time for recess when compared with African American and other minority students (Jarrett, 2013). In addition to the influence of racial inequalities on youth access to play, other factors that have impacted student recess time include the growing emphasis on academics and the use of reduced recess as a disciplinary strategy to manage negative classroom behavior (Stegelin, Fite, and Wisneski, 2015).

Out-of-school time (OST) is another important context for play. Youth spend between 6 and 8 hours of their waking time in formal classroom settings, leaving much of their day for OST programs and experiences (Weiss and Lopez, 2015). Play during OST has changed considerably over the past several decades. Children are spending more time indoors. They are less likely to ride their bikes to or from school due to population, traffic, and distance. Furthermore, many children come home after school and have no one to play with, are responsible for taking care of siblings, or have not grown up in a home where active play was modeled or observed. In those cases, active play is often ignored in favor of passive activities such as watching television or using computer or mobile devices (Stegelin, Fite, and Wisneski, 2015).

The reduction of play during OST has been influenced by movements toward organized and adult-led activities. One longitudinal study on children's play found that because many children have experienced reduced opportunities for free and unstructured play, young people increasingly rely on adults to organize or scaffold their play experiences (Miller and Almon, 2009). Many of these structured, adult-facilitated OST experiences are youth sports. In the United States, sports participation is a major activity for youth with approximately 45.7 out of 52 million children participating in at least one sports program annually (Sports and Fitness Industry Association, 2014), making it one of the most ubiquitous types of OST activities among youth today (Zarrett, Fay, Li, Carrano, Phelps, and Lerner, 2009).

Youth sports are attractive to parents looking for adult-supervised activities for their children. In this context, many parents place a high priority on sports because they occur under the control of coaches and/or teachers. This prioritization of highly controlled experiences is influenced by several factors, including a media-inspired perception among parents that the world outside of one's home can be a dangerous place for children, a belief that sport participation automatically builds character, and a general fear that children will get into trouble if they are not controlled by adults (Coakley, 2005). Youth sports also provide parents with predictable schedules and an easy way to measure their children's development and achievements. Many parents feel that youth sports provide a way to keep their children busy and out of trouble during OST as well as build character and other life skills (Coakley, 2011). Another reason that youth sports are attractive to parents is related parents' perceptions of their parenting abilities. Child development expert Michael Thompson (2009) has suggested that many parents feel uncertain about the quality of their parenting, and whether or not they are being successful. In this environment of uncertainty, youth sports can provide parents with an indicator of their own competence.

Parents also define and manage their children's time and OST experiences due to parental perceptions of social risks to their children, such as being threatened or bullied, being exposed to drugs or drug use, and being associated with negative role models (Prezza, Alparone, Cristallo, and Luigi, 2005). In this risk averse society (Scott, Jackson, and Backet-Milburn, 1998), parents are highly attuned to identifying, assessing, and reducing potential risks that could physically or emotionally harm their children. When parents impede their child's OST experiences because of their anxiety toward potential risk, a child's healthy development may be impeded (Fredricks and Eccles, 2005). This results in increasing dependence on adults. Unfortunately, adult-controlled spaces and experiences tend to exclude features that maximize the potential for active play (Matthews and Limb, 1999). As Stephen Wallace, director of the Center for Adolescent Research and Education, points out, "children used to go outside and play, make stuff up, goof around and generally have a good time, all the while learning important skills, such as sharing, group decision-making and conflict resolution. When we structure the activities, set the ground rules and determine the time, place and nature of just about every aspect of their day, kids lose pieces of their childhood bit by bit" (Wallace, 2015, 9).

Declines in Youth Sport

A curious trend in youth sports participation has emerged, one that mirrors what has happened with youth play. A 2015 report from PHIT America highlighted the drastic decline in youth team sports participation by children ages 6–17. These statistics not only suggest a drop in overall participation in youth sports, but also reveal a drop in the number of youth who are participating in the top 10 major team sports: baseball, basketball, cheerleading, court volleyball, fast-pitch softball, field hockey, ice hockey, outdoor soccer, tackle football, tennis, and track and field. According to PHIT America, the reasons for this decline in youth involvement in team sports include the decline and lack of physical education in schools; the emphasis on "travel" ball at any early age, which focuses young athletes on one versus several activities; and heavy use of electronics and social media by youth. Also, the movement toward a pay-to-play structure in schools makes sports too expensive for many families.

As it does with childhood play, extreme forms of overvigilant and overcontrolling parenting can reduce youth participation in sports (Janssen, 2015), which can cause children to miss out on roughly 20 different physical activity experiences each week, including activities such as outdoor play, walking, biking, and sports (PHIT America, 2015). In addition, parents are taking youth sports experiences—once designed to be fun and recreational—too seriously, which is detracting from the primary purpose of these experiences—to enhance youth development through fun (PHIT America, 2015).

The bottom line appears to be that the number of children who spend a lot of time every year being physically active in play and sport experiences is dropping. Play can be a conduit to sport, and encouraging kids in healthy play also prepares them to be athletes. To save sport, save play. How can parents engage children in play at a young age that can support them in becoming more successful in sports, while also developing in them an understanding of sportsmanship, an ability to cope with failure or loss, and an ability to be physically prepared for life?

Relationships between Play and Sports

Since the 1980s there has been increasing interest in mapping settings and experiences that contribute to positive developmental outcomes in young people. From a child development perspective, play and sport have much in common (Frost, Wortham, and Reifel, 2001), and the relationship between them can help people understand how experiences can contribute to positive outcomes for youth. The associations between play and sport are exemplified in the following points:

1. **Play is fun:** It may come as little surprise that young athletes identify fun as the most important motivator for participation in youth sports (Smoll, Cumming, and Smith, 2011). *Fun, the essence of play, constitutes the central element of successful youth sport experiences.* Children thrive when playing, and in fact are most creative when they play (Gray, 2013). Play experiences, during which youth are not being judged and are able to practice a wide range of behaviors, are a good contrast to sport experiences, in which youth may be compared to other peer athletes or judged on the quality of their own performance.

2. **Play makes children physically capable for sport:** Children need to be active. Brain research suggests that when young people sit for more than 20 to 30 minutes at a time, over 80 percent of the blood in their bodies pool in the hips, when they really need to have that oxygenated blood flowing to their brains (Blaydes, 2000). Furthermore, children are increasingly demonstrating poor strength and balance due to a lack of physical activity (Hanscom, 2014). In fact, according to the American Heart Association, youth over the age of 2 need at least an hour of moderate, enjoyable physical activity daily (Pappas, 2011). Play provides a mechanism for physical activity, and evidence suggests that active children grow into active adults. Thus *play prepares youth to become athletes* because play improves physical development that may make children better conditioned and prepared for sport. At a time when youth face increasing rates of childhood obesity, weight-related health problems, and sedentary routines in school, play combined with sport provides a developmentally appropriate strategy for preventing obesity and increasing the physical development of children. Researchers have noted that "the physical benefits of active play include large muscle skills as children reach, grasp, crawl, run, climb, skip and balance, and develop hand-eye coordination as the child handles objects in play. There is no substitute for active physical play and activity in order for these developmental milestones to occur" (Stegelin, Fite, and Wisneski, 2015, 3). In this way, play builds stronger youth who may be physically better prepared to play and excel in sports.

3. **Play improves behavior and teaches nuances of rules for sport:** Studies of the impact of free play on the behavior of 8- to 9-year-olds find that youth who had more than 15 minutes of breaks behaved better during academic time (Pappas, 2011). In addition to improving behavior, *play also helps children understand rules and rule breaking.* Thomas Henricks, professor of sociology at Elon University, points out that while play can often involve rules, play can also be varied and unexpected in a way that encourages children to create order followed by chaos. He also suggests that the function of this type of play is for children to develop "abilities related to conceiving

ends of action, forming and implementing strategies, evaluating the world's reaction to these, then trying something different" (*American Journal of Play*, 2015, 292). In this way, children who learn to make and break rules during play may be better prepared to grasp and negotiate the many rules and strategies that can accompany sports participation. It may also be that youth demonstrate better behavior because of their involvement in play and then have more time for sports. For example, a student who avoids trouble during the school day does not have to spend time on behavioral consequences and will have more time for other activities such as sports.

4. **Play increases youth resilience and prepares them for competition:** When children reach the age of 4 or 5, and they become adept at categorizing, they quickly learn how to make comparisons such as fastest, biggest, strongest, and so on (Klein, 2014). At this point in a child's development, concepts of winning and losing begin to take on a concrete meaning and children become more competitive. Unfortunately, the part of the brain that helps young people learn how to accept losing is the last to develop, so they need help in appropriately coping with both success and failure. Competition can be beneficial for youth. As explained by Nim Tottenham, associate professor of psychology at Columbia University, "when we're in competition, we are balancing the positive feelings of reward and positive feedback about ourselves against potentially daunting frustration" (Turner, 2014). *Through play, children experience competition and practice winning and losing*, skills that translate well to other activities such as sports and are vital for adulthood.

5. **Play helps children develop emotional self-regulation:** Building on the previous point, play also teaches young people to regulate their own emotions. During play, negative emotions that may arise (such as anger) have to be controlled or used in a more constructive way through self-assertion so children can keep playing (Gray, 2013). Sergio Pellis, a researcher at the University of Lethbridge in Canada, pointed out that the executive control system in a child's brain that regulates emotions needs plenty of free play in order for the system in the brain to develop properly (Turner, 2014). Aggression-management learned through self-regulation during play may translate to more sportsmanlike behavior during youth sports. An important benefit of play for children's self-regulation is gaining experience solving their own problems and managing their own issues without interference from adults.

6. **Play facilitates youth social skills during sport:** For many, youth play is a deeply social experience, and in order to succeed at play children have to master social rules. Research reveals that both adult-guided as well as free play helps children become more aware of other people's feelings. As children become aware of others' feelings during play, they also begin to practice

negotiation and compromise (Hirsch-Pasek and Golinkoff, 2008). One researcher called play the "academy for learning social skills" (Gray, 2013, 28). Social development during play prepares children to be better team players and to pay attention to social elements of sports. Mastering social elements of play may also assist in preparing youth for leadership positions on their sports teams.

7. **Play facilitates higher level thinking in youth:** In addition to physical development, play is important for cognitive development. Jean Piaget, a Swiss developmental psychologist known for his epistemological studies with children, found that stimulating play environments facilitated progress to higher levels of thought throughout childhood (Piaget and Inhelder, 1962). Studies of children's brains during play show that play establishes specific pathways in the brain between the systems that control the frontal lobe (our thinking) and the limbic system (our physical movements) (Hannaford, 2005). When children are encouraged to play in open and creative ways, they take on diverse roles, show imaginative behaviors, and strengthen their ability to problem solve (Stegelin, Fite, and Wisneski, 2015). Such diversity in roles, behaviors, and problem solving can have important benefits for successful youth sport participation.

As these points suggest, play can be a conduit to sport. Preparing kids for healthy play also prepares them to be youth athletes.

The Interwoven Futures of Play and Sport

The world is home to more than 2 billion children. Now is the time for supporters of children and play to join together to promote a unified message about the importance of play for children's healthy development (Steglin, Fite, and Wisneski, 2015). As this entry described, the reinvigoration of youth play can help youth sports thrive. There are reasons to be hopeful for the future of youth involvement in both play and sport. One, schools are recognizing the benefits of children's access to recess. For example, some Atlanta area districts have reversed their "no recess" policies. In addition, Chicago public schools have lengthened the school day to include 20 minutes for play (Stegelin, Fite, and Wisneski, 2015). Congressional legislation has also been introduced in recent years calling for mandatory recess among children in kindergarten to fifth grade (U.S. Play Coalition, 2015). Two, technology is shaping a range of games and other practices that are integrating physical movement and activity, which may influence youth to experiment with new kinds of play and sport experiences (Stegelin, Fite, and Wisneski, 2015). Although technology use and access must be balanced with other childhood experiences, technology can be a bridge for youth who are unaccustomed to freely chosen and self-directed play.

The future of play is full integration into a child's day. Through physical education, recess, and after-school sports, opportunities for play can be enhanced as well as intentionally and thoughtfully incorporated into a child's daily life. Parental involvement in, and support of, youth play and sport experiences must also mature (Coakley, 2005). The changing roles of parents may create different opportunities for both structured and unstructured play in sport. For example, parents who practice sports or sport-related play with their children in order to have meaningful "quality time" with them may also be facilitating in their children an overall interest in play. Parents can also become more mindful of the risk anxiety that they associate with childhood play and youth sports, and recognize that there are ways to give children time and space for play and sport-related development, yet still ensure their safety. Parents can also encourage their children to play in a variety of ways both at home and away from home, and to let play be emergent rather than constrained. Children need to play, and parents hold the key.

Barry A. Garst and Stephanie P. Garst

Further Reading

American Journal of Play. 2015. "Play as a Basic Pathway to the Self: An Interview with Thomas S. Henricks." *American Journal of Play, 7*(3): 271–297

Blaydes, J. 2000. *Thinking on Your Feet.* Richardson, TX: Action Based Learning.

Chudacoff, H. 2007. *Children at Play: An American History.* New York: New York University Press.

Coakley, J. 2005. "The Good Father: Parental Expectations and Youth Sport." *Leisure Sciences, 25*(2): 153–163.

Coakley, J. 2011. "Youth Sports: What Counts as 'Positive Development'?" *Journal of Sports and Social Issues, 35*(3): 306–324.

Fredricks, J. A., and J. S. Eccles. 2005. "Family Socialization, Gender, and Sport Motivation and Involvement." *Journal of Sport and Exercise Psychology, 27*(1): 3–31.

Frost, J., L. Bowers, and S. Wortham. 1990. "The State of American Preschool Playgrounds." *Journal of Physical Education, Recreation, and Dance, 61*(8): 18–23.

Gray, P. 2013. *The Play Deficit.* Accessed at http://aeon.co/magazine/culture/children-today-are-suffering-a-severe-deficit-of-play.

Hamilton, J. 2014, August 6. *Scientists Say Child Play Helps Build a Better Brain* [Radio broadcast episode]. National Public Radio.

Hannaford, C. 2005. *Smart Moves: Why Learning Is Not All in Your Head* (2nd ed.). Salt Lake City, UT: Great River Books.

Hanscom, A. 2014, August. "The Real Reason Why Kids Fidget." *The Huffington Post.* Accessed at http://www.huffingtonpost.com/angela-hanscom/the-real-reason-why-kids -fidget_b_5586265.html.

Hirsch-Pasek, K., and R. M. Golinkoff. 2008. "Why Play=Learning." *Encyclopedia on Early Childhood Development.* Accessed at http://www.ecswe.org/wren/documents /Hirsh-Pasek-Why-Play=Learning.pdf.

Janssen, I. 2015. "Hyper-Parenting Is Negatively Associated with Physical Activity among 7–12 Year Olds." *Preventive Medicine, 73*: 55–59.

Jarrett, O. S. 2013. *A Research-Based Case for Recess.* U.S. Play Coalition. Accessed at http://www.playworks.org/sites/default/files/US-play-coalition_Research-based-case -for-recess.pdf.

Jensen, E. 2001. *Arts with the Brain in Mind.* Alexandria, VA: Association for Supervision and Curriculum Development.

Karsten, L., W. Van Vliet. 2006. "Children in the City: Reclaiming the Street." *Children, Youth and Environments, 16*(1): 151–167.

Kim, K. H. 2011. "The Creativity Crisis: The Decrease in Creative Thinking Scores on the Torrance Tests of Creative Thinking." *Creativity Research Journal, 23*: 285–295.

Klein, T. P. 2014. *How Toddlers Thrive: What Parents Can Do Today for Children 2–5 to Plant the Seeds of Lifelong Success.* New York: Touchstone.

Matthews, H., and M. Limb. 1999. "Defining an Agenda for the Geography of Children: Review and Prospect." *Progress in Human Geography, 23*(1): 61–90.

Miller, E., and J. Almon. 2009. *Crisis in the Kindergarten: Why Children Need to Play in School.* College Park, MD: Alliance for Childhood.

Morrongiello, B. A., and K. Major. 2002. "Influence of Safety Gear on Parental Percep-tions of Injury Risk and Tolerance for Children's Risk Taking." *Injury Prevention, 8*: 27–31.

National Association for the Education of Young Children. 2009. *Developmentally Appro-priate Practice in Early Childhood Programs Serving Children from Birth through Age 8.* Accessed at http://www.naeyc.org/files/naeyc/file/positions/PSDAP.pdf.

Pappas, S. 2011. *The Top 5 Benefits of Play.* Accessed at http://www.livescience.com/15541 -top-5-benefits-play.html.

PHIT America. 2015. *Hyperparenting in Sports: It's Keeping Your Kid Inactive.* Accessed at http://www.phitamerica.org/News_Archive/Hyperparenting.htm.

Piaget, J., and B. Inhelder. 1962. *The Psychology of the Child.* New York: Basic Books.

Prezza, M., F. R. Alparone, C. Cristallo, and S. Luigi. 2005. "Parental Perception of Social Risk and of Positive Potentiality of Outdoor Autonomy for Children: The Development of Two Instruments." *Journal of Environmental Psychology, 25*(4): 437–453.

Roth, J. L., and J. Brooks-Gunn. 2003. "What Is a Youth Development Program? Identifi-cation and Defining Principles." In F. Jacobs, D. Wertlieb, and R. M. Lerner (Eds.), *Enhancing the Life Chances of Youth and Families: Public Service Systems and Public Policy Perspectives: Vol. 2. Handbook of Applied Developmental Science: Promot-ing Positive Child, Adolescent, and Family Development through Research, Policies, and Programs* (pp. 197–223). Thousand Oaks, CA: Sage.

Scott, S., S. Jackson, and K. Backett-Milburn. 1998. "Swings and Roundabouts: Risk Anxiety and the Everyday Worlds of Children." *Sociology, 32*(4): 689–705.

Smoll, F. L., S. P. Cumming, and R. E. Smith. 2011. "Enhancing Coach-Parent Relationships in Youth Sports: Increasing Harmony and Minimizing Hassle." *International Journal of Sports Science & Coaching, 6*(1): 13–26.

Sports and Fitness Industry Association. 2014. *2014 Sports, Fitness, and Leisure Activities Topline Participation Report.* Silver Spring, MD: Author.

Stegelin, D. A., K. Fite, and D. Wisneski. 2015. *The Critical Place of Play in Education.* U.S. Play Coalition and the Association of Childhood Education International. Accessed at http://www.hehd.clemson.edu/downloads/PRTM-Play-Coalition-White-Paper.pdf.

Thompson, M. 2009. *Managing the Anxious and Intervening Parents. American Camp Association.* Accessed at https://www.acacamps.org/staff-professionals/events -professional-development/recorded-webinar/managing-anxious-intervening-parent.

Turner, C. 2014, August 14. *When Kids Start Playing to Win* [Radio broadcast episode]. National Public Radio.

U.S. Play Coalition. 2015, Spring. *Play Pulse.* Accessed at https://usplaycoalition.org/wp -content/uploads/2015/09/0000Final-Play-Pulse-Spring-2015.pdf.

Wallace, S. 2015, June. "Used to Be." *The Huffington Post.* Accessed at http://www.huff ingtonpost.com/stephen-gray-wallace/used-to-be_b_7558414.html.

Weiss, H. B., and M. E. Lopez. 2015. *Engage Families for Anywhere, Anytime Learning. Phi Delta Kappan, 96*(7): 14–19.

Zarrett, N., K. Fay, Y. Li, J. Carrano, E. Phelps, and R. M. Lerner. 2009. "More Than Child's Play: Variable- and Pattern-Centered Approaches for Examining Effects of Sports Participation on Youth Development. *Developmental Psychology, 45*(2): 368–382.

Sexual and Physical Abuse

Millions of people around the United States are involved in youth sport as athletes, coaches, volunteers, referees, and organizers. Most of these individuals perceive sport as a positive influence on health and well-being of young people. The world of youth sports, however, is also sometimes clouded by coaches and other authority figures who take advantage of their positions to sexually or physically abuse youth athletes. Indeed, it is difficult for many young athletes experiencing such abuse to speak up against such abuse or inform other adults of what they are enduring. The pressure to perform and progress as an athlete is often just too high. In addition, many young people doubt that they will be believed if they come forward with accusations against their coaches or trainers, many of whom are respected, long-standing members of their communities, clubs, or school programs. As a result, these experiences may cause an athlete to suffer from depression and other forms of psychological distress, dependence on substance abuse to ward off feelings of anger and guilt, and long-term difficulties with trust and intimacy. Complicating the issue is that the negative outcomes youth athletes face from sexual and physical abuse are typically ignored or overlooked as symptoms that might be stemming from some other element of their lives (such as academics or romantic relationships), or even just the general turbulence of adolescence. The challenge of addressing sexual and physical abuse in youth sports is further exacerbated by schools, clubs, and parents who have only a limited understanding of the potential factors leading to sexual and physical abuse in the context of youth sports, as well as precautions that can be taken to prevent young athletes from becoming victimized.

What Are Sexual and Physical Abuse?

The definitions of sexual harassment, sexual abuse, and physical abuse are not universally agreed on, but they are broadly aligned with the following terms. Sexual harassment refers to any unwanted acts of sexualized verbal, nonverbal, or physical behaviors from individuals who are in positions of power or trust over the athletes (IOC, 2007). While the International Olympic Committee (IOC) Consensus Statement (2007), further extended by Margo Mountjoy in 2016, defined sexual abuse as the act of any sexual contact, penetrative, or noncontact behaviors where consent is forced or manipulated. To be more specific, contact sexual abuse involves sexual touching, fondling, and masturbation, while penetrative involves oral, vaginal, or anal penetration with the use of objects or body parts (Leahy, Pretty, and Tenenbaum, 2002;) while noncontact sexual abuse refers to acts such as exhibitionism, exposing athletes to sexual intercourse and pornographic materials, engaging athletes in pornographic photography and sexually explicit conversation (Leahy, Pretty, and Tenenbaum, 2002; Matthews, 2004).

Researchers led by sports medicine physician and youth advocate Margo Mountjoy have extended the consensus statement by adding several other types of harassment and abuse, including physical abuse. They defined physical abuse as "a non-accidental trauma or physical injury of an athlete caused by punching, beating, kicking, biting and burning or otherwise harming an athlete." To be more specific, physical abuse includes instances in which individuals are forced to do inappropriate physical activities, such as age-inappropriate or physical capability-inappropriate training loads and/or training when injured or in pain. Other acts of physical abuse include forcing athletes to consume alcohol or systematical doping practices (Mountjoy et al., 2016).

Further, research has referred to child physical abuse in the context of sport in three ways: (1) the act of physical assault caused by an adult or peer on the youth athlete, (2) forcing a youth athlete to overtrain in ways that lead to high risk of injury, and (3) forcing a youth athlete to train when he or she is injured or exhausted (Alexander, Stafford, and Lewis, 2011). Of those three types of physical abuse, forcing youth athletes to train when injured or exhausted was found to be the most common behavior. Identifying these kinds of abuse is challenging, however, due to the level of subjectivity involved; some may find an act to be physical abuse while others might consider it as reasonable physical discipline in a sport setting (McPherson et al., 2017).

Severity of Sexual and Physical Abuse of Young Athletes

The prevalence of sexual and physical abuse is difficult to determine for children as they are often scared or embarrassed to step forward and report the crime. In addition, these crimes have been given relatively little attention by sport clubs, organizations, schools, and government agencies until relatively recently. However, more broadly, according to the U.S. Department of Health and Human Services'

Children's Bureau report *Child Maltreatment 2015,* it was determined that 683,487 (0.92 percent) of the estimated 74,382,502 children under age 17 living in 50 states had experience with some form of maltreatment. The percentages for both boys (48.6 percent) and girls (50.9 percent) were similar. Of the child victims, 8.4 percent were sexually abused, while 17.2 percent were physically abused. Researchers warn, though, that the actual number of children and teens suffering from such treatment might be higher, as child abuse has historically been significantly underreported (Fasting, 2015).

Sexual Abuse in American Youth Sports

As of 2017, few empirical studies have been undertaken with regard to the extent of sexual abuse on youth athletes in the United States, although some policy has been studied or scales developed for measurement (Baker and Byon, 2014; Lopiano and Zotos, 2015). One of the few studies conducted in the United States that partially covers this subject was conducted by Karin Volkwein and several colleagues in 1997 to examine the perceptions and experiences of sexual harassment by female student-athletes at higher learning institutions. Studies on sexual abuse in youth sports have been conducted in other countries such as Australia, Canada, Norway, and the United Kingdom, however.

Sexual abuse in youth sports is a sensitive topic, but it has been gradually exposed in American news media in a series of high-profile scandals that have rocked respected and image-conscious institutions ranging from Penn State University to Olympic swimming and gymnastics programs. Marvin Sharp, who was named 2010 coach of the year by USA Gymnastics was arrested for child molestation and possession of child pornography. A year later, Lawrence G. Nassar, a long-time USA Gymnastics team doctor, was accused of sexual abuse by Jamie Dantzscher, a 2000 Sydney Olympics bronze medalist, and Jeanette Antolin and Jessica Howard, who also competed on the U.S. national gymnastics team. Eventually, more than 225 girls and women came forward to accuse Nassar of sexual abuse. He was then arrested and charged with sexually abusing the athletes during their medical appointments and possession of thousands of child pornographic images. The Oakland County Register reported in 2017 that according to Antolin's attorney, "Nassar's abuse of top U.S. female gymnasts was so widespread that there have been victims of his abuse on every U.S. Olympic team from the 1996 gold medal triumph in Atlanta to record-setting victories in London and last summer [2016] in Rio de Janeiro." These incidents have created an air of anxiety for current young female gymnasts and their families and underscored the potential vulnerability of all young female athletes.

However, researchers, law enforcement experts, and youth advocates all emphasize that boys can be the victims of sexual predations from coaches and other adult authority figures in the world of sports as well.

Jerry Sandusky, a former Penn State assistant football coach, was sentenced in 2012 for sexually abusing 10 young boys over a period of at least 15 years. He is currently serving 30–60 years in state prison for his crimes. Similarly, Dennis Hastert, a former Yorkville High School wrestling coach in Illinois who served as speaker of the U.S. House of Representatives from 1999 to 2007, pleaded guilty in 2015 to charges that he engaged in bank fraud to cover up his sexual abuse of at least four young male wrestlers during his coaching years at Illinois (he was not charged with sexual abuse crimes since the statute of limitations had expired).

In the great majority of documented cases of sexual abuse of youth athletes, the abusers are male coaches, teachers, and other men in positions of influence or authority. Other countries report that males account for virtually all abusers in youth sports settings as well. In Norway, for example, 15 court reports were analyzed, and it was found that all the incidents reported a male coach as the perpetrator of youth athletes in sport (Fasting, Brackenridge, and Kjølberg, 2013). This is not to say that only male coaches or administrators commit sexual abuse in sport, but to date there have been few confirmed cases in which female coaches sexually abused young athletes in their charge.

Physical Abuse in American Youth Sports

Although physical abuse has often been more prevalent than sexual abuse, research on the issue within the unique context of youth sport has been limited (Stafford, Alexander, and Fry, 2013; Vertommen et al., 2016). The reason behind this is probably due to the widespread acceptance of the "no pain, no gain" mentality that individuals have in mind in order to achieve performance goals in the competitive sporting environment (McKay et al., 2000). In addition, there exists a blurred line between competitive training and physical abuse where many find it difficult to distinguish the two (Brackenridge et al., 2007).

In the context of youth sports, coaches are often viewed as parental figures for young athletes. Therefore, young athletes may be more susceptible to physical abuse as they are more likely to trust and respect their coaches' authority. This is especially typical for young athletes who participate in elite sports where they are trained in more pressured conditions (Lang, Hartill, and Rulofs, 2016). Dominique Moceanu, a gold medal Olympian gymnast, revealed that she and her other elite gymnasts were physically abused by their coaches in order to secure success at their highest performance level (Moceanu, 2017). As an elite athlete, it was not easy for

Dominique and her peers to report the ongoing abuse to the authorities who had so much power over their success in the sport. If a culture of abuse is prevalent within an organization, it is difficult to seek out someone outside the organization who will be supportive or help verify that abuse is taking place.

Studies regarding physical abuse in youth sports assert that coaches are most often reported as perpetrators (Lang, Hartill, and Rulofs, 2016). However, there have also been documented cases in which young athletes experience the abuse by their peer athletes. Research has demonstrated that peer athletes were most often reported as perpetrators in team sports (Alexander, Stafford, and Lewis, 2011).

Risk Factors for Sexual and Physical Abuse in Youth Sports

To more fully understand the risks of young athletes falling victim to sexual or physical abuse from coaches or other sport-related authority figures, scholar Celia Brackenridge looked at situational risk factors in sport and found that there were two unique elements: normative risk factors and constitutive risk factors. Normative risk factors are factors that relate to the culture and ethos of the activity or sport organization. To be more specific, normative organizational culture has a (1) autocratic authority system; (2) involves close personal contact with athletes; (3) sets up clear power imbalance between athlete and coach; (4) gives scope for separation of athlete from peers in time and space; (5) gives scope for development and maintenance of secrecy; (6) involves mixed sexes and ages sharing room on away trips; (7) condones sexual relationships between all ages (8) sexualizes athletes' idiocultural traditions (songs, jokes, nicknames, hazing ritual, pranks); (9) provokes intense peer group competition/jealously; and (10) supports collective silence on matters of sexuality (Brackenridge, 2003).

On the other hand, constitutive risk factors are structurally embedded factors that include (1) involving hierarchical status system; (2) gives awards based on performance; (3) links rewards to compliance with the authority system; (4) has rules and procedures that omit/exclude consultation; (5) has no formal procedures for screening, hiring, and monitoring staff; (6) involves intense training regimes to acquire necessary technical skill; (7) makes technical/task demands that legitimate touch; and (8) subsumes individuality within competitive structure (Brackenridge, 2003).

In addition to these risk factors, some observers have speculated that revealing and/or form-fitting sport clothing might be a significant contributor to sexual abuse acts, but surprisingly, studies have thus far found that the amount of body and/or skin revealed due to sport clothing, like swimmers in bathing suits or gymnasts in their suits, has little or no influence on the likelihood of sexual abuse (Fasting, Brackenridge, and Sundgot-Borgen, 2004).

Researchers have found, however, that risks of child abuse are greater in less supervised environments (Brackenridge, 2003). Understanding the risk factors in youth sports on child abuse can significantly help families and professionals working with youth athletes to reduce vulnerability to predation. Parents should stay around to watch practice or be involved in helping with training or traveling with the team when possible so as to avoid situations where the child is left alone with an adult in a position of authority.

Preventing Sexual and Physical Abuse in Youth Sports

Awareness and discussion of sexual abuse in youth sports increased in the United States and in a number of other countries during the 1990s (Lang, Hartill, and Rulofs, 2016). In recent years, major organizations such as the IOC and UNICEF have also been paying close attention in order to prevent abuse and support children who are victimized by abuse (Lang, Hartill, and Rulofs, 2016). However, in the field of academia, knowledge of the extent of sexual abuse in youth sport remains incomplete. This is especially true of the United States, as most studies on the subject have been conducted in European countries or are only estimates of the numbers of youth both physically and sexually abused in the United States (Parent and Demers, 2011; Shattuck, Finkelhor, Turner, and Hamby, 2016). Therefore, with the restrictions faced by scholars, immediate action is needed by sport governing bodies to step forward and take the issue of child abuse seriously. Sports like USA Swimming and USA Gymnastics have found out all too quickly that things like this cannot simply be swept under the rug but rather must be dealt with.

The following are prevention strategies recommended by the IOC to all sport organizations, which might increase the efficacy of child abuse protection (IOC, 2007). The strategies include (1) develop policies and procedures for the prevention of sexual harassment and abuse; (2) monitor the implementation of these policies and procedures; (3) evaluate the impact of these policies in identifying and reducing sexual harassment and abuse; (4) develop an education and training program on sexual harassment and abuse in their sport(s); (5) promote and exemplify equitable, respectful, and ethical leadership; (6) foster strong partnerships with parents/caregivers in the prevention of sexual harassment and abuse; and (7) promote and support scientific research on these issues.

Sexual *and* Physical Abuse Policies in Youth Sports

Spearheaded by organizations like the IOC, protecting youth athletes has become an increasingly prominent concern in policy making and research communities around the world (Lang, Hartill, and Rulofs, 2016). With the implementation of policies in various sport organizations, numerous past cases of sexual and physical abuse have emerged. Thus, in the United States, it has become a much higher priority for sport organizations at both elite and nonelite levels to conduct an independent review of their bylaws, policies, procedures, and practices to ensure that young athletes are protected from sexual or physical abuse. Although this independent process is clearly more cost prohibitive, it is seen by some observers as a way to prevent cases like the Sandusky one, where internal cover-ups of abuse are undertaken to protect the organizational image. Other schools and clubs, meanwhile, have become more proactive in establishing policies based on guidance from state and/or federal agencies and youth welfare organizations.

In recent years, sport organizations and researchers have been gradually focusing more on the development of policies aimed to decrease the crime rates in sport. For example, Margo Mountjoy and colleagues extended the 2007 IOC consensus statement on sexual harassment and abuse in sport by adding the psychological, physical, and neglect consensus statement to their statements (Mountjoy et al., 2007). In 2012, meanwhile, the United Nations International Children's Fund (UNICEF) hosted a safeguarding workshop for international youth, sport, and development organizations to draft standards and implementation methods to protect youth athletes in their sport (Paramasivan, 2012). The so-called International Standards were piloted in 2013–2014 in several sport organizations across the globe prior to being introduced worldwide (Lang et al., 2016).

In the United States, MomsTEAM Institute, one of the sport and development organizations among the 40 selected global organizations by UNICEF UK, with support from UNICEF International, is implementing the International Safeguards for Children in Sport across the country. The safeguards aim to (1) help create a safe sporting environment for children wherever they participate and at whatever level; (2) provide a benchmark to assist sports providers and funders to make informed decisions about child safety in sport; (3) promote good practice and challenge practice that is harmful to children; and (4) providing clarity on safeguarding children to all involved in sport.

With so much interest from the world's most influential sport organizations, it is important that youth sports organizations ensure policies, practices, and procedures are in place to eradicate both sexual and physical abuses. In most cases, a simple background check of prospective coaches just isn't enough anymore (although such checks should definitely be undertaken); more stringent fact checking and no child left alone policies need to be put in place as well. Also, it is significantly important that safe measures be put in place to report, investigate, and deal with reported incidents to establish a safe and protected environment for youth athletes both on and off the field.

It is crucial for parents to check on sport clubs and sport organizations to ensure that there are child abuse policies, practices, and procedures in place before sending their children to participate in the sport. Also, parents should know the exact definitions of all child abuse acts in order to better understand and notice the assault at a glance.

Young Suk Oh and Skye G. Arthur-Banning

Further Reading

Alexander, K., A. Stafford, and R. Lewis. 2011. *The Experiences of Children Participating in Organised Sport in the UK*. Edinburgh: University of Edinburgh/NSPCC Centre for UK-wide Learning in Child Protection.

Baker T. A., III, and K. K. Byon. 2014. "Developing a Scale of Perception of Sexual Abuse in Youth Sports (SPSAYS)." *Measurement in Physical Education and Exercise Science*, *18*(1): 31–52.

Brackenridge, C. 1999. "Managing Myself: Investigator Survival in Sensitive Research." *International Review for the Sociology of Sport*, *34*(4): 399–410.

Brackenridge, C. 2003. "Dangerous Sports? Risk, Responsibility and Sex Offending in Sport." *Journal of Sexual Aggression,* *9*(1): 3–12.

Brackenridge, C. H., A. Pitchford, K. Russell, and G. Nutt. 2007. *Child Welfare in Football: An Exploration of Children's Welfare in the Modern Game*. London: Routledge.

Donnelly, P., G. Kerr, A. Heron, and D. DiCarlo. 2016. "Protecting Youth in Sport: An Examination of Harassment Policies." *International Journal of Sport Policy and Politics*, *8*(1): 33–50.

Fasting, K. 2015. "Assessing the Sociology of Sport: On Sexual Harassment Research and Policy." *International Review for the Sociology of Sport*, *50*(4–5): 437–441.

Fasting, K., and C. Brackenridge. 2009. "Coaches, Sexual Harassment and Education." *Sport, Education and Society*, *14*(1): 21–35.

Fasting, K., C. H. Brackenridge, and G. Kjølberg. 2013. "Using Court Reports to Enhance Knowledge of Sexual Abuse in Sport: A Norwegian Case Study." *Scandinavian Sport Studies Forum*, *4*: 49–67.

Fasting, K., C. Brackenridge, and J. Sundgot-Borgen. 2004. "Prevalence of Sexual Harassment among Norwegian Female Elite Athletes in Relation to Sport Type." *International Review for the Sociology of Sport*, *39*(4): 373–386.

International Olympic Committee. 2007. *IOC Consensus Statement on Sexual Harassment & Abuse in Sport*. Accessed August 17, 2017, at http://www.olympic.org/search?q=consensus+statement&filter=documents.

Lang, M., M. Hartill, and B. Rulofs. 2016. "Child Abuse in Sport: From Research to Policy and Protection." In K. Green and A. Smith (Eds.), *Routledge Handbook of Youth Sport*. (pp. 505–514). London: Routledge.

Leahy, T., G. Pretty, and G. Tenenbaum. 2002. "Prevalence of Sexual Abuse in Organised Competitive Sport in Australia." *Journal of Sexual Aggression*, 8(2): 16–36.

Lopiano, D. A., and C. Zotos. 2015. "Athlete Welfare and Protection Policy Development in the USA." In M. Lang and M. Hartill (Eds.), *Safeguarding, Child Protection and Abuse in Sport* (pp. 97–106). London: Routledge.

McKay, J., M. Messner, and D. Sabo. 2000. *Masculinities, Gender Relations and Sport*. Thousand Oaks, CA: Sage.

McPherson, L., M. Long, M. Nicholson, N. Cameron, P. Atkins, and M. E. Morris. 2017. "Secrecy Surrounding the Physical Abuse of Child Athletes in Australia." *Australian Social Work*, 70(1): 42–53.

Moceanu, D. 2017. *A Gold Medal Olympian Says That Youth Athletes Need to Hear Our Voice*. Accessed August 17, 2017, at https://sports.good.is/features/dominique-oceanu.

MomsTEAM Institute. *UNICEF International Safeguards for Children in Sport*. Accessed July 18, 2017, at http://www.momsteaminstitute.org/unicef-international-safeguards-children-sport.

Mountjoy, M., C. Brackenridge, M. Arrington, C. Blauwet, A. Carska-Sheppard, K. Fasting, S. Kirby, T. Leahy, S. Marks, K. Martin, K. Starr, A. Tiivas, and R. Budgett. 2016. "International Olympic Committee Consensus Statement: Harassment and Abuse (Non-Accidental Violence) in Sport." *British Journal of Sports Medicine*, 50(17): 1019–1029.

Mountjoy, M., D. J. A. Rhind, A. Tiivas, and N. Leglise. 2015. "Safeguarding the Child Athlete in Sport: A Review, a Framework and Recommendations for the IOC Youth Athlete Development Model." *British Journal of Sports Medicine, 49*: 883–886.

Paramasivan, M. 2012. *UNICEF Takes Safeguarding Procedures beyond Paper*. Accessed July 18, 2017, at https://www.sportanddev.org/en/article/news/unicef-takes-safeguarding-procedures-beyond-paper.

Parent, S., and G. Demers. 2011. "Sexual Abuse in Sport: A Model to Prevent and Protect Athletes." *Child Abuse Review*, 20(2): 120–133.

Reid, S. 2017, February 20. "Former Gymnast Jeanette Antolin Speaks about Sexual Abuse Allegations against U.S. Team Doctor." *Orange County Register*.

Sand, T. S., K. Fasting, S. Chroni, and N. Knorre. 2011. "Coaching Behavior: Any Consequences for the Prevalence of Sexual Harassment?" *International Journal of Sports Science & Coaching*, 6(2): 229–241.

Shattuck, A., D. Finkelhor, H. Turner, and S. Hamby. 2016. "Children Exposed to Abuse in Youth-Serving Organizations: Results from National Sample Surveys." *JAMA Pediatrics, 170*(2). doi:10.1001/jamapediatrics

Stafford, A., K. Alexander, and D. Fry. 2013. "Playing through Pain: Children and Young People's Experiences of Physical Aggression and Violence in Sport." *Child Abuse Review*, 22(4): 287–299.

Statistic Brain. (2017). Accessed July 5, 2017, at http://www.statisticbrain.com/youth-sports-statistics.

Stirling, A. E., and G. A. Kerr. 2009. "Abused Athletes' Perceptions of the Coach-Athlete Relationship." *Sport in Society, 12*(2): 227–239.

Timpka, T., S. Janson, J. Jacobsson, J. Ekberg, Ö. Dahlström, J. Kowalski, V. Bargoria, M. Mountjoy, and C. G. Svedin. 2015. "Protocol Design for Large-Scale Cross-Sectional Studies of Sexual Abuse and Associated Factors in Individual Sports: Feasibility Study in Swedish Athletics." *Journal of Sports Science & Medicine, 14*(1): 179.

Vertommen, T., N. H. Schipper-van Veldhoven, M. J. Hartill, and F. Van Den Eede. 2015. "Sexual Harassment and Abuse in Sport: The NOC*NSF Helpline." *International Review for the Sociology of Sport, 50*(7): 822–839.

Vertommen, T., N. Schipper-van Veldhoven, K. Wouters, J. K. Kampen, C. H. Brackenridge, D. J. Rhind, K. Neels, and F. Van Den Eede. 2016. "Interpersonal Violence against Children in Sport in the Netherlands and Belgium." *Child Abuse & Neglect, 51*: 223–236.

Volkwein, K. A., F. I. Schnell, D. Sherwood, and A. Livezey. 1997. "Sexual Harassment in Sport: Perceptions and Experiences of American Female Student-Athletes." *International Review for the Sociology of Sport, 32*(3): 283–295.

Sexual Orientation and Inclusion

This entry will address many of the issues facing the lesbian, gay, bisexual, and queer (LGBQ) community within sport. Although the community is often listed as LGBTQ, or LGBTQIA, to be inclusive of transgender and intersex individuals, the issues around sexual orientation in sport are different than those around gender identity. As such, this entry will focus on the LGBQ community. (For an overview of transgender and intersex access to sport, please see the entry "Gender Identity and Inclusion.") This entry will begin with some definitions of terms and a general discussion of the LGBQ community, before moving on to the stereotypes and stigmas faced by different segments of the community within youth sport. The entry will then close by focusing on issues regarding LGBQ access, integration, and segregation within sport communities.

Definitions

The LGBQ umbrella encompasses many different identities. Although there are similarities, there are also many differences in how members of the distinct identity groups experience the world, and sport specifically. As such, it is important to know some of the differences between the identities in order to understand their experiences within the sport community. It is important to note as well that while the acronym covers a large swath of identities and serves as an umbrella identifier for the community, there can be factions, disagreements, and stereotypes within the community itself.

Lesbian: A woman who is primarily physically, romantically, and/or emotionally attracted to other women.
Gay: A man who is primarily physically, romantically, and/or emotionally attracted to other men.

Bisexual: A person who is physically, romantically, and/or emotionally attracted to both men and women.

Queer: A term used by some, usually younger members of the community, to describe themselves or their community. It can be used as an umbrella term such as "the queer community" rather that "the LGBT community" in order to be more inclusive of the entire extended acronym. It can also be used as an identity descriptor that seeks to transcend binaries—the assumption that sex and gender can only be classified as two distinct, and opposite, entities of male or female. Individuals may identify their sexual orientation as queer in that they are not gay or straight but queer; or they may identify as gender-queer, which challenges the male-female gender binary. It is a reclaimed term; queer has often been used as a pejorative insult. Due to this, some individuals are still uncomfortable with the term. This entry will utilize queer to reference the broader community, including those who fall outside the standard societal parameters of binaries and the limiting terms or LGBT.

Stigma and Stereotypes

LGBQ athletes often face stigmas and stereotypes in participating in sport, but lesbian athletes frequently face different stereotypes than gay athletes. Due to this, the identities will be addressed separately. However, there are some stereotypes and stigmas that are experienced by LGBQ youth in general. Queer youth face more harassment and bullying in school than their straight peers and feel less safe within the sport community. In respect to everyday life of queer youth, the 2013 National School Climate Survey found that 74.1 percent of LGBT students reported being verbally harassed in school because of their sexual orientation, and 55.5 percent felt unsafe at school because of their sexual orientation (GLSEN, 2013). According to the study, 68.1 percent of LGB students avoided certain school functions and/or extracurricular activities because they felt unsafe or uncomfortable due to both interpersonal and structural reasons. This could include school-sponsored sports.

The school locker room is a contentious place for LGB athletes and can serve as a structural site of discomfort. There is a stigma that LGB athletes might take advantage of being in the locker room to "check out" or make sexual advances on their teammates. However, several former male professional athletes who came out as gay after retirement have pointed out that there have been gay athletes in all the major sports for years that chose to hide their sexual orientation—a decision commonly known as "staying in the closet." There have not been any issues of that sort reported, and LGB athletes do not expect athletes "coming out of the closet" to change that. If anything, out athletes have a vested interest in showing the public that those are not relevant concerns (Bruni, 2014). However, the concern of being targeted by teammates in the locker room, or facing stigmas about their behavior, can impact LGBQ youths' experience in sport. Some may avoid participating in sports because of the stigmas and stereotypes that they believe they will face in the locker room and on the field.

Lesbians

The stereotype of lesbians in sport is long held and widely known. Due to the cultural association between sport and masculinity and the link between lesbianism and a lack of "appropriate" femininity, athletic girls have often risked being called a lesbian (whether or not they identify as one). Although it is slowly becoming more acceptable to be gay or lesbian in society, this risk has served as a deterrent to girl's participation in sport. Being labeled as lesbian has historically been a significant threat to one's social capital. It could mean the loss of friends and family, diminished interest from college programs, and increased difficulty in securing scholarships or sponsorships. Until relatively recent, the professional level has often been most visibly represented by traditionally feminine female athletes, often with visible husbands or boyfriends, when it comes to endorsement deals. As such, being openly lesbian or presenting onself in a manner that does not meet traditional standards of femininity could result in a loss in media attention or sponsorships. In response, some girls have avoided playing sports altogether, avoided playing certain sports that are viewed as more masculine or that carry a strong association with lesbianism, or presented themselves in ways that fit the social expectations of heterosexual femininity. Being lesbian has often been associated with being overly masculine, or not sufficiently feminine. Certain sports contain more of a lesbian stigma (such as softball, basketball, ice hockey) than others (figure skating, gymnastics). In order to combat the label within these sports, athletes often present themselves as hyperfeminine both on and off the field to dispel the stereotypes of "butch," "unfeminine," or "lesbian" in their sport. This hyperfemininity can take the form of always maintaining long hair, wearing bows in their hair while playing, wearing a full face of makeup on the field, and always wearing skirts, dresses, and other clothing that are identifiably feminine off the field. These actions have facilitated women's participation in sports while lessening the likelihood of attracting the lesbian label. However, the actions simultaneously breed an environment where those who do identify as lesbian and/or do not present as traditionally feminine may not feel welcome, even while women's sport is stereotyped as a refuge for lesbians.

Many women's sports have tried to dispel the lesbian label of their sport. For example, team photos will often present very feminine images of the players, as of 2017, only one Division I head coach of women's basketball is openly lesbian. Beyond that, college recruiters of high school athletes sometimes participate in negative recruiting through the use of coded words to actively discourage players from going to teams that are thought to have lesbian coaches or many lesbians on the team. Women's basketball is an often-cited perpetrator of these tactics. Coaches will talk about a team being "family friendly" or having good "family values" to indicate that neither their coaching staff nor their players are lesbians (Cyphers and Fagan, 2013). Lists of coaches that are suspected of being lesbian are circulated to recruits in an effort to scare players and their parents away from attending those programs. The Women's Basketball Coaches Alliance has materials on combating negative recruiting and creating an inclusive team environment. Due to negative recruiting, as well as fear of departmental homophobia, many lesbian coaches choose to not be open about their sexuality. Some teams, both at the youth and college level, impose no lesbian policies for their players. Rene Portland at Penn State became famous for her three-team rules: "No drinking, no drugs, and no lesbians." She was known to have benched and subsequently kicked women off the team if she suspected they were lesbians (see the film *Training Rules* for more on this). More recently, while at Baylor University, Britney Griner, who currently plays in the WNBA for the Phoenix Mercury, was not allowed to come out to the public as lesbian while still on the team. She came out shortly after her final season ended.

Although the stereotype of women's sports as being lesbian friendly has allowed many lesbian women to find safety and community, it also can create a toxic and unfriendly environment when it leads to homophobic rules or practices within teams and sport cultures. This can lead to players staying closeted for fear of being shunned by their teammates, losing their roster spots, or not being accepted by the public at the professional level. However, female athletes who are out are becoming more common. For example, there were four out lesbian members of the 2015 U.S. Women's National Soccer Team, compared with zero during the 2011 Women's World Cup team. After winning the FIFA Women's World Cup, Abby Wambach was shown live on national television kissing her wife and fellow soccer player, Sarah Huffman, in celebration. These players serve as role models for young lesbian athletes, signaling that they can succeed in sport while being their true selves.

Gay Men and Boys

While female athletes fight the stereotype that if they are good at sports, they must be lesbians, the association of sports with masculinity often means there is an assumed heterosexuality of men in sports. Particularly in stereotypically masculine sports such as hockey, football, and wrestling, gay boys and men have historically been treated as if they were not tough enough to compete in these sports. Since gay males are often stereotyped as lacking appropriate masculinity to thrive in sports settings, homophobic insults are often used to reinforce masculine norms on the field and court, as well as in the locker room.

This assumed heterosexuality of male athletes also breeds homophobia within the sport. Since gay has often been associated with weakness and femininity in society, it is often used as an insult toward other males. Gay, fag, and queer are often words that get used as insults to question an individual's masculinity. According to the National School Climate Survey, 71.4 percent of LGBT students reported hearing the word *gay* used derogatorily frequently or often, and 64.5 percent reported hearing other homophobic words such as *dyke* or *faggot* frequently or often (GLSEN, 2013). These insults are used to retain the masculine culture of sports. Thus, although male athletes are often assumed heterosexual, those who are gay may live in fear of being outed or being called gay, which could lead to further bullying or mistreatment within their sport. With Jason Collins (basketball), Michael Sam (football), Robbie Rogers (soccer), and others that have come out, however, there is a growing understanding that there are gay players in all types of sport—and that their sexual orientation does not make them less skilled players or less worthy teammates. Many gay athletes report, in fact, that when they come out, the language of teammates changes and they show more respect. The language is learned and part of the culture youth athletes are brought up in, but it can change. As Cyd Zeigler, owner of Outsports.com, said, "There is an atmosphere and language that's used, but when an LGBT athlete comes out, people apologize and change their behavior. Because what is behind the behavior is not homophobia, it's just learned language" (Gleeson and Brady, 2015). As long as gay and fag are used as insults, young athletes will question their safety and their acceptance by teammates if they choose to come out. It is challenging to come out when the homophobic language is ever present, and an athlete cannot be sure the language will change or that he will be accepted by teammates who appear to be homophobic.

Integration of LGBQ in Sport

With increased acceptance of LGBQ people in the United States, their visible presence and integration into mainstream sport are becoming more common. However, there are still issues that need to be addressed by sport organizations to be fully inclusive of queer youth. In terms of integration of LGBQ athletes into mainstream sports, it has less to do with their ability to participate, but rather the acceptance and inclusion of the individuals and their ability to participate openly and safely. Integration for LGBQ athletes means that they are able to be out and proud of who they are, without worrying about being kicked off of a team, shunned, or bullied by teammates, coaches, parents, or fans. However, this is not always the case. The stereotypes and stigmas mentioned earlier still have the power to prevent youth from either participating in sport or from being open about their sexual orientation.

There have been LGB individuals in every sport, but many have chosen not to come out until after they retire, citing safety and acceptance concerns. The decisions by Jason Collins, Robbie Rogers, and Michael Sam to come out while still active players, though, has given younger male athletes role models showing that it is possible to be a gay male player in contact sports at a high level. Despite the stigma of being a gay male athlete and the fears about locker room issues, those that have come out have talked about the support they received from their teammates. Michael Sam, for instance, recalled that "I was kind of scared, even though they already knew. Just to see their reaction was awesome. They supported me from Day One. I couldn't have better teammates" (Connelly, 2014). Many athletes come out to their teammates well before they come out publicly and mention similar levels of support, despite their fears. Since their coming out, there have been more high school and college players coming out publicly while still playing, even before reaching the professional draft level where athletes have been concerned about impacts on their draft status. In 2014, Michael Martin, a high school soccer player in West Virginia, came out first to his team and then to his entire school, by attending Homecoming with his boyfriend during his senior season (Martin, 2014). He said that Rogers inspired him to come out, and that although he did face some homophobia in school, his teammates and friends were very supportive.

On the women's side, there has long been knowledge of lesbian players and even some who were publicly out. However, in the last few years, the number of out players has increased as social acceptance of lesbian and gay individuals has increased. Players have also cited a desire to be role models, helping move society toward acceptance, as a reason for coming out publicly. Brittney Griner explained why it was important for her to come out: "I didn't have a real role model that I could look up to that was out openly, I knew there were a lot of younger girls that needed someone."

Lesbians such as Abby Wambach (soccer), Megan Rapinoe (soccer), Brittney Griner (basketball), and Seimone Augustus (basketball), among others, are not only actively playing their sports on the women's side, but are household names with endorsement deals (all four are with Nike, and Wambach has additional endorsement deals with Gatorade and other brands). Historically, even those who were on teams that accepted their sexual orientation (many of the athletes mentioned were out to their teams long before being out to fans) were afraid that coming out would hurt their careers, but these athletes are showing that they can build fan bases and gain endorsements while being openly lesbian athletes. These athletes not only open the door for queer youth to follow in their footsteps, but they also act as role models for young athletes, showing that they can succeed while still being their authentic selves.

LGB Issues and Coaching

Many LGB coaches do not come out publicly (even if they are out to their players) for fear of losing their jobs due to homophobic athletic departments (it is legal in 29 states to be fired based on sexual orientation), or losing players because parents do not want their child playing for an LGB coach. This occurs at all levels from youth to college. It not only prevents coaches from being their true, honest selves, but it also prevents them from serving as role models to their queer players. If there are LGB players on their team, by remaining closeted, the coaches are not able to be an example of how it is OK to be an LGB adult and succeed; instead they are in a position in which their sexual orientation is treated as something to be ashamed of and hide.

Many observers believe, however, that coaches are becoming more sensitive to the need to create a welcoming environment for players of all sexual orientations. Michael Martin, the soccer player in West Virginia, discussed the importance of coaches creating an inclusive environment, even when they do not know they have a gay player on the team, as it makes the environment feel more welcoming and less hostile. "My coach for my traveling soccer team laid down the law that there was not going to be any racism or discrimination based on sexuality, which made me feel safe. I still did not have the guts to tell anyone I was gay. My travel coach never knew that I was gay, nor did I tell him, but he was determined to create a safe environment on the team" (Martin, 2014). Coaches, whether or not they are LGB themselves, can make a significant difference on the inclusion of queer athletes. If the coach can create an inclusive environment that does not tolerate discrimination, they will create a space that is more welcoming of queer athletes, even if the athletes are not ready to come out.

The openly gay and lesbian professional athletes can serve as role models for LGBQ youth that it is OK to be themselves, and be proud of who they are, while still participating in sport. It also shows that LGBQ individuals can be successful and healthy and provide an image beyond what TV shows and movies present of LGBQ people in the public eye. This helps increase acceptance, which is the key aspect when talking about LGBQ integration in youth sport.

LGBQ Specific Participation

Although integration into mainstream sport is vital, having their own space is often important for minority communities, including the LGBTQ community. When people have minority identities and face stigma, stereotyping, and harassment on a daily basis, having a community where they are unquestioningly accepted for who they are is important to psychological well-being. Sport can help build this sense of community and provide a place where people with shared interests or shared histories can come together and create community. Due to this, lesbian and gay sports leagues have been created in cities across the country. For example, LGB softball leagues exist in Chicago, San Francisco, Fort Lauderdale, Portland, and many other cities. There are also gay hockey leagues in Chicago, New York, Colorado, Minneapolis, and elsewhere; and lesbian softball leagues have been established in a number of large cities around the country. LGBTQ advocacy groups and even some city park districts have now created gay and lesbian sports leagues across the country in a myriad of sports from softball, to kickball, to volleyball, and hockey, among others.

There also larger scale events, including the Gay Softball World Series (GSWS) and the Gay Games, which allow LGBTQIA athletes from around the country and world to come together as a community and compete. The Gay Games has been around since 1982, and during that time it has grown steadily. The 2014 Gay Games held in Cleveland, Ohio, for example, included 10,000 participants from 60 countries. The Gay Games prides itself on inclusion and is open to all adults regardless of sexual orientation or athletic ability. They also allow transgender participants to compete as the gender that is either on their legal documentation or is the gender they live and present as, even if that does not match their legal documentation.

The Gay Softball World Series (GSWS) has existed since 1977 and is supported by the North American Gay Amateur Athletic Alliance. It has 5,000 participants from 44 cities. In order to meet their mission of providing a space for the LGBT community, teams are only allowed to have two heterosexual players per roster. In 2008 there was an incident where a team was stripped of their second place award for having three players that the league deemed to be straight; however, the players identified as bisexual (Bishop, 2011). This case serves as an example of an LGBT organization also struggling with issues of identity and inclusion that are faced by mainstream organizations. The organization has since updated its identity definitions to be more accepting of bisexual and transgender athletes rather than solely lesbian and gay athletes. However, it has maintained the two players per team cap on heterosexual players. Events like the GSWS and the Gay Games help to create community and give LGBT athletes a place to gather and build community with one another.

There are few leagues specifically crafted for LGBT youth; however, these adult organizations serve as examples to queer youth that there is space and acceptance for them within society and within sport. Creating queer specific spaces for youth and adults is important to give people a community with whom they may share certain similar experiences and can support one another. LGBTQ sports leagues or tournaments can help do this, both at the local as well as national level. These leagues can serve to not only build community among athletes but can also show youth or adults who may be struggling with their identity or with negotiating being LGBQ that there are others like them. It may give individuals who are struggling hope. Events like the Gay Games can also provide a space for people who have to hide their identity in their hometowns—a space to participate and be out and among similar people for a small amount of time. Although the queer community needs to be integrated and seamless within mainstream sport, the continued presence of separate spaces is also important for the community.

Conclusion

Although queer athletes still face stigmas and issues in society and sport, the landscape is becoming more accepting and inclusive. As society becomes more accepting, and as more players continue to come out as LGBQ, sports will continue to become more accepting and welcoming. Open athletes, coaches, and administrators are helping with this, as are teammates who serve as vocal allies. With society as a whole being more supportive of the queer community, vocal allies are becoming increasingly present, and this is a necessary step toward inclusion. With only roughly 10 percent of the population being LGBQ, allies are an important asset to creating an inclusive and welcoming environment. As more athletes come out, and as more allies express their support, it will continue to be easier for queer youth to feel comfortable in the sporting environment and to continue to gain the benefits of sport without having to hide an aspect of themselves.

Nonprofit organizations are also working to help support LGBQ athletes through advocacy, resources, and general promotion of inclusive teams. GLSEN provides information for athletes, coaches, parents, and schools about coming out, and about creating supportive environments. You Can Play is an initiative started within hockey in order to promote inclusion of LGBQ athletes in hockey and in other sports. They have counseled athletes through the coming out process, partnered with professional and college teams and leagues to create diversity and inclusion initiatives, and their founders and board members often talk to leagues, schools, and teams about inclusion in sport. Meanwhile, Go Athletes! is a network of current and former LGBTQ athletes that seeks to create safe spaces in sport through education, advocacy, and visibility. These are just some of the organizations that are working to promote inclusion and acceptance of LGBTQ athletes in all levels of sport. They play an important role in supporting athletes in their coming out process as well as in teaching other athletes, teams, and leagues about acceptance and how to foster inclusion within their organizations. With the current events and trends in society, it is becoming more common to see collegiate and professional LGBQ athletes, and that will continue. As this continues, more youth athletes may feel comfortable coming out, not only because society as a whole is more accepting but also because they have athletic role models who are similar to themselves.

Erin L. Morris

Further Reading

Azzopardi, C. 2014, December 9. "Q&A: Robbie Rogers on Why Athletes Won't Come Out, ESPN's 'Ridiculous' Locker Room Coverage." *Pride Source*. Accessed at http://www.pridesource.com/article.html?article=69300.

Bishop, G. 2011, June, 29. "Three Straights and You're Out in Gay Softball League." *The New York Times*. Accessed at http://www.nytimes.com/2011/06/30/sports/softball-case-raises-question-who-qualifies-as-gay.html.

Bruni, F. 2014, February 10. "Panic in the Locker Room." *The New York Times*. Accessed at http://www.nytimes.com/2014/02/11/opinion/bruni-panic-in-the-locker-room.html?_r=0.

Connelly, C. 2014, February 10. "Mizzou's Michael Sam Says He's Gay." *ESPN*. Accessed at http://espn.go.com/espn/otl/story/_/id/10429030/michael-sam-missouri-tigers-says-gay.

Cyphers, L., and K. Fagan. 2013. "Unhealthy Climate." *ESPN*. Accessed at http://sports.espn.go.com/ncw/news/story?page=Mag15unhealthyclimate.

Gleeson, S., and E. Brady. 2015, June 4. "Catch-22: Coming Out Can Quell Gay Slurs, but Fear of Homophobia Hinders Closeted Athletes." *USA Today*. Accessed at http://www.usatoday.com/story/sports/2015/06/04/homophobia-international-study-openly-gay-athletes-jason-collins-michael-sam/28434159.

GLSEN. 2013. *The 2013 National School Climate Survey, Executive Summary*. Accessed at http://www.glsen.org/sites/default/files/NSCS_ExecSumm_2013_DESIGN_FINAL.pdf.

Martin, M. S. 2014, December 16. "Gay W. Virginia High School Soccer Player Comes Out by Dancing with Homecoming King." *Out Sports*. Accessed at http://www.outsports.com/2014/12/16/7378317/michael-martin-gay-soccer-west-virginia-high-school-coming-out.

Mosbacher, D., and F. Yacker. (Producer, Director). 2009. *Training Rules* [Motion picture]. USA: A Woman Vision.

Parents, Families, and Friends of Lesbians and Gays. 2015. *The PFLAG National Glossary of Terms*. Accessed at http://community.pflag.org/glossary.

Rohlin, M. 2013, July 17. "WNBA's Brittney Griner Has Learned to Rise Above It All." *LA Times*. Accessed at http://articles.latimes.com/2013/jul/17/sports/la-sp-brittney-griner-20130718.

Women's Basketball Coaches Association. (2015). Accessed at http://www.wbca.org/files/2015_Convention_LGBTQ_Handouts_for_Roundtable_Sessions.pdf.

Websites

CAAWS. http://www.caaws-homophobiainsport.ca/e/resources_caaws/index.cfm

Gay Games. https://gaygames.org/wp

Gay, Lesbian, & Straight Education Network (GLSEN). www.glsen.org

Gay Softball World Series. http://www.gsws2015.org

GLAAD. www.glaad.org

GO! Athletes. http://www.goathletes.org

North American Gay Amateur Athletic Alliance. http://www.nagaaasoftball.org

Out Sports. http://www.outsports.com

Parents, Families, and Friends of Lesbians and Gays (PFLAG). http://community.pflag.org

You Can Play Project. http://youcanplayproject.org

Single-Sport Specialization versus Sampling

Youth sports are central to many young people's lives. Most current athletes began their careers in youth sports, and organized youth sports are everywhere in the United States, regardless of community size or location. Although participation rates vary, it is estimated that three out of every four households have at least one child participating in some youth sport (Swanson, 2016). Youth sports can provide many benefits to boys and girls, including improvements in leadership development, communication skills, work ethic, and overcoming adversity. Participation in organized activities, like youth sports, is associated with a variety of positive outcomes in adolescence and may lead to more regular physical activity as young adults (Kjønniksen, Anderssen, and Wold, 2009).

However, youth sports can also be problematic when improperly structured. Although many participate, many youth will also drop out of their sport in any given year. This dropout can be due to involvement in other activities; however, it is often due to parental overinvolvement, poor coaching, excessive training, and increased stress. Youth often perceive such environments as "occupations" that are no longer fun, motivating activities in which they feel that they are building skills, experiencing excitement, and meeting friends.

One current trend in youth sport is single-sport specialization. In recent decades, specialization has become more common and sometimes problematic (Gould, 2010), especially when parents make the decision for their child to specialize, or when specialization occurs too young. This entry will focus on sport specialization in contemporary youth sport. As such, it will examine differences between so-called youth sport "specializers" and "samplers" (multisport participants), noting benefits and drawbacks of each. It will also cover topics that better contextualize specialization, including major youth sport trends, and also distinguish between deliberate practice and deliberate play in youth sport. Finally, the entry will conclude with some recommendations for adults working with young athletes to successfully navigate issues related to youth sport specialization. It should also be noted that there is an important distinction between *youth sport* and *interscholastic sport*. Youth sport is generally defined as organized sport programs designed for children 14 and younger (National Association for Sport and Physical Education, 2010), whereas interscholastic sport typically refers to organized high school sports. This distinction is important because youth sport settings are more likely characterized by coaches who have less formal training, more direct parent involvement, and younger athlete involvement. By contrast, interscholastic sports are characterized by more structured organizations (e.g., state high school athletic associations), more formally trained coaches, and more developmentally mature athletes who are better able to handle the physiological and psychological demands of their sport.

Defining Sport Specialization and Diversification (Sampling)

Youth sport specialization is best described as intense, year-round training in a single sport to the exclusion of other sports and activities. Increased pressure to specialize in one sport can come from parents, coaches, and even athletes themselves. This is in contrast to multisport participation, sometimes referred to as sampling or diversification that is characterized by involvement in multiple sports, especially during early to middle childhood (ages 6 to 12). The distinction between youth sport specializers and nonspecializers is not simply the number of sports participated in, but the emphasis of sport participation as well.

The Rationale for Sport Specialization

Numerous examples can be found of famous athletes who began competing exclusively within one sport at a very young age. These include Lindsey Vonn (who began skiing at age 2), Michael Phelps (an Olympic swimmer by age 15), the Williams's sisters in tennis (Venus and Serena, who both began training at age 3), and Tiger Woods (who was displaying his golf skills on national television at age 8). In particular, Tiger Woods's story captured people's attention in describing success through early specialization. Earl Woods (Tiger's father) published an influential book titled *Training a Tiger: A Father's Guide to Raising a Winner in Both Golf and Life* (1997) that provided what many felt was a "blueprint" for early specialization success.

There is some evidence supporting early sport specialization as a path to increased athletic success. Research indicates that early specialization through *deliberate practice* (described as effortful practice lacking enjoyable qualities and performed specifically to improve one's performance levels) was important in developing skill expertise and that in order to become an expert, beginning early in that skill was necessary (Ericsson, Krampe, and Tesch-Römer, 1993). Other support for early specialization came from the "10-year rule" (Simon and Chase, 1973) and the "power law of practice" (Newell and Rosenbloom, 1981).

The 10-year rule refers to the idea that approximately 10 years (or 10,000 accumulated hours) of deliberate practice are needed to reach an expert status in a given skill. This guideline was first identified in chess, where experts were found to possess superior information-processing skills compared to less-elite players. However, support for the 10-year rule has also been found in music, academics, and sports. Subsequent researchers found that the earlier regular deliberate practice begins the better, because accumulation of such training needs to occur gradually; when young athletes begin deliberate practice, initial durations must be limited because increasing the intensity or duration of deliberate practice too quickly leads to overuse and overtraining. In short, optimal long-term deliberate practice is characterized by slow, regular progressions in amount and intensity of practice, which allows for adaptations to increased sport demands (Ericsson et al., 1993). In sport, it is thought that an early beginning is required to obtain an early expert status and reach a competitive level with older athletes. Application of this rationale to youth sport would mean that if an athlete began a regiment of deliberate practice at age 6, and became elite in that sport by 16, another child might have an advantage (theoretically) by beginning intensive training in that sport at 5 years of age.

The "power law of practice," meanwhile, is the idea that there is a relationship between accumulated practice in a given sport and rate of learning. Specifically, this means that the relative rate of learning and skill development is initially rapid for a beginner, but this rate of learning and improvement slows down as one improves in that skill over time. For example, the more time a tennis player invests in deliberate practice (i.e., drills, rote practice), the better the athlete becomes in terms of tennis skills (and potential achievement), but the more difficult it becomes to make further improvements over time. In other words, early dramatic improvement gives way to more incremental improvements as skills become more advanced.

Deliberate Play and the Developmental Model of Sport Participation

In order to understand the difference between specialization and diversification in youth sports, one needs to understand the distinction between deliberate practice and *deliberate play*. As previously noted, deliberate practice is a form of sport practice that requires effort, is often not perceived as enjoyable (such as when athletes are engaged in strenuous physical conditioning or static, monotonous drills for sport skill development), and is performed with the goal of improving performance. This would be akin to sport-specific drills or rote practice (when a tennis player serves a basket of balls or a basketball player repeats a specific shooting drill). Conversely, *deliberate play* activities are developmental sport activities that athletes tend to experience as enjoyable and intrinsically motivating. These settings are more informal (often without adults present), have flexible contexts, and offer youth freedom to experiment with their skills. In short, they possess a spontaneous "play" element even as they develop sport skills. Common examples of deliberate play include sandlot baseball, backyard soccer, or driveway basketball. These settings allow youth to use their imagination ("I'll be LeBron James and you can be Kobe Bryant"), develop important self-regulation skills (e.g., calling your own basketball fouls requires knowing what counts as a foul), and social negotiation skills (e.g., participants agreeing to modify rules for a less-skilled athlete). Deliberate play is thought to strengthen motivation by providing enjoyable sport experiences that form a foundation for sustained motivation later in adolescence when sport training becomes more intense (Soberlak and Côté, 2003). Given that lack of enjoyment is a main reason for youth sport dropout, deliberate play activities are important in strengthening intrinsic motivation for sport participation. In his book *Game On: The All-American Race to Make Champions of Our Children*, Tom Farrey (2008) presents an illustrative contrast of deliberate practice and deliberate play within soccer by contrasting American organized youth soccer with youth soccer in other countries. Although typical American soccer programs are characterized by highly structured, competition-based, and adult-run programs, in countries like France and Brazil there is more emphasis on unstructured play at younger ages. The sports cultures in these latter countries encourage youth to develop passion and improvisational skills through unstructured play, and as a result, the rewards for playing soccer are more intrinsic. In contrast to early specialization, Jean Côté and several colleagues (Côté, 1999; Côté, Baker, and Abernathy, 2007) developed the Developmental Model of Sport Participation (DMSP) as a framework to understand youth sport through different developmental tracks. The DMSP contains two pathways to youth sport skill development. These pathways include (1) early diversification (sampling multiple sports) and (2) early specialization. In the sampling track, athletes pass through three consecutive phases as they develop in their sport: (1) the sampling years (6–12 years of age), (2) the specializing years (13–15 years of age), and (3) the investment years (age 16 and older).

During the early sampling years, youth experience less intensive training (deliberate practice) and are more likely to participate in more deliberate play across multiple sports, where skill development and enjoyment are emphasized. In the specializing years, youth experience similar amounts of deliberate play, deliberate practice, and have likely narrowed participation to one or two sports. Finally, in the investment years, athletes (now adolescents) are more likely to devote many hours to deliberate practice in their chosen sport. In the early specialization track, youth immediately specialize in one sport and devote extensive time and energy to deliberate practice in that sport, with little to no other sport participation. Due to differences in deliberate play and deliberate practice, early specialization sport settings are often more serious, regimented, goal-directed, and "work-like" settings. The DMSP also notes that within all three phases (sampling, specializing, investment), youth athletes may also drop out of sport, or choose to progress to only a recreational participation in sport for a variety of reasons (e.g., the child may not be good enough to progress to the next level or may decide his or her motivations for being involved in the sport are not highly competitive, but more recreational in nature).

From this model, it is known that many elite athletes actually did not begin their sport careers through specialization. Instead, they were introduced to active lifestyles, played multiple sports, and primarily participated for fun and enjoyment, especially during their early sport years. It was only later in childhood that they specialized in one sport after developing more serious aspirations. There are numerous examples of successful professional athletes who played multiple sports before specializing in their career sport: basketball's Steve Nash (who played soccer and ice hockey before starting basketball at age 12), LeBron James (who played football as well), and football's Tom Brady (who excelled in both baseball and football). The DMSP emphasizes the importance of not specializing too early and instead recommends an early emphasis on fundamental motor skill development and enjoyment, with a supportive (but not overinvolved) parental presence in youths' sport involvement. Since the DMSP provides a contrast of youth athlete development through phases rather than direct, early specialization, it also provides a contrast between deliberate play (prominent in early sampling) and deliberate practice qualities (prominent in early specialization).

Parents and Sport Specialization

Parents often play a key role in youths' sport specialization. In fact, they often make this decision for their child. They provide financial support for everything from equipment and private lessons, to club fees to sports camps and year-round training facilities where youth may train and go to school. Coaches (who may also be the child's parent) also promote specialization by reinforcing the importance of year-round competition in one sport in order to develop more rapidly, get recognized, win championships, attract athletic scholarships, and become professional athletes. However, these expectations are often unrealistic given that less than 1 percent of high school athletes go on to play their sport professionally (National Collegiate Athletic Association, 2004). Youth sports are socially valued as productive activities and are visible within the community. Many parents (and athletes), though, value winning and advancing to the next level over skill development and having fun. Overinvolved parents who develop a mindset that they are investing in their child's future sometimes fall victim to a "return on investment" expectation that children will "reward" outlays of time and money by earning a college athletic scholarship. When youth athletes perceive such parental expectations, the result can be extreme pressure on the child.

Benefits of Sport Specialization

Youth sport specialization has become popular because many parents, coaches, and athletes believe that more practice, physical conditioning, and playing time devoted to a single sport will lead to more (and earlier) success.

Specialization benefits, for example, can be seen within motor skill acquisition. There is support for deliberate practice accumulation in developing sport talent (Ford et al., 2009; Helsen, Starkes, and Hodges, 1998), and Ericsson and colleagues (1993) found that youth who begin early deliberate practice routines have an advantage over those who do not. However, this advantage is largely sport-specific as it is likely that other motor skills in a different sport might not become as refined; a swimmer, for example, might be less likely to develop hand-eye coordination. In regard to youth sport, these findings make sense. The earlier a child begins specialized sport training, and the more time devoted to deliberate practice in that sport, the more likely his or her performance outcomes will improve, surpassing those kids who do not devote as much practice time to that specific activity. Younger, more talented athletes often receive more attention from the most experienced coaches, which is one reason athletes are led to early specialization. The push to specialize also depends on the sport, as some sports like gymnastics and figure skating have complex skills that need to be mastered before maturation (Judge and Gilreath, 2009). Youth who specialize early often benefit from better coaching and instruction because experienced coaches often want to work with athletes choosing to specialize, and scout for young prodigies. Finally, it is often out of necessity that specializers, who devote many hours of practice to it, develop better time management skills in childhood.

Drawbacks

Most would agree that positive youth development requires diversified experiences across different life areas. For example, most parents would agree that a well-rounded education is characterized by learning a variety of academic subjects like math, English, and sciences. If, for example, a young child was very talented in math, most would question the decision to eliminate all other academic subjects from that child's academic schedule so that he or she could maximize his or her potential and skills in math to the exclusion of other subjects. Such an academic regimen would not constitute a well-rounded education. Yet, that is precisely the logic of youth sport specialization. Critics of early specialization suggest that it does not justify the results since such a small percentage of youth athletes reach an elite status. Increased stress, emotional exhaustion, and burnout are linked to early sport specialization (Strachan, Côté, and Deakin, 2009), and early specialization may be associated with social isolation because intensive, year-round sport involvement separates youth from their peers and can interfere with normal identity development.

Aside from psychological concerns, physical concerns exist with specialization. In terms of motor skill development, it has been noted that children who specialize in one sport may not develop a solid base of fundamental motor skills, which could hamper their ability to be active as adults (Branta, 2010). An example of this concern, as mentioned above, might be seen with a child who specializes in swimming and never develops hand-eye skills needed for ball sports like tennis, baseball, or volleyball. Single sport participation is also linked to increased injury risk (Kaleth and Mikesky, 2010), especially overuse injuries. Specialization advocates note that early-specialized training improves the functioning of the body's various physiological systems. Although systems like the cardiovascular and muscular system will develop, they do so more because of natural growth and maturation and are not tied to early specialization. Physiologically, many youth sports experts believe that the drawbacks of early sport specialization outweigh the advantages due to injury and that youth who begin to specialize in a single sport at an early age are more likely to succumb to burnout.

Support for Youth Sport Diversification (Sampling)

Diversification refers to multisport participation, especially during early to middle childhood (6–12 years of age). Diversification may be advantageous because it allows for multifaceted social, psychological, and motor skill development (Wiersma, 2000). An argument frequently employed against diversification is that it may ultimately prevent youth from devoting the necessary time and practice to reach an elite status in their primary sport. However evidence actually contradicts this claim. For example, multisport participation has historically been found to be the norm for professional baseball players (Hill, 1993), and elite soccer players have been found not to specialize until after age 16 (Ward et al., 2007). More recently, youth competing in three sports between ages 11 and 15 were found by researchers to be more likely to compete at a national level in their sport between ages 16 and 18 than specializers (Bridge and Toms, 2013). Such findings have led advocates of sport sampling to assert that young athletes actually have a greater chance of achieving higher performance standards when they diversify their sport participation. In addition, studies indicate that sampling different sports provides benefits to overall fitness and gross motor coordination (Fransen et al., 2012). Such findings challenge the notion that early sport specialization is a prerequisite to an athletic scholarship or a professional sport career.

There may be a trade-off in that improvements in a given sport occur more slowly for samplers compared to specializers (Bompa and Haff, 2009); however, samplers may be more likely to reach eventual elite status. Also related to the notion of early diversification is the *timing* of specialization. Although Ericsson and colleagues (1993) have noted that early specialization is important, Côté and colleagues (2007) have argued, through the DMSP, that later specialization is more appropriate. More recently, European researchers (Moesch et al., 2011) compared elite and near-elite athletes to determine whether early or late specialization was associated with greater elite status in objectively timed or measured sports (e.g., swimming, weightlifting). They found that elite athletes specialized later in adolescence and trained less in their sport in early childhood, but had more intense training routines later in adolescence compared to less-elite athletes. It should also be noted that as long as a play-like component (deliberate play) is present in sport environments, such a sampling/deliberate play combination may be more likely to sustain intrinsic motivation when training becomes more difficult in a primary sport later in adolescence (Baker, 2003), thereby benefiting necessary long-term persistence in reaching elite athlete status. Thus, not only does it appear sampling is beneficial, but may ultimately allow kids to reach higher levels in their sport by delaying single-sport specialization until their later teens.

Conclusions and Recommendations

Based on existing information on specialization and diversification, several conclusions can be offered. Although adults often emphasize and prioritize winning and outcomes, these are less important to youth than having fun, developing skills, and being with friends (Ewing and Seefeldt, 1996). Hall of Famer and youth baseball organizer Cal Ripken Jr., for example, contended that prioritizing winning in youth sports should be postponed until at least middle childhood because if competition is overemphasized too early, kids will not develop the necessary confidence to be competitive later in their athletic journeys (Farrey, 2008). Adults within youth sport must realize that few young athletes will become elite, yet all youth athletes have a right to participate, which includes both practice and competitive contexts. Youth are motivated by active involvement; lack of participation is a main reason why they drop out of sport, so regardless of whether or not they specialize, youth need opportunities to actively participate within their chosen sport(s).

Early diversification does not appear to hurt elite athlete status attainment where peak performance is reached after physical maturation. Early diversification is also linked to longer sport careers and more positive sport involvement because youth who take this path are less likely to suffer from injury or burnout. Regardless of whether or not youth specialize, experts emphasize that early youth sport contexts characterized by high amounts of deliberate play are important because they build kids' intrinsic motivation through involvement in activities perceived as enjoyable, and in doing so promote intrinsic regulation. This is important because intrinsically motivated youth athletes become more self-directed in their later sport involvement. By late adolescence (age 16), athletes have developed the physical, social, emotional, and motor skills necessary to invest in highly specialized training in one sport, so it is recommended that youth wait until late adolescence to specialize because by this age, they can fully understand and weigh the costs and benefits of more intense, single-sport investment. Finally, in 2010, the National Association of Sport and Physical Education published a position statement on multiple-sport participation versus single-sport specialization. The organization concluded that while early specialization *may* be linked to earlier athletic success, it is more often associated with risks such as reduced motor skill development, loss of motivation, injury, and burnout. They therefore indicated that positive overall development was more likely when youth diversified sport participation. This statement echoed a similar recommendation from the American Academy of Pediatrics (2000), which discouraged single-sport specialization before adolescence.

Recommendations

Youth sport specialization is a hotly debated topic, and the social, physical, and psychological risks must be weighed against any potential benefits. However, based on what is known regarding early youth sport specialization versus early sampling, there are several recommendations based on academic research, medical professionals who deal with youth and youth injuries as well as youth sport administrators:

- Youth athletes should be encouraged to sample multiple sports so that they can discover what *they* enjoy rather than strictly follow adults' recommendations.
- Regardless of whether or not youth specialize, adults should establish sport environments where youth participate out of their own free will, and can

develop positive peer relationships and a sense of competence through their involvement, as these three factors are instrumental in producing long-term, self-regulated sport involvement.

- Parents should look for and support youth sport programs that emphasize participation and development of fundamental motor and sport skills, rather than exclusively emphasize competitive outcomes at an early age.
- Regardless of whether or not youth specialize, adults directly involved in youth sport should ensure athletes experience a range of deliberate play activities and informal games, where athletes can develop sport skills in safe, enjoyable settings.
- Because of the noted risks of specializing early, sport specialization should be discouraged until approximately age 15 or 16 when youth are capable of making independent decisions on their sport future.

In considering these recommendations, Cal Ripken Jr. provides useful insights, regardless of whether youth decide to specialize or diversify. In his 2006 text, *Parenting Youth Athletes the Ripken Way,* Cal Ripken discusses the "3 P's" of youth sport: *passion, praise, and patience. Passion* relates to intrinsic motivation and drive that fuels youths' love of the game. *Praise* refers to providing youth positive, accurate, and timely feedback about their sport skills and progress. Finally, *patience* refers to the idea that adults must remember that youth need lots of time to master sport skills and progress to higher levels. Ripken's 3 P's are relevant to the topic of sport specialization because regardless of whether youth specialize or diversify, adults involved in youth sport directly impact these three areas which, in turn, ultimately influence youths' continued sport involvement. In short, if youth sport environments do not include these three elements, it is not a matter of if, but when youth will drop out from their sport.

William Russell

Further Reading

American Academy of Pediatrics. 2000. "Intensive Training and Sports Specialization in Young Athletes." *Pediatrics, 106*: 154–157.

Baker, Joseph. 2003. "Early Specialization in Youth Sport: A Requirement for Adult Expertise?" *High Ability Studies, 14*: 85–94.

Bompa, Tudor, and Gregory Haff. 2009. *Periodization: Theory and Methodology of Training* (5th ed.). Champaign, IL: Human Kinetics.

Branta, Crystal F. 2010. "Sport Specialization: Developmental and Learning Issues." *Journal of Physical Education, Recreation, and Dance, 81*: 19–28.

Brenner, Joel S. 2007. "Overuse Injuries, Overtraining, and Burnout in Child and Adolescent Athletes." *Pediatrics, 119*: 1241–1245.

Bridge, Matthew W., and Martin R. Toms. 2013. "The Specialising or Sampling Debate: A Retrospective Analysis of Adolescent Sports Participation in the UK." *Journal of Sport Sciences, 31*: 87–96.

Coakley, Jay. 2015. *Sport and Society: Issues and Controversies* (11th ed.). New York: McGraw-Hill.

Côté, Jean. 1999. "The Influence of the Family in the Development of Talent in Sport." *The Sport Psychologist, 13*: 395–417.

Côté, Jean, Joseph Baker, and Bruce Abernathy. 2007. "Practice and Play in the Development of Sport Expertise." In Gershon Tenenbaum and Robert C. Eklund (Eds.), *Handbook of Sport Psychology* (pp. 184–202). Hoboken, NJ: Wiley.

Côté, Jean, and Ronnie Lidor. 2013. *Conditions of Children's Talent Development in Sport.* Morgantown, WV: Fitness Information Technology.

Côté, Jean, Ronnie Lidor, and Dieter Hackfort. 2009. "ISSP Position Stand: To Sample or Specialize? Seven Postulates about Youth Sport Activities That Lead to Continued Participation and Elite Performance." *International Journal of Sport and Exercise Psychology, 9*: 7–17.

Ericsson, K. Anders, Ralf Krampe, and Clemens Tesch-Römer. 1993. "The Role of Deliberate Practice in the Acquisition of Expert Performance." *Psychological Reviews, 100*: 363–406.

Ewing, Martha E., and Vern Seefeldt. 1996. "Patterns of Sport Participation and Attrition in American Agency-Sponsored Sports." In Frank L. Smoll and Ronald E. Smith (Eds.), *Children and Youth in Sport: A Biopsychological Perspective* (pp. 31–45). Madison, WI: Brown & Benchmark.

Farrey, Tom. 2008. *Game on: The All-American Race to Make Champions of Our Children.* New York: ESPN Books.

Fish, Joel. 2003. *101 Ways to Be a Terrific Sports Parent: Making Athletics a Positive Experience for Your Child.* New York: Simon & Schuster.

Ford, Paul R., Paul Ward, Nicola J. Hodges, and A. Mark Williams. 2009. "The Role of Deliberate Practice and Play in Career Progression in Sport: The Early Engagement Hypothesis." *High Ability Studies, 20*: 65–75.

Fransen, Job, Johan Pion, Joric Vandendriessche, Barbara Vandorpe, Roel Vaeyens, Matthieu Lenoir, and Renaat M. Philippaerts. 2012. "Differences in Physical Fitness and Gross Motor Coordination in Boys Aged 6–12 Years Specializing in One versus Sampling More Than One Sport." *Journal of Sport Sciences, 30*: 379–386.

Gould, Daniel. 2010. "Early Sport Specialization: A Psychological Perspective." *Journal of Physical Education, Recreation, and Dance, 81*: 33–37.

Helsen, Werner F., Janet L. Starkes, and Nicola J. Hodges. 1998. "Team Sports and the Theory of Deliberate Practice." *Journal of Sport and Exercise Psychology, 20*: 12–34.

Hill, Grant. 1993. "Youth Sport Participation of Professional Baseball Players." *Sociology of Sport Journal, 10*: 107–114.

Judge, Lawrence, and Erin Gilreath. 2009. "The Growing Trend of Early Specialization: Why Can't Johnny Play Three Sports?" *Indiana AHPERD Journal, 38*: 4–10.

Kaleth, Anthony S., and Alan E. Mikesky. 2010. "Impact of Early Sport Specialization: A Physiological Perspective." *Journal of Physical Education, Recreation, and Dance, 81*: 29–37.

Kjønniksen, Lise, Norman Anderssen, and Bente Wold. 2009. "Organized Youth Sport as a Predictor of Physical Activity in Adulthood." *Scandinavian Journal of Medicine and Science in Sports, 19*: 646–654.

Moesch, Karin, A. M. Elbe, T. Hauge, and J. M. Wikman. 2011. "Late Specialization: The Key to Success in Centimeters, Grams, or Seconds (cgs) Sports." *Scandinavian Journal of Medicine and Science in Sports, 21*: e282–e290.

National Association for Sport and Physical Education. 2010. *Guidelines for Participation in Youth Sport Programs: Specialization versus Multi-Sport Participation [Position statement].* Reston, VA: Author.

National Collegiate Athletic Association. 2004. *A Career in Professional Sports: A Guide for Making the Transition.* Indianapolis: Author.

Newell, Alan, and Paul S. Rosenbloom. 1981. "Mechanisms of Skill Acquisition and the Law of Practice." In J. R. Anderson (Ed.), *Cognitive Skills and Their Acquisition* (pp. 1–55). Hillsdale, NJ: Erlbaum.

Ripken, Cal. 2006. *Parenting Youth Athletes the Ripken Way: Ensuring the Best Experience for Your Kids in Any Sport.* New York: Gotham Books.

Simon, Herbert A., and William G. Chase. 1973. "Skill in Chess." *American Scientist, 61*: 394–403.

Soberlak, Peter, and Jean Côté. 2003. "The Developmental Activities of Elite Ice Hockey Players." *Journal of Applied Sport Psychology, 15*: 41–49.

Strachan, Leisha, Jean Côté, and Janice Deakin. 2009. "'Specializers' versus 'Samplers' in Youth Sport: Comparing Experiences and Outcomes." *The Sport Psychologist, 23*: 77–92.

Swanson, Beth, 2016. *Youth Sport Participation by the Numbers.* Accessed August 1, 2017, at www.activekids.com.

Ward, Paul, Nicola J. Hodges, Janet Starkes, and Mark Williams. 2007. "The Road to Excellence: Deliberate Practice and the Development of Expertise." *High Ability Studies, 18*: 119–153.

Wiersma, Lenny D. 2000. "Risks and Benefits of Youth Sport Specialization: Perspectives and Recommendations." *Pediatric Exercise Science, 12*: 13–22.

Woods, Earl. 1997. *Training a Tiger: A Father's Guide to Raising a Winner in Both Golf and Life.* New York: Harper Collins.

Sports-Based Youth Development (SBYD) Movement

It's almost a cultural phenomenon in the United States to pay lip service to the social and economic divisions in the country without taking the action that is necessary to address them. This is no less true for youth sports. Costs of participation in sports have risen during the past decade and, as a result, more and more youth, especially in low-income communities, have found themselves shut out of the game. It is in part to address these inequalities in youth sports that the sports-based youth development (SBYD) movement began. However, it is not the only reason. Supporters of the SBYD movement contend that the intrinsic values derived by playing sports, such as teamwork, leadership, and discipline, have been impeded upon by a multi-billion-dollar sports industry and its never-ending thirst for talent, scholarships, and merchandizing, all of which have further monetized play and driven the expectations of the child athlete to excess.

During the past decade, an unprecedented number of young athletes have been forced to play more games annually than professional athletes play, and many youth feel pressure to specialize in specific sports before they even hit middle school. As a result, adolescents are experiencing physical injuries (e.g., torn tendons and ripped ACLs) that once only afflicted adults (Musinski, 2014). Other youth are finding sports to be so mentally stressful that they are simply dropping out of sports entirely, as evidenced by the steady decline in participation rates across all four major youth sports (Wallerson, 2014). In this context, youth advocates concluded that sports needed a facelift. Not just reforms to address the equity issues among the "haves and have-nots," but also ones that return sports to their fundamental role in society as an inclusive activity that teaches values and encourages youth to explore their potential in a fun and engaging setting. Supporters assert that whether it is viewed as a derivative of sports or the next phase of its evolution, SBYD is rapidly becoming the remediation that youth sports desperately needs.

What Is Sports-Based Youth Development?

At its broadest, SBYD, as a *movement,* is an effort to reform youth sports. Depending on the goals and tactics of the reformer, SBYD can be defined as an emerging field of child development, a rallying cry to demand more from youth sports, and/or a social movement to engage the wider community in undoing negative trends that have emerged in youth sports over the past two decades.

First, SBYD can be viewed as a newly emerging field of child development that integrates the best practices of positive youth development into a sport setting. During the last few decades, a tremendous amount of work has focused on how protective factors embodied by positive youth development contribute to successful outcomes in young people. These outcomes include the ability to make healthier life choices, to set long-term goals such as graduating from high school and attending college, and to avoid risk behaviors such as smoking, substance abuse, and gang participation (Search Institute, 2015).

Fostering positive youth development requires creating an informal setting in which children are encouraged to explore new skills, interests, and abilities. It requires caring adults to play the role of mentors or guides and/or establish an atmosphere in which peers can exert a similar positive influence. The academic mentoring movement during the past two decades is one example of the impact of the youth development movement. Mentors, as role models, have provided children with a less structured environment to ask questions, explore new topics, and seek advice from a trusted adult outside of their everyday classroom and home environments. Studies have suggested that the presence of mentors in children's lives increase their likelihood of academic success and reduce their participation in negative social behaviors (Bruce and Bridgeland, 2014).

In recent years, finding new ways to promote positive youth development has gained momentum as issues such as youth violence, dropout rates, and childhood obesity have garnered national attention. Using sports as a methodology for youth development seems like a "no brainer," and many have gravitated to this medium as a way to engage youth in positive change. Sports provide unique characteristics that fit into a youth development framework, including an informal setting to tackle challenges and develop self-efficacy, the presence of positive adult role models, the opportunity to build social connections in a prosocial peer setting, and the lure of participation in something that is fun.

Sports, however, also offer a new dimension to the youth development framework: an emphasis on physical activity. Physical activity is not only correlated with health benefits, such as reduction in childhood obesity, but is also correlated with improved functioning. Research has shown that regular physical activity contributes to brain function that is tied to stronger academic outcomes. Studies have also found that physical activity reduces anxiety and depression, which are highly correlated with substance abuse, gang participation, and other risky behavior. As this connection between physical activity and brain development becomes more evident, SBYD holds promise as an emerging field in child development that can directly address dropout rates, gang participation, teen pregnancy, and childhood obesity.

Secondly, SBYD may be viewed as a rallying cry for those interested in reasserting the importance of youth sports in the United States. A rallying cry is a word or phrase that unites people to action, and SBYD has become the term that inspires those who want to see sports become accessible and affordable in communities and schools again. These advocates are frustrated by those who view sports as simply an athletic activity without recognizing the cognitive skills and life lessons that sports uniquely develop in children. Advocates have also expressed frustration with the rising costs that have made sports accessible only to those with resources and the potential for athletic success. In this context, these youth advocates are rallying to make SBYD programs a core component of public education.

This rallying cry could not have come at a more opportune time. Since the recession in 2008, the costs associated with youth sports have skyrocketed for most American families. Public schools, the staple for athletic programming for decades, have been forced to cut sports in order to address other priorities, such as extending classroom hours and/or transforming gyms into classrooms. To counter the outright elimination of sports activities, many schools have implemented pay-to-play schemes. Proponents argue that waivers exist to counter any detrimental effects of pay-to-play. However, studies have shown that schools that charge fees have lower rates of participation. Reasons for less participation include the perceived social stigma associated with having to ask for the waiver form; the hesitation of youth with tenuous legal status to apply; and the qualification that links these waivers to certain levels of poverty (often eligibility for free and reduced lunch) that may not accurately reflect a family's financial situation.

By emphasizing that SBYD addresses child development more than simply athletic development, SBYD proponents challenge school boards and administrators to understand that by cutting these programs, and/or making them unaffordable, they are actually undermining student performance, reducing academic motivation, and weakening the school atmosphere.

Lastly, youth practitioners are embracing SBYD as a social movement that returns sports to one of its core characteristics: fun. A social movement is a large group of people who organize to promote a social change or to undo a social change. Arguably, SBYD fits either definition. Thousands of organizations are joining forces to promote a new way of seeing the value of sports through a child development context, while at the same time they are uniting to undo the morphing of sports in

the last decades into a highly pressurized and exclusive activity aimed at only promoting the very elite child athlete.

Many older Americans are surprised by the present-day "business" of youth
sports that includes buying the right equipment, focusing on winning, and specializing early enough in one sport to increase the odds of a scholarship and/or professional career. Older Americans are also baffled that pickup sports have seemingly
disappeared and that the concept of playing sports just to be part of the neighborhood group has become obsolete. These changes in sports culture have become so
entrenched today that some of the most glaring proponents of this new status quo
are in fact coaches, parents, and onlookers whose aggressive behavior emphasizes
victory at all costs. As a result, young people are not having fun, and when presented with less stressful alternative activities, such as virtual and online gaming,
they drop out of sports entirely.

To bring traction to their movement, SBYD leaders are building a broad coalition of stakeholders that includes parents, teachers, and coaches who want to
undo these negative developments in youth sports. They are doing so armed with
research that demonstrates the value of SBYD to youth and society at large. The rise
in childhood obesity alone during the past quarter century provides enough evidence
of the harm being caused by youth who are becoming more sedentary because traditional sports no longer appeal to them. Leaders of the SBYD movement are calling on all sectors to reform sports so that they are once again viewed as a socially
engaging experience for all youth. Supporters emphasize that this effort will require
schools, parks, nonprofits, faith-based institutions, and most importantly, parents
to become advocates for SBYD and its promise to once again engage a wider
umbrella of youth in sports that are both skills-building and fun.

How Did Sports-Based Youth Development Evolve?

Sports have always been valued for the positive impact they can have on the physical and mental health of youth. It was largely for this reason that sports were integrated into public school curricula in the early 20th century. This public health
measure ensured the benefits of physical activity to a growing nation of immigrants,
many of whom lived in squalid and overcrowded urban neighborhoods.

The modern SBYD movement had its origins, not in the schools, but in nonprofit organizations that were focused on serving a similar population of disadvantaged youth. These nonprofits discovered that simply by adding a sports component
to their academic and social services (e.g., mentoring, violence prevention, teen
pregnancy prevention, and substance abuse prevention), they were able to attract
and to retain more youth in their programming. Eventually this "carrot and stick"

methodology of using sports as leverage for engaging youth in other beneficial activities became labeled "Sports Plus." Examples of Sports Plus include homework-help programs where the participant must complete his or her homework in order to play basketball.

During the first decade of this century, a major shift started to take place in the mindset of youth practitioners. Nonprofit leaders conducting Sports Plus programs noticed that youth participants were learning important life skills from the sports activity itself. In many of these cases, they witnessed how the benefits gleaned from the sports activity were accelerating the aptitude of young people in other program components, particularly when guided by a trained coach. For example, programs that used sports in tandem with teaching literacy discovered that students were more focused on reading and writing if they played sports *before* the academic exercise rather than playing it as a reward for completing the exercise. America SCORES, for example, is a national soccer and literacy program that challenges students from largely low-income urban neighborhoods to participate in soccer and writing courses that alternate throughout the week. Students do not perceive soccer as a reward for writing; rather, they tackle each component in tandem with one another. Being part of the soccer team, in fact, "develops a sense of trust and confidence on the field that is actually a motivator for the youth to excel in the creative writing program and in school," commented Holly O'Donnell, executive director of America SCORES (interview with author).

Similarly, program leaders have observed a correlation between skills-building through sports and achieving prosocial outcomes. Leaders of Row New York, a girl's rowing program, found that participants were more likely to graduate from high school and matriculate into college because of the confidence and self-esteem they developed on the racing shell. Program directors of Harlem RBI, a baseball program, observed that boys were much more academically motivated, and girls much more likely to avoid teen parenthood, because of the leadership skills and passion they developed for the baseball diamond. And, leaders of Tenacity, a tennis program, discovered that participants were much less likely to drop out of school (tenacity.org).

These programs have the following in common: (1) they serve underrepresented youth; (2) they use youth sports as the primary methodology for engaging youth; and (3) their missions do not focus exclusively on athletic excellence but also on achieving some social or academic outcome. These are some of the common characteristics shared by many SBYD programs, but prior to the beginning of the SBYD movement, what they also had in common was that they were operating in silos from one another. In many cases, SBYD programs in the same cities (even the same neighborhoods) did not know that the others even existed. They also lacked standards on how to operate their programs, design their curriculum, and train their staff and coaches. The field of SBYD had not yet been defined, and many of these programs were simply figuring it out day by day.

Perhaps the greatest detriment to the growth and sustainability of these programs was that even though they fully recognized the role of sports in enhancing character development and life skills, the outside world still thought of their organizations as traditional "sports" programs. Even at present, many foundations and corporate donors explicitly state that they do not fund "youth sports." This may be because the philanthropic community has been reticent to believe that "sports" fit into the larger youth development framework. As a result, SBYD pioneers found themselves in a dilemma: they feared that if they continued to emphasize the role of sport as a primary component of their logic model for youth development, it could jeopardize their financial security.

In June 2006, nonprofit leaders who were using sports to foster positive youth development in programs around the country assembled in Vail, Colorado, to discuss the state of youth sports. The summit was led by Harvard professor Gil Noam and a private school headmaster, Jeff Beedy. Although the purpose of the summit was to discuss a newly emerging trend in which an increasing number of youth were dropping out of sports entirely, the assembled group of leaders found themselves drawing a distinction between "traditional sports" and sports that incorporated life skills and youth development. "Kids were dropping out of highly competitive sports because of issues like stress and burnout," stated Aaron Dworkin, a conference attendee and president of the National Network of After School All-Stars. "That's not what we were. We were programs that were much more intentional on using sports to create engaging experiences that were inclusive of all kids." Jai Nanda, founder and executive director of Urban Dove and Urban Dove Team Charter School, a basketball program in New York, added, "We were increasingly realizing that our programs had a lot in common. While we embraced our sports for their competitive nature, we also were much more intentional about how we executed our programs so that kids learned lessons that would help them on and off the court. And, of course, we never lost track of the fact that sports are supposed to be fun and not stressful" (interview with author). It was at this summit that bonds first started developing in linking SBYD program leaders.

The participants recognized that in order to achieve credibility for how they were using sports in this context of youth development, they needed to organize. Within a year, Up2Us Sports was established as a nonprofit coalition to develop and advocate for the newly labeled field, SBYD, or sports-based youth development. The first task of the Up2Us Sports coalition was to conduct a needs assessment on what obstacles and challenges SBYD programs faced in terms of sustainability and growth. This assessment pointed to several challenges.

First, for these programs to become sustainable, they needed to educate funders that SBYD could effectively address major challenges facing youth in this country including child obesity, violence, and academic failure. This would require that supporters gather proof via developing evaluation instruments to study the impact of SBYD.

Up2Us Sports created an evaluation team to both launch studies and develop assessment tools to help program leaders determine their social return on investment (SROI). Up2Us Sports staff helped youth sports leaders learn how to collect and analyze data on a wide range of outcomes from levels of physical activity, to understanding of nutrition, to development of cognitive skills that are associated with children making better life choices. For youth sports, this practice of evaluation was entirely new and required considerable training on how to administer surveys, conduct focus groups, and levy actual physical assessments to determine SROI. What's more, these evaluation tools also needed to be flexible enough for programs to use across different age groups, cultures, genders, and sports.

A second need of SBYD practitioners was to define a common set of inputs, or "best practices," that would enable them to achieve the outcomes they desired. Up2Us Sports launched a team of program experts to create standards that distinguished an SBYD program from traditional sports programs. These standards addressed areas such as program design, youth engagement, coach training, safety, and program context.

Third, programs wanted training to help them achieve standards and demonstrate their effectiveness. In response, Up2Us Sports built a workforce of trainers to help program leaders design their sports activities within the SBYD framework. A large part of this training focused on helping coaches to incorporate SBYD into their everyday practice. This involved training coaches on positive youth development, trauma sensitive coaching (i.e., for youth living in low-income communities), health and nutrition, youth leadership and voice, gender in sports, diversity and inclusion, and prosocial connections. Ultimately, this training would lead to the Up2Us Sports Coach Certification, a multilevel professional course to maximize the effectiveness of the coach practitioner.

Other critical challenges also emerged from the needs assessment that were less about defining the SBYD field and more about the common struggles these programs faced in terms of operations and financial stability. These included finding sufficient funds to maintain staff and coaches, having enough product and equipment for kids to play, finding access to affordable spaces for practices and game days, and finding affordable transportation for transporting youth to game days and tournaments. As many SBYD programs operate in low-income communities, the solutions to these challenges would necessitate explaining to potential donors, including corporations, foundations, and government agencies, that investments in these resources were not simply about "funding sports" but about "funding youth development."

With the needs assessment serving as a "call to action," Up2Us Sports was officially chartered as a 501(c) nonprofit organization in 2010. At the time of its incorporation, the coalition had roughly 40 member organizations. In five short years it would have 1,300 member organizations, all of whom were committed to SBYD in their communities. Although the vast majority of member organizations remained local, nonprofits that embraced the SBYD philosophy, schools, charter schools, parks departments, and other government-led youth programs also joined the movement, as they experienced greater pressure to demonstrate that their sports activities were contributing to the mental, physical, and social health of their youth participants.

One of the flagship programs launched by Up2Us Sports was Coach Across America (CAA). Coach Across America is a national service and workforce development program that challenges adults to spend a year as an SBYD coach in a low-income community. The program serves multiple purposes for both Up2Us Sports and its member organizations. It provides a platform for attracting more practitioners to the SBYD field. Much as the nonprofit, Teach for America engages young adults in the field of education, CAA focuses on hiring and training adults to be role models through sports. Many CAA coaches are identified from the same communities in which they serve and, as a result, the program has become a platform for these young adults to discover careers in nonprofits, sports, and recreation. Coach Across America also provides SBYD organizations with trained coaches who help them achieve SBYD standards and, as a result, increase their impact on the community. In addition, CAA is a grant-making program of Up2Us Sports and, as such, provides the organization an additional vehicle for supporting its members, particularly those fledgling programs in poorer neighborhoods that need resources to hire staff. Lastly, CAA enables Up2Us Sports to measure the effectiveness of its training and evaluation tools through a centrally managed workforce of coaches who are committed to the SBYD field.

What Promise Does SBYD Have for Youth Sports?

Youth sports, in its current state, is losing participants as well as financial support. Sports-based youth development promises to turn this around by showing that sports are critical to child development and that SBYD should be incorporated into the core curriculum of public education. This is even more critical today as many public schools have eliminated and/or severely reduced their physical education programs. Advocates of sports-based youth development assert that it cannot only revive important content from physical education in a more engaging and inclusive format, but also broaden the potential of recreational programs to address major challenges facing youth: health, violence, and academic preparedness.

SBYD and Health

With the CDC's report that one in three children in the United States are obese or overweight, SBYD will be a critical tool for engaging youth in regular physical activity. Trained coaches in SBYD engage all youth during most of their practice time in moderate to vigorous physical activity (MVPA). The CDC recommends at least 60 minutes of MVPA daily for every child in the United States. SBYD coaches are also trained to make the sports experience engaging and fun, which is critical for retaining youth in programming throughout their childhood and adolescence. Studies have shown that youth who play sports are much more likely to develop lifelong habits of physical exercise. Ironically, traditional sports do not hold the same promise as SBYD as either an obesity deterrent or solution. SBYD advocates attribute this to the exclusivity of traditional sports and the fact that coaches focused mainly on winning games tend to favor the more athletic members of the team. Even within the traditional sports teams themselves, many athletes spend a good deal of time physically idle (i.e., sitting on the bench).

SBYD and Violence

Youth violence rates have captured the headlines with cities like Chicago experiencing epidemic rates of juvenile homicide. SBYD coaches are trained to use "trauma-sensitive" approaches to sports. By intentionally interweaving sports activities with opportunities to develop positive social connections, leadership skills, self-confidence, and self-efficacy, coaches provide youth with a platform to develop grit and resiliency to negative social behaviors like substance abuse and violence. SBYD programs are already demonstrating that youth with trained coaches develop cognitive skills associated with making better life choices. Studies have also demonstrated that youth who participate in sports are much less likely to join gangs and/or participate in violence.

SBYD and Academics

With nearly 50 percent of African American and Hispanic students not completing high school on time (America's Promise Alliance, 2009), SBYD programs provide a platform for character development that contributes to young peoples' academic preparedness and performance. Trained coaches teach life skills through sports, like goal setting and "Plan-B" thinking, that help children establish a greater focus on their futures and academic success. The presence of SBYD coaches, as consistent role models who incorporate informal time (i.e., outside of practice) as an opportunity to ask about school and encourage academic engagement, is also associated with greater student attendance. Even physical activity, itself, is correlated with greater brain functioning and academic focus. As a result, studies have shown that student athletes are more likely to graduate school and matriculate to college.

How Will SBYD Fulfill Its Promise?

To achieve its full potential impact in the field of youth development, observers indicate that SBYD will need to address the following:

SBYD Coach Certification

Coaches will need to be certified in SBYD to maximize their impact on the youth they serve. Up2Us Sports has already begun to develop partnerships with schools, parks, nonprofits, and even professional sports leagues and teams to implement SBYD certification. Parents and other caretakers should demand that this certification be a requirement of the coaches to whom they entrust their children daily.

SBYD Coach Employment

Supporters describe SBYD as a pathway of workforce development that is both needed and cost effective. SBYD defines the job of coaching of not only one that encourages athletic development through community-based leagues and teams, but also one that addresses challenges facing communities by hiring adults who are trained to encourage more positive pathways for youth. Up2Us Sports estimates that the costs of hiring one coach to serve at-risk youth in a disadvantaged community may save as much as 25 times that amount based on societal costs of reduced youth violence and increased health of participants. To address the promise of coaching as a career path, Up2Us Sports launched Coach Across America. Since the program's inception in 2009, the program has not only engaged more than 170,000 disadvantaged youth in regular sports activities, but nearly 65 percent of its alumni coaches have gone on to careers in SBYD and/or higher education.

SBYD Program Accreditation

Advocates of sports-based youth development encourage schools, parks departments, and nonprofits to accredit themselves in SBYD. This designation is the only way to assure parents and youth that a program incorporates the best practices in youth development and safety as well as athletic development. Parents and other caretakers should seek out programs that are SBYD accredited with the confidence that these programs are more likely to engage their youth in a positive experience in sports that contribute to their child's success on and off the field. Up2Us Sports is rolling out SBYD accreditation to its member organizations and is seeking to educate parents about its value.

SBYD Impact Studies

Although current studies have established a significant library of data on the positive impact of SBYD, practitioners will need to continue to collect data as the field becomes more defined in the years ahead. Data will help to inform best practices in coach training and program accreditation as well as establish an even more solid basis for funding SBYD as a health promotion strategy, academic enrichment program, and violence prevention alternative.

Mandatory SBYD in Schools

It is critical that schools address character development in order to more fully prepare their students to succeed academically, socially, and economically. SBYD advocates describe their programs as a cost-effective platform for doing this. They believe that mandating SBYD programs as a supplement to physical education and/ or as an alternative to traditional "gym" class provides schools a platform for engaging students in activities that reinforce their commitment to education and promote the pride and safety of the school community. SBYD programs can be incorporated before, during, and after school. They can also be launched in partnership with accredited community-based SBYD programs to alleviate some of the administrative and financial costs on the schools.

SBYD Funding

Ultimately, supporters of sports-based youth development acknowledge that it will take a recognition of the value of SBYD to entice further private and public investment in the field. As initial studies continue to demonstrate the impact of SBYD, however, they hope that foundations will prioritize SBYD as a youth development strategy and invest in SBYD in the school and community settings. "SBYD Empowerment Zones" can blanket neighborhoods with trained coaches so that parks, schools, and nonprofits can engage all children in sports activities that develop character, reduce crime, and promote graduation. They also urge that SBYD be incorporated into wider collective impact initiatives with public health, education, violence prevention, economic development, and community planning as part of a more coherent framework for encouraging the health and well-being of this nation's next generation of leaders and sports enthusiasts.

Organizations Supporting Sports-Based Youth Development

Coaching Corps; website: coachingcorps.org
Positive Coaching Alliance; website: positivecoach.org
The Women's Sports Foundation; website: womenssportsfoundation.org
The Aspen Institute's Project Play; website: aspenprojectplay.org
Laureus Sport for Good Foundation; website: laureususa.com
Up2Us Sports; website: up2us.org

Paul Caccamo

Further Reading

America's Promise Alliance. 2009. *Cities in Crisis 2009: Closing the Graduation Gap.* Accessed August 17, 2015, at http://www.americaspromise.org/cities-crisis.

Anxiety and Depression Association of America. 2015. *Substance Use Disorders.* Accessed August 17, 2015, at http://www.adaa.org/understanding-anxiety/related-illnesses/sub stance-abuse.

The Aspen Institute Project Play. 2006. *Sport for All, Play for Life: A Playbook to Get Every Kid in the Game.* Accessed August 17, 2015, at http://youthreport.projectplay.us.

Bruce, Mary, and John Bridgeland. 2014. *The Mentoring Effect: Young People's Perspectives on the Outcomes and Availability of Mentoring. Civic Enterprises with Hart Research Associates for MENTOR: The National Mentoring Partnership.*

Coid, Jeremy, Simone Ullrich, Robert Keers, Paul Bebbington, Bianca DeStavola, Constantinos Kallis, Min Yang, David Reiss, Rachel Jenkins, and Peter Donnelly. 2013. "Gang Membership, Violence, and Psychiatric Morbidity." *The American Journal of Psychiatry, 170*(9): 985–993.

Crime Lab. 2012. *BAM–Sports Edition.* Accessed August 11, 2015, at https://crimelab .uchicago.edu/sites/crimelab.uchicago.edu/files/uploads/BAM_FINAL%20 Research%20and%20Policy%20Brief_20120711.pdf.

Musinski, Robert. 2014. "ACL Injuries on the Rise but Evidence Based Programs Can Reduce the Risk: Clinical Report." *AAP News, 35*(5). doi:10.1542/aapnews.2014355-11

Nike, Inc. 2012. *Designed to Move: A Physical Activity Agenda.* Accessed August 17, 2015, at www.designedtomove.org.

Perkins, Daniel F., and Gil G. Noam. 2007. "Characteristics of Sports-Based Youth Development." *New Directions for Youth Development*, (115), 75–84.

Ratey, John. J., and Eric Hagerman. 2008. *Spark: The Revolutionary New Science of Exercise and the Brain*. New York: Little, Brown and Company.

Rosewater, A. 2009. *Learning to Play and Playing to Learn: Organized Sports and Educational Outcomes*. Prepared for Team Up for Youth, Oakland, CA.

Rowe, Claudia. 2012, January 7. "Higher Fees to Play Sports Leaves Kids on Sidelines." *The Seattle Times*. Accessed August 11, 2015, at http://www.seattletimes.com/seattle -news/higher-fees-to-play-sports-leaves-kids-on-sidelines.

Search Institute. 2015. *The Power of Developmental Assets*. Accessed August 11, 2015, at http://www.chicagomanualofstyle.org/tools_citationguide.html.

Sportanddev.org. 2015. *Healthy Development of Children and Young People through Sport*. Accessed July 10, 2015, at http://www.sportanddev.org/en/learnmore/sport_education _and_child_youth_development2/healthy_development_of_children_and_young_people _through_sport.

Tenacity. *Pathway to Post-Secondary Success*. Accessed February 1, 2018, at https://tenacity .org/about-us.

Tomporowski, Phillip D., Catherine L. Davis, Patricia H. Miller, and Jack A. Naglieri. 2008. *"Exercise and Children's Intelligence, Cognition, and Academic Achievement." Educational Psychology Review, 20*: 111–131. doi:10.1007/s10648-007-9057-0

Trost, Stewart, Richard Rosenkranz, and David Dzewaltowski. 2008. "Physical Activity Levels among Children Attending After-School Programs." *Medicine & Science in Sports & Exercise, 40*(4): 622–629.

Up2Us Sports. *Up2Us Center for Sport Based Youth Development*. Accessed February 12, 2018, at http://www.asandaces.org/uploads/4/3/2/4/43244011/front_runners_of_sbyd _report.pdf.

Wallerson, Ryan. 2014, January 31. "Youth Participation Weakens in Basketball, Football, Baseball, Soccer." *The Wall Street Journal*. Accessed August 11, 2015, at http://www .wsj.com/articles/SB10001424052702303519404579350892629229918.

Substance Abuse

Participation in youth sport is regarded by many as a positive developmental experience. Youth sport promotes physical activity, establishes meaningful social connections with teammates and coaches, and provides unique learning experiences that are typically not provided in classroom settings (e.g., opportunities to engage in leadership/mentoring roles). Many parents and educators believe that involvement in sport also has the potential to deter youth from engaging in delinquent activities such as the consumption of alcohol and drugs. The deterrent effect of sport participation on delinquency is based on the understanding that this activity places youth in a structured environment with influential peers and adults. Moreover, youth who participate in sport often develop strong bonds with teammates and coaches within this conventional social arena, reducing the likelihood of engaging in delinquent activities. Although some studies have found that involvement in sport reduces violent forms of delinquency, various studies have found that participation in youth sport actually has the potential to increase other nonviolent forms of delinquency like substance use, specifically, alcohol abuse (Kwan, Cairney, Faulkner, and Pullenayegum, 2012). In particular, there is a large amount of evidence that indicates that youth who participate in sport are at greater risk of underage drinking, use of smokeless tobacco, and performance-enhancing drugs.

The association between substance use and involvement in sport among youth reveals a troubling health paradox: despite athletes engaging in many health-promoting behaviors (e.g., physical activity), they are at a greater risk of engaging in certain types of substance use. Although this appears contradictory, previous research has noted that participation in sport may put some youth at risk for substance use because of increased access to different types of substances (e.g., prescription pain medication). The exposure to normative behaviors that can facilitate the use of different types of substances (e.g., using steroids to gain a competitive edge), and the stress associated with managing a competent athletic identity (e.g., self-medicating with drugs and alcohol due to the stress of being an athlete) are cause for concern as youth sport continues to grow in exposure and pressure mounts for young athletes to perform.

Increased Access to Drugs and Alcohol among Athletes

Athletes who participate in sport have greater access to drugs and alcohol. For instance, many adults and youth who participate in sport sustain injuries that may require certain types of drugs to manage pain. It is estimated that every year, nearly 20 percent of interscholastic sport participants in the United States (about 1.4 million athletes) sustain an injury that requires medical attention by a team physician, certified athletic trainer, personal physician, or emergency department physician (Comstock, 2012). Although interscholastic sport injury rates dropped slightly between 2005 (2.51 injuries per 1,000 exposures) and 2012 (2.17 injuries per 1,000 exposures), the percentage of sports-related injuries that required surgery among interscholastic sport participants increased from 5.3 percent to 8.2 percent during this same time period (Comstock, 2012).

Several studies have found that youth who are highly involved in competitive sport are at a greater risk of being prescribed painkillers, misusing painkillers to "get high," and being approached to divert (e.g., give away or sell) these medications. A national study found that youth who participated in high-injury sports like football and wrestling were at an increased risk of misusing prescription painkillers (Veliz, Boyd, and McCabe, 2013). It is possible that the greater risk to misuse painkillers may be related to the fact that football players and wrestlers have the highest severe injury rate among high school athletes and may be more likely to have been prescribed painkillers by a physician. Moreover, youth who participate in high-injury sports may be surrounded by peers who are more likely to have leftover prescription painkillers, making it easier to receive diverted prescription painkillers to ease injuries without having to acknowledge to parents and coaches that they need medical attention. Although prescription painkillers can be effective in helping athletes deal with acute pain, increased access to prescription painkillers frequently provides opportunities for youth athletes to illegally divert these medications or use them in a manner not intended by the prescriber. Problematically, participation in sport can also indirectly place athletes within groups of peers who have greater access to other types of substances like alcohol, tobacco, or performance-enhancing drugs.

One clear example of sport providing a context in which participants have greater access to certain substances is the case of alcohol use. One of the most consistent findings among studies examining the association between sport participation and substance use is that athletes are more likely to consume alcohol when compared to their nonparticipating peers. One potential explanation is that sport provides a context in which youth come into contact with a distinct group of peers who share a similar orientation to engage in certain types of behaviors like alcohol use. In other words, participation in sport may introduce youth to a group of peers who have greater access to alcohol and who view underage alcohol consumption as an acceptable behavior (e.g., senior football players inviting their freshmen teammates to a keg party).

Particularly, peers influence one another, and adolescents conform to the expectations and demands of peers in order to make and sustain these relationships. Alcohol use is no exception. Conformity in engaging in underage alcohol consumption is driven to a large extent by an anticipated social payoff—increased popularity within different types of peer groups. Given that athletes tend to occupy higher levels of social status within their peer group, athletes may feel a higher level of pressure to consume alcohol during social gatherings in order to gain or maintain a certain level of popularity among their peers. Moreover, younger athletes may feel an additional burden to engage in alcohol consumption in order to establish meaningful relationships with older teammates and prove that they are truly committed to their team.

Exposure to Norms That Facilitate Substance Use

The notion of sport being a positive aspect in the lives of adolescents has been an ongoing debate in the sociology of sport. One side of the debate views sport as a mechanism to help socialize adolescents to a set of values and behaviors that promote positive physical, cognitive, and emotional development. The other side of the debate views youth sport as a distraction from full engagement in academics, or as a potentially harmful developmental experience that socializes participants to a set of norms that facilitates health-compromising behaviors (e.g., using steroids to gain an advantage).

Although many studies have found sport to be beneficial in promoting positive social behaviors, some researchers have pointed out that sport socializes youth into a hypermasculine orientation that facilitates deviant or risk-taking behaviors. There is consistent support that athletes are more likely to drink alcohol and engage in problem drinking as well as take steroids, fail to wear seat belts and motorcycle helmets, and speed. Studies that have asked students to self-identify their athletic identity have found that these forms of risk taking tend to be more prevalent among those who consider themselves to be athletes (Kokotailo, Henry, Koscik, Fleming, and Landry, 1996). It should also be acknowledged that certain types of sports provide vastly different socialization experiences for participants. The athletic experiences of youth wrestlers, for example, are often much different than those of soccer players. Sports that involve high levels of physical contact, such as football, ice hockey, lacrosse, and wrestling, tend to socialize youth to view pain, violence, and risk as normative features within the sporting context. Participants in contact sports are more likely to come to view their body as an instrument that can be easily gambled with, even if it might result in permanent damage. Conversely, sports that involve minimal to no contact with opponents, such as cross-country, swimming, tennis, and track, are valorized for their sustainability for participants across the life course. These types of sports emphasize a more self-disciplined lifestyle that cultivates a normative orientation that values moderation and self-control in order to sustain long-term health. Accordingly, certain types of sports may foster attitudes and behaviors favorable to drug use (or unfavorable to drug use) due to the social norms and practices embedded within these sporting contexts. In fact, high-contact sports may be more capable of socializing participants to a set of normative behaviors that can facilitate substance use given the pervasive norms that surround risk taking, concealing pain, and the unending pursuit of being the best.

Several recent national cross-sectional studies in the United States have examined the association between substance use and involvement in certain types of sport among youth. For instance, Bryan Denham (2011) found that youth who participate in baseball, football, and weightlifting have higher levels of alcohol consumption when compared to their peers. Denham suggests that these types of athletes may believe that their athletic performance will not be hindered by alcohol consumption because the sports that they participate in require more power than endurance. Interestingly, several of these recent studies have also considered categorizing the type of sport adolescents participate in by the amount of physical contact that is embedded within the sport. Data collected from nationally representative samples of youth find that athletes who participate in different types of high-contact sports (e.g., football, lacrosse, ice hockey, and wrestling) are more likely to engage in various types of substance use (e.g., binge drinking, cigarette use, marijuana use, and prescription drug misuse) when compared to their peers who do not participate in these sports. Moreover, athletes who participate in noncontact sports (e.g., cross-country, gymnastics, swimming, tennis, track, volleyball, and weightlifting) are less likely to engage in cigarette and marijuana use when compared to their peers who do not participate in these sports (Veliz, Boyd, and McCabe, 2015).

These studies provide some evidence that certain types of sport may teach and reinforce behaviors that facilitate substance use. Although it is difficult to untangle whether certain types of sport may attract participants who are more likely to engage in risky behavior or substance use, this research does show consistent patterns that can indicate which sports should be highly monitored with respect to providing interventions and potential types of drug counseling for athletes. Accordingly, prevention efforts should be directed toward athletes who may find it more difficult to seek help for potential substance use disorders.

The Stress of Successfully Managing an Athletic Identity

Participation in competitive youth sport in the United States drops significantly over the course of high school. One study, for example, found a decline in participation from 83.5 percent in 8th grade to 68.9 percent in 12th grade (Sabo and Veliz, 2014). The most common reason cited by youth for dropping out of sports is that they were no longer having fun. Part of the reason for this diminishment in enjoyment is directly related to the high level of competition that is embedded within sport during the middle and high school years. Despite the large number of youth who exit sport, however, the majority of youth continue to participate under a model that values winning and excellence in performance over participation to have fun and socialize.

The majority of youth who participate in sport subscribe to a performance ethic that stresses that athletes should always "strive to be the best," "play through pain," and "win-at-all-costs." This dominant ethic has the potential to create a stressful context that can place a physiological toll on participants. For instance, athletes may conceal injuries from teammates and coaches in order to keep their position on a team and may resort to using illicit substances to self-medicate the pain and stress associated with their injuries. In fact, a recent study found that male athletes who were highly involved in youth sports were more likely to misuse prescription painkillers (Veliz et al., 2014). Although the ostensible relationship between sports participation and medical use and misuse may be driven by opportunity and access, sports is a pivotal force in male adolescent development and has the potential to influence various types of substance use like prescription painkiller misuse. In particular, adolescent boys often depend on sports to elevate their social status, maintain relationships with teammates and family members (especially fathers), and project a tough and competent masculine identity to their peers. In other words, sport is a powerful context for boys to prove they are men, and boys may sacrifice their bodies through athletic performances to prove their masculinity. Consequently, substance use among boys may be influenced by the stress associated with managing a masculine identity within the context of sport. Interestingly, the difference between female athletes and nonathletes and substance abuse is minimal with the exception of some diuretic types of medications or techniques.

Although the institution of sport still rests on an ethic that is firmly based on heterosexual norms of masculinity and femininity, it must be acknowledged that there is greater acceptance of gay and other nontraditional sexual identities (i.e., sexual minorities) both within the United States and the larger social arena of sport than in years past. Despite this progress, studies that examine sexual minority athletes who are open about their sexual orientation have found that these athletes felt pressure to maintain a heterosexual framework that involved a self-silencing of their sexual orientation among their teammates and coaches. Moreover, acceptance of gay and other sexual minority athletes within the context of sport has been found to be contingent on their performance on the playing field; sexual minority athletes must use their athletic prowess to mediate the stigma associated with their sexual orientation.

Given that gay and other sexual minority athletes face multiple layers of stress in managing a stigmatized identity within the social context of sport while dealing with the pressure of being an athlete competing at a high level of competition, it is not surprising that they have been found to be at higher risk of substance use disorders than heterosexual athletes, heterosexual nonathletes, and sexual minority nonathletes. Male sexual minority athletes have the highest rate of being diagnosed with a substance use disorder. Consequently, this elevated level of stress may contribute to male sexual minority athletes misusing various types of substances to cope with the myriad stressors of being a gay male in the hypermasculine context of sport.

These studies suggest that a greater effort should be placed on developing preventative measures and providing outlets for athletes to receive treatment for either substance use or mental health. Therapist-led support groups, for example, have been identified as resources that can help mitigate the likelihood of substance abuse issues. Problematically, the culture of sport is based on the notion of self-reliance, mental and physical toughness, and the avoidance of acknowledging mental or physical pain; this culture prevents athletes from seeking help to manage these problems with substance use or mental health before they escalate to a point of severe emergency. This may even be more burdensome for sexual minority athletes, since they experience unique stressors and may feel that any acknowledgment of their sexual identity to team counselors, coaches, or teammates might jeopardize their position on their team or endanger highly valued relationships with team members. Future research needs to examine this subpopulation of youth athletes in greater detail to understand the underlying causes for the increased risk of substance use disorders. Such information could help inform the development of services to minimize stressors among sexual minority athletes and reduce substance use disorders and other mental health issues.

Conclusion

Although many people commonly accept sport as a valuable and necessary experience for youth, some aspects of sport can hinder the positive development of adolescents and encourage lifestyles that can jeopardize both short- and long-term health, such as alcohol and drug consumption. Such findings are inconsistent with narratives provided by youth sports organizations such as the National Federation of State High School Associations, which view sport as only promoting positive experiences and encouraging "healthy lifestyles" among participants rather than seeing that sport has the potential to be both good and bad depending on the lessons and behaviors that can come from participation.

Although many researchers who study youth sport understand that participation can provide both positive and negative outcomes with respect to health and physiological development, many parents may be unaware of the negative consequences of participating in this type of extracurricular activity. It is important to openly communicate that participation in competitive sports during elementary, middle, and high school may put some individuals at risk to engage in substance use. Accordingly, parents, coaches, counselors, and educators need to be aware that not all sports protect youth from engaging in unhealthy practices, and should also consider the possible risks as youth transition into young adulthood. Moreover, school administrators and coaches should consider in-season counseling for athletes or require athletes to be screened for potential substance use or mental health disorders during yearly physicals.

Philip Veliz

Further Reading

Anderson, Eric. 2009. *Inclusive Masculinity: The Changing Nature of Masculinities.* New York: Routledge.

Balsa, Ana, Jenny Homer, Michael French, and Edward Norton. 2011. "Alcohol Use and Popularity: Social Payoffs from Conforming to Peers' Behavior." *Journal of Research on Adolescence, 21*: 559–568.

Coakley, Jay. 2010. *Sports in Society: Issues and Controversies.* Colorado Springs, CO: McGraw-Hill.

Comstock, Dawn, Christy Collins, Jill Corlette, and Erica Fletcher. 2012. *National High School Sports-Related Injury Surveillance Study: 2011–2012 School Year.* Columbus, OH: Center for Injury Research and Policy. Accessed May 15, 2015, at http://www .nationwidechildrens.org/cirp-rio-study-reports.

Cottler, Linda, Arbi Ben Abdallah, Simone Cummings, John Barr, Rayna Banks, and Ronnie Forchheimer. 2011. "Injury, Pain, and Prescription Opioid Use among Former National Football League (NFL) Players." *Drug and Alcohol Dependence, 116*: 188–194.

Darrow, Cory, Christy Collins, Ellen Yard, and Dawn Comstock. 2009. "Epidemiology of Severe Injuries among United States High School Athletes: 2005–2007." *American Journal of Sports Medicine, 37*: 1798–1805.

Denham, Bryan. 2011. "Alcohol and Marijuana Use among American High School Seniors: Empirical Associations with Competitive Sports Participation." *Sociology of Sport Journal, 28*: 362–379.

Farb, Amy, and Jennifer Matjasko. 2012. "Recent Advances in Research on School-Based Extracurricular Activities and Adolescent Development." *Developmental Review, 32*: 1–48.

Hughes, Robert, and Jay Coakley. 1991. "Positive Deviance among Athletes: The Implications of Overconformity to the Sport Ethic." *Sociology of Sport Journal, 8*: 307–325.

Kokotailo, Patricia, Bill Henry, Rebecca Koscik, Michael Fleming, and Gregory L. Landry. 1996, July. "Substance Use and Other Health Risk Behaviors in Collegiate Athletes." *Clinical Journal of Sport Medicine, 12–38*.

Kwan, M., J. Cairney, G. E. Faulkner, and E. E. Pullenayegum. 2012. "Physical Activity and Other Health-Risk Behaviors during the Transition into Early Adulthood: A Longitudinal Cohort Study." *American Journal of Preventive Medicine, 42*: 14–20.

Lisha, Nadra, and Steve Sussman. 2010. "Relationship of High School and College Sports Participation with Alcohol, Tobacco, and Illicit Drug Use: A Review." *Addictive Behaviors, 35*: 399–407.

Miller, Kathleen. 2009. "Sport-Related Identities and the 'Toxic Jock.'" *Journal of Sport Behavior, 32*: 69–91.

Miller, Kathleen, Joseph Hoffman, Grace Barnes, Michael Farrell, Don Sabo, and Merrill Melnick. 2005. "Jocks, Gender, Race, and Adolescent Problem Drinking." *Journal of Drug Education, 33*: 445–462.

Reardon, Claudia, and Shane Creado. 2014. "Drug Abuse in Athletes." *Substance Abuse and Rehabilitation, 5*: 95–105.

Sabo, Don, and Philip Veliz. 2008. *Go Out and Play: Youth Sports in America.* East Meadow, NY: Women's Sports Foundation.

Sabo, Don, and Philip Veliz. 2014. "Participation in Organized Competitive Sports and Physical Activity among U.S. Adolescents: Assessment of a Public Health Resource." *Health Behavior & Policy Review, 1*: 503–512.

Veliz, Philip, Carol Boyd, and Sean E. McCabe. 2013. "Playing through Pain? Sports Participation and Nonmedical Use of Opioid Medications among Adolescents." *American Journal of Public Health, 103*: e28–e30.

Veliz, Philip, Carol Boyd, and Sean E. McCabe. 2015. "Competitive Sport Involvement and Substance Use among Adolescents: A Nationwide Study." *Substance Use & Misuse, 50*: 156–165.

Veliz, Philip, Quyen Epstein-Ngo, Elizabeth Meier, Paula Ross-Durow, Sean E. McCabe, and Carol Boyd. 2014. "Painfully Obvious: A Longitudinal Examination of Medical Use and Misuse of Opioid Medication among Adolescent Sports Participants." *Journal of Adolescent Health, 54*: 333–340.

Veliz, Philip, Quyen Epstein-Ngo, Jennifer Zdroik, Carol Boyd, and Sean E. McCabe. 2016. "Substance Use among Sexual Minority Collegiate Athletes: A National Study." *Substance Use & Misuse, 51*(4): 517–532.

Veliz, Philip, and Sohaila Shakib. 2012. "Interscholastic Sports Participation and School Based Delinquency: Does Participation in Sport Foster a Positive High School Environment?" *Sociological Spectrum, 32*: 558–580.

Travel-Club Teams

Youth sport used to conjure a picture of children from the local community getting together on a Saturday to play against other teams from the community. The stands were populated by neighbors, and most spectators knew one another. That scenario exists today, but it is only a very small part of the overall youth sport landscape. It is still common for children to get their start in sport through community recreation leagues. However, it is increasingly common for children to move from these recreation leagues to more competitive settings. In fact, travel teams are taking over youth sport. In Minnesota, for example, Minneapolis Parks and Recreation sport programs lost 600 participants from 2009 to 2015. At the same time, the growth in travel basketball teams has increased exponentially, with more than 1,400 boys and girls teams participating in the state tournament in 2015 (McCoy, 2015).

The Draw of Travel Teams

The most obvious difference between playing for a recreational team and playing for a travel team is the extent and cost of travel to tournaments. Recreational teams play against other teams in the same community or nearby communities. Competition typically consists of league play over a set period of time (i.e., the season). Practice schedules vary but average once or twice per week with a single game scheduled on the weekend. Some recreational programs may also include a midweek game. Travel teams, on the other hand, require a more intense commitment with more practice time, overnight travel to competitions, and tournament-based competitions rather than single games. The intensity of travel team participation is at the core of its influence and its impact on young athletes and their families. Participation on travel teams affects family interactions, as well as the social lives of players, parents, and siblings. The costs involved can be significant, affecting families' ability to provide travel team opportunities for their children and limiting some parents' ability to participate in their children's sport. Still, travel teams remain popular venues for sport participation and can be beneficial to athletes and their parents. Their value depends on the manner in which they are implemented.

Travel teams can and often do take over family time. Families invest time traveling to practices and competitions (many of which require overnight stays), watching their children play, planning travel, and even fund-raising (Hoefer et al., 2001; Wiersma and Fifer, 2008). This can have both beneficial and detrimental effects on the family. Importantly, it can affect some family members more than others.

Effects on Parents

Consider, for example, the case of Pat. Pat and her husband were former athletes and had two sons. Both of Pat's sons were year-round swimmers. Like other club sports, swim competitions were weekend events and most often involved travel and overnight stays. Pat was lucky that both of her children competed with the same club, and the family was able to travel together to competitions. Pat noted, "We spent a LOT of time together. It was great! We had an activity that everyone in the family enjoyed; one that we could share. Not only did we share time at meets, we had something we could talk about with the kids at home—even when they were in their teen years and didn't want anything to do with us most of the time" (Green, 2011). Because of the downtime at swim meets and the extensive travel with the club, Pat's family became close with the other swimmers' families. The swim club families had much in common and became an important part of the family's social world. Then it happened. Pat's boys decided they didn't want to swim anymore. It was no longer fun. Pat was devastated. As she put it, "I didn't really care whether the boys swam or not, but I was about to lose my social life. I had spent years with the parents of the other swimmers. They were our friends. We rarely had time to socialize outside of swimming. Now I was losing all of it." Pat's story highlights several ways in which club sports impact the family—sometimes beneficially, sometimes not. For Pat and many other club sport parents, participation increased both the quantity and the quality of interactions that Pat and her husband had with their children. As one of her sons put it, "It's what we did. My parents came to everything. I never felt like it was 'my thing.' It was always 'our thing.' I have great memories of our family trips to swim meets." Youth travel teams are, at least for some parents, an important part of their social world, providing them with a community of like-minded others that share their values and interests (Green, 1997). For others, it's a chance to learn more about their child's interests and to get to know their child's friends (Dorsch, Smith, and McDonough, 2014). In both cases, parents report increased communication and an enhanced relationship with their child.

Most travel team parents lament the time commitment required for club participation. At the same time, few feel the need to pull their child out of these high-commitment clubs. Instead, families accommodate increasing time and travel requirements by incorporating it into their view of family life. It becomes part of the routine. Youth sport slowly and gradually takes over weekends, evenings, and family vacation time. A report by the Minnesota Youth Sport Research Consortium (LaVoi, 2011) asked parents how often youth sport interfered with five common family functions: religious services, sleep, homework, vacations, general family time, and meals. Parents reported that sport most often interfered with meals. Parents of children on travel teams reported more interference in all aspects of family life, with particular emphasis on meals, family time, and vacations. Yet these same parents considered the interference as normal and unproblematic. Further, a study by *ESPN The Magazine* revealed that more than half of parents feel that youth sport has strengthened their marriages. As one dad admitted, "About the only time my wife and I are totally focused on the same thing is at the kids' games. It's nice to feel that we are on the same page, at least for a little while" (Clemmons et al., 2013).

Effects on Siblings

Not all children in a family choose to participate in sport, and those that do may or may not participate in the same sport or in the same club as their siblings. These situations can result in a great deal of stress and conflict among family members (Fraser-Thomas, Strachan, and Jefferey-Tosoni, 2013), and guilt and anguish among parents (Lindstrom Bremer, 2012). At best, parents are forced to choose which child's activity each will attend. One parent goes to the basketball tournament; the other goes to indoor soccer practice. All that togetherness and quality family time is now fraught with perceptions of favoritism and fairness as parents have no choice but to choose one child's activities over the other. These feelings and the resulting tensions are exacerbated when one child is selected to a travel team and the other is not, or when one child does not play sports at all. Interviews with the family of Susan, a 15-year-old club volleyball player, illustrate this point. Susan's younger brother no longer plays organized sport. He prefers video gaming with his friends. However, their parents want the family to do things together. William, Susan's brother, feels like his interests don't matter. He explains it this way, "Susan is the son my father always wanted. She's the jock. I'm just a joke. Even worse, I get dragged around to all her tournaments so we can have 'family time'" (Green, 2011).

Clearly, not all siblings are jealous or resentful of their brother's or sister's travel team participation. In fact, there is strong evidence to suggest that siblings play an important role in socializing one another into sport (Partridge, Brustad, and Babkes

Stellino, 2008). In fact, it is likely that attending practices and competitions and traveling to tournaments with siblings and family members can potentially motivate younger siblings to take up the sport. As with the social lives of parents, many siblings find friendships and community through their participation in the extended experience of their sibling's travel sport participation. For this to occur, however, families must have the financial resources and work flexibility to support their children's travel team participation. Not all families have this capability.

Financial Costs

Travel teams offer a wide array of potential benefits to athletes and their families. However, these benefits come with a hefty price tag (Hyman, 2012). The cost of travel team participation has been estimated anywhere from $1,500 to more than $10,000 per child per year depending on the sport, the club, and the frequency and distance traveled (Butler, 2011; Riddle, 2014; Sullivan, 2015). That's just the cost for the athlete; travel costs for other family members who accompany their child or sibling to tournaments can make the total expense much higher for families. And those are just the explicit costs: club dues, equipment and uniforms, tournament fees, and travel-related expenses such as hotels, automobile rentals, train or plane fares, or gasoline purchases for car travel. An entire industry has emerged, seemingly designed to assist parents to provide everything possible to help their child achieve athletic success (and, hopefully, a college scholarship). Swing coaches, personal trainers, nutritionists, skill camps, exposure opportunities, videographers, and a host of other services are all available to support young athletes in their quest to make it to "the next level." None of these costs are included in club dues. It is fair to say that none of these extra costs are required, yet competition for roster spots, playing time, and the elusive college scholarship drive many athletes and their parents to invest heavily in any service that can conceivably provide a competitive advantage. In actuality, however, fewer than 2 percent of high school athletes obtain an athletic scholarship (Scholarshipstats.com, n.d.), and almost no one gets a full scholarship other than Division I basketball and football players. In fact, few high school athletes will ever play organized college sports, with or without a scholarship. Indeed, although a college scholarship is an often cited goal that motivates investment in club sports, few club team players will actually obtain a scholarship. Those that do are likely to obtain only minimal support (e.g., the average scholarship for Division I athletes was $14,270 in 2015/16) (Scholarshipstats.com, n.d.).

It is not surprising, given the costs of travel teams, that they are heavily populated by upper-middle-class suburban families. Club sport participation is increasingly limited to families with income of $75,000 or more (Project Play, n.d.). Forty to 44 percent of youth tackle football, baseball, and basketball players come from families with household income of $75,000 or more. The percentages are higher for soccer (52 percent), swimming (64 percent), and lacrosse (70 percent) (Project Play, n.d.). These figures are particularly disturbing when you consider that sport is popularly considered a meritocracy. Although it is true that some clubs are able to provide scholarships to a few athletes without the financial means to otherwise participate, the club systems that prevail across both boys' and girls' sports are generally so expensive that they are beyond the reach of players from families from lower socioeconomic levels.

Effects on the Young Athlete

Whether the travel team experience is good for young athletes or bad for them has been hotly debated. There seem to be some straightforward benefits, a least in the short term, such as enhanced quality of training and competition. On the other hand, the social and psychological stresses associated with travel team participation may have negative consequences, at least for some young athletes.

Quality Competition and Training

Travel teams are normally intended to bring the best local athletes together to train and then to compete with similar quality athletes from other jurisdictions. The athletes must be good enough to make the team and must train hard enough to stay on it. The focus is on improvement and winning. In such an environment, athletes are challenged to keep up with one another both within the team and across the teams against which they compete. This raises the bar and sets a premium on striving and competitive excellence.

In social psychology, any environment of this type is known as one that is characterized by "social comparison." In other words, the individual compares himself or herself to others and is aware that coaches, family members, and others may also be comparing them to others. Social comparison can enhance the pace and level of skill and performance development (Mussweiler and Strack, 2000) because it fosters ever-more-ambitious group and individual goals as well as the group and individual commitments necessary to attain those goals.

In the case of travel teams, this occurs on the team and also across the radius of competition. Athletes must excel sufficiently to be good enough to remain on the team and compete for it, so they are constantly endeavoring to be as good as or better than teammates. The team becomes a venue for constant improvement. This same process is occurring on other teams, as well—teams against which the athlete will later compete. So, it is not sufficient to be as good as or better than local athletes; it is necessary to be able to excel against athletes from other teams. So the process becomes intensified.

In short, the travel team is designed to be a place that nurtures excellence through constant social comparison. Consider Ernesto, who played baseball on a travel team. He observes, "I wanted to be the best hitter on the team, and I wanted us to win because I could hit. I thought all the time about how to do it better, and then I'd practice it. And soon I was the best hitter we had, and I had the highest batting average of anyone we played against. That's how it works." Of course, Ernesto relied on his coaches to help him develop his hitting. Coaching plays a pivotal role in the pursuit of sporting excellence.

An Expectation for Excellent Coaching

Local-level recreational teams typically rely on parents to coach—parents who do so to enable their children to participate in a sport. Those parents may mean well, but they often lack coaching expertise. Indeed, the inadequacy of much recreational sport coaching has caused most national governing bodies (i.e., the organizations responsible for running each sport in the country) to develop systems for coach training and certification. Many local recreation departments also require coaches to receive some training.

Things change, however, when coaching becomes a profession, as is increasingly the case for travel teams. When families are paying handsomely to enable their children to travel to compete, and to provide them with high-quality uniforms and gear, they also expect quality coaching to be provided. As a result, coaches of travel teams are increasingly expected to have undergone training and even to be certified. In many instances coaches are paid. The result is that the coaching is at a higher standard than can be found for children outside the travel team context. As one young volleyball protégé put it, "We are the best because we have the best coaches."

Early Specialization

No aspect of the travel team phenomenon has engendered more debate and angst than has the growth of early specialization. If a young athlete is going to have the opportunities associated with high-quality social comparisons and qualified coaching, then it may help to commit to a sport at a young age so that the athlete doesn't have to play catch-up to make the team or to excel relative to other players. In the intensified competitive atmosphere of the travel team, it simply makes sense to choose a sport and specialize in it early.

However, many experts decry early specialization and worry that travel teams may be doing more harm than good. Medically, it may increase the risk of injury, especially because particular movements are repeated over and over, causing increased stress to muscles and joints (American Academy of Pediatrics, 2000). On the other hand, it has been argued that with close attention to diet and appropriate training, early specialization may not pose an unusual level of risk (Malina, 1994).

The apparent advantage of early specialization is that more hours of deliberate practice in a sport can be obtained than if specialization occurs later. It is expected that many hours of deliberate practice are necessary to enable sporting excellence (Ericsson, Kramer, and Tech-Romer, 1993). However, recent advocates of long-term athlete development (Balyi, Way, and Higgs, 2013) suggest that the amount of deliberate practice required can be reduced if athletes first develop fundamental physical capacity and movement skills. It is also suggested that enjoyment and greater complexity of skill capability will be fostered. Thus, advocates of long-term athlete development systems recommend programs for young athletes that encourage training in a variety of sport skills and participation in multiple sports and games. It is expected that so doing will provide a foundation for higher levels of sport skill than would be obtained through early specialization, and that young athletes can find the sport they like best and at which they might be most likely to excel. Such systems are antithetical to the travel team model.

Athlete Burnout

The timing of specialization does not alter the fact that the training, competition, and travel associated with travel teams can be demanding to the point of being stressful. Although there has been very little direct research on travel teams versus alternative structures, the conditions thought to be associated with travel teams have been shown to be conducive to burnout. For example, the perfectionism associated with travel team coaching and competition can cause burnout among some participants (Madigan, Stobeber, and Passfield, 2015). When athletes find the constant social comparisons of elite programs to be overly demanding, they feel stressed, and so become likely to quit permanently (De Francisco et al., 2016).

The issue is not that travel teams necessarily cause participants to burnout. The issue is that participants experiencing the intense demands associated with travel teams are more likely to burn out. Some will; some will not. In fact, it depends greatly on the ways that parents, coaches, and administrators on the team behave. In other words, how severe the problem becomes depends in no small measure on the ways that expectations and demands are interpreted and communicated to young athletes (Coakley, 1992). Nevertheless, the very nature of travel teams elevates the risk of turning some participants sour on sport, thereby causing some loss of participation and future excellence. For those who do experience burnout, there are consequences such as lowered self-esteem (Cresswell and Eklund, 2006), withdrawal from friendships (Gustafson et al., 2015), and increased long-term risk for cardiovascular disease (Melamed et al., 2006).

Anecdotal reports of athlete burnout abound. Consider the case of Roger, a young soccer player. Roger began soccer at a very young age on a team run by his local parks and recreation department. He enjoyed the sport, and became skilled for his age as he practiced dribbling and kicking in his backyard after school. His parents joined Roger to a local soccer club that offered several levels of increasingly demanding travel squads. After his second season, Roger complained about his coaches' yelling and about the ways his teammates criticized him if he made a mistake. He said that soccer wasn't fun anymore. When the next season ended, Roger quit soccer altogether, and refused to spend time with any of his old teammates. Roger seemed unhappy, and his parents worried that he would never play sport again.

Yet, for every story about an athlete who burned out during his or her travel team experience, there are others about athletes who have thrived in it. As a soccer player from Roger's team put it, "The travel and the great competition are what makes this fun. We are a team. It's great!"

Opportunity Costs

The time spent in training, competition, and travel is time not spent on other activities. The participating athlete's peer group is often the team itself. Friendships outside the sport become difficult or sometimes impossible to sustain. As a young swimmer put it, "My friends don't understand why I can't go out with them because I'm training or at a meet. They get annoyed. So, it's easiest to hang out with other swimmers."

Developing other skills can also be a challenge. A gymnast described it by noting, "I love music. It's even part of my sport. I used to take piano lessons, but I had to quit to keep up with my [gymnastics] training."

There is no inventory of what athletes on travel teams trade away in order to be on the team. Yet, the fact remains that the commitment of time required by travel teams is substantial. The commitment implies that the sport and its associated training, competition, and travel are more important than the activities that are supplanted. It is a trade-off that warrants better evaluation than has been forthcoming so far.

The Excluded

The aspiring athlete who rides the bench but rarely plays is a common motif in popular media. What has been ignored is the athlete who doesn't even get that chance. Some, but not all, travel teams are selected. That is, only some athletes get onto the team. What is the effect of simply being left out entirely? As with any other form of social exclusion (Byrne, 2005), one would expect negative social and psychological repercussions. Whether those occur, when they might occur, and what they might be is not yet well understood.

Conclusion

The stakes and demands in youth sport continue to escalate. Travel teams are a palpable manifestation of that escalation. For some children, they may be beneficial; for others, perhaps not. It is significant that many who have spent their lives at the pinnacle of their sport worry about where this escalation is taking us. Joe Maddon, manager of the 2016 World Series champion Chicago Cubs, said, "That's why I hate the specialization with kids, when they're playing on these travel squads when they're like 12, 13, 14 years old, only dedicated to one thing. Traveling all the time. Paying exorbitant amounts of money to play baseball with hopes they're going to become a professional baseball player. I think that's crazy" (Finley, 2015). We should not take the travel team phenomenon at face value. Ultimately, we are talking about the well-being of our children. How we provide sport to them matters.

B. Christine Green and Laurence Chalip

Further Reading

American Academy of Pediatrics. 2000. "Intensive Training and Sports Specialization in Young Athletes." *Pediatrics, 106*: 154–157.

Aspen Institute. 2015. *Sport for All Play for Life: A Playbook to Get Every Kid in the Game.* Washington, D.C.: Aspen Institute. Accessed at http://aspeninstitute.org.

Balyi, I., R. Way, and C. Higgs. 2013. *Long-Term Athlete Development.* Champaign, IL: Human Kinetics.

Butler, S. 2011, April 29. "$4,000 for Youth Baseball: Kids' Sports Costs are Out of Control." *CBS News: Moneywatch.* Accessed at http://www.cbsnews.com/news/4000-for -youth-baseball-kids-sports-costs-are-out-of-control.

Byrne, D. S. 2005. *Social Exclusion* (2nd ed.). Maidenhead, UK: Open University Press.

Clemmons, A. K., M. Ehalt, D. Friedell, T. Manahan, M. Muench, and K. O'Hara. 2013, July 8. "Parent Confidential." *ESPN The Magazine, Kids in Sports Issue.* Accessed at http://www.espn.com/espn/story/_/id/9421568/parent-surveys-show-youth-sports-improve -family-dynamics-academics-espn-magazine.

Coakley, J. 1992. "Burnout among Adolescent Athletes: A Personal Failure or a Social Problem?" *Sociology of Sport Journal, 9*: 271–285.

Cote, J., and R. Lidor. (Eds.). 2013. *Conditions of Children's Talent Development in Sport.* Morgantown, WV: Fitness Information Technology.

Cresswell, S. L., and R. C. Eklund. 2006. "The Nature of Player Burnout in Rugby: Key Characteristics and Attributions." *Journal of Applied Sport Psychology, 18*: 219–239.

De Francisco, C., C. Arce, M. de Pilar Vilachez, and A. Vales. 2016. "Antecedents and Consequences of Burnout in Athletes: Perceived Stress and Depression." *International Journal of Clinical and Health Psychology, 16*: 239–246.

Dorsch, T. E., A. L. Smith, and M. H. McDonough. 2014. "Early Socialization of Parents through Organized Youth Sport." *Sport, Exercise, and Performance Psychology, 4*(1): 3–18.

Ericsson, K. A., R. T. Kramer, and C. Tech-Romer. 1993. "The Role of Deliberate Practice in the Acquisition of Expert Performance." *Psychological Review, 100*: 363–406.

Farrey, T. 2009. *Game On: How the Pressure to Win at All Costs Endangers Youth Sports, and What Parents Can Do about It.* Storrs, CT: ESPN.

Finley, P. 2015, March 17. "'Cubs University' Features Football, Hoops Experience." *Chicago Sun Times.* Accessed at http://chicago.suntimes.com.

Fraser-Thomas, J., L. Strachan, and S. Jefferey-Tosoni. 2013. "Family Influence on Children's Involvement in Sport." In J. Cote and R. Lidor (Eds.), *Conditions of Children's Talent Development in Sport* (pp. 179–196). Morgantown, WV: Fitness Information Technology.

Green, B. C. 1997. "Action Research in Youth Soccer: Assessing the Acceptability of an Alternative Program." *Journal of Sport Management, 11*: 29–44.

Green, B. C. 2011. [Parents' Views of Youth Sport.] Unpublished raw data.

Gustafson, H., P. Davis, T. Skoog, G. Kentta, and P. Haberl. 2015. "Mindfulness and Its Relationship with Perceived Stress, Affect and Burnout in Elite Junior Athletes." *Journal of Clinical Sport Psychology, 9*: 263–281.

Hoefer, W. R., T. L. McKenzie, J. F. Sallis, S. J. Marshall, and T. L. Conway. 2001. "Parental Provision of Transportation for Adolescent Physical Activity." *American Journal of Preventative Medicine, 21*: 48–51.

Hyman, M. 2012. *The Most Expensive Game in Town: The Rising Cost of Youth Sports and the Toll on Today's Families.* Boston: Beacon Press.

LaVoi, N. M. 2011. *Youth Sport Report: Parent Perceptions of How Frequently Youth Sport Interferes with Family Time.* Minneapolis: Minnesota Youth Sport Research Consortium.

Lindstrom Bremer, K. 2012. "Parental Involvement, Pressure, and Support in Youth Sport: A Narrative Literature Review." *Journal of Family Therapy Review, 4*: 235–248.

Madigan, D. J., J. Stobeber, and L. Passfield. 2015. "Perfectionism and Burnout in Junior Athletes: A Three-Month Longitudinal Study." *Journal of Sport & Exercise Psychology, 37*: 305–315.

Malina, R. M. 1994. "Physical Growth and Biological Maturation of Young Athletes." *Exercise and Sport Science Review, 22*: 389–434.

McCoy, D. 2015, November 16. "As Competition Rises, Team Sports Decline but Traveling Teams Soar." *CBS Minnesota.* Accessed at http://minnesota.cbslocal.com/2015/11/16/as-competition-rises-team-sports-decline-but-traveling-teams-soar.

Melamed, S., A. Sharon, S. Toker, S. Berliner, and J. Shapira. 2006. "Burnout and Risk of Cardiovascular Disease: Evidence, Possible Causal Paths, and Promising Research Findings." *Psychological Bulletin, 132*: 327–353.

Mussweiler, T., and F. Strack. 2000. "Consequences of Social Comparison: Selective Accessibility, Assimilation, and Contrast." In J. Suls and L. Wheeler (Eds.), *Handbook of Social Comparison* (pp. 253–270). New York: Springer.

O'Sullivan, J. 2013. *Changing the Game: The Parent's Guide to Raising Happy, High Performing Athletes, and Giving Youth Sports Back to Our Kids.* New York: Morgan James Publishing.

Partridge, J., R. Brustad, and M. Babkes Stellino. 2008. "Social Influence in Sport." *Advances in Sport Psychology, 3*: 269–291.

Project Play. n.d. "Facts: Sports Activity and Children." *Project Play: Reimagining Youth Sports in America.* Washington, D.C.: Aspen Institute. Accessed at http://www.aspen projectplay.org/the-facts.

Riddle, G. 2014. "Club Sports Offer Exposure—But at a Steep Price." *The Dallas Morning News.* Accessed at http://res.dallasnews.com/interactives/club-sports/part3.

Scholarshipstats.com. n.d. *College Athletic Scholarship Limits.* Accessed at http://www .scholarshipstats.com/ncaalimits.html.

Sullivan, P. 2015, January 16. "The Rising Costs of Youth Sports, in Money and Emotion." *The New York Times.* Accessed at http://nyti.ms/1Cw02Bv.

Wiersma, L. D., and A. M. Fifer. 2008. "The Schedule Has Been Tough but We Think It's Worth It: The Joys, Challenges, and Recommendations of Youth Sport Parents." *Journal of Leisure Research, 40*: 505–530.

Appendix

Popular Youth Sports in the United States

Baseball

The sport of baseball originated in the United States before the American Civil War (1861–1865). It was developed from earlier folk games in England, but the version that spread across American sandlots and fields featured distinctive rules and rhythms. It eventually became so popular with children and adults that it earned the nickname "America's pastime."

Amateur leagues began playing under the modern rules during the 1840s. In 1857, 16 New York amateur teams formed the first organization to govern the sport, the National Association of Baseball Players (NABBP). The first professional baseball league was established in 1871. Youth leagues formed gradually across the nation, including the foundation of Little League in 1939. Traditionally, baseball in the United States has been a male-oriented sport from youth leagues through professional levels. Although there are many large-scale tournaments, the three most popular baseball tournaments for adults are the Major League Baseball (MLB) World Series, the Premier 12 World Championship, and the World Baseball Classic. The World Baseball Classic, the first major baseball tournament to feature professional players from across the world, began in 2006 and is held every four years.

Among younger American athletes, baseball remains a very popular sport, although some reports have documented a gradual decrease in participation rates:

- 486,567 male and 1,203 female high school students, and 56,878 total college students played baseball during the 2015 season.

- 2.1 percent of high school players continue participating in the sport and compete as NCAA Division I college athletes.
- Baseball is the third most popular high school sport for boys, with 15,899 schools fielding teams in 2015.
- The state of Texas held the most high school male participation in baseball in 2015 with 46,638 youth, followed by California with 44,325.

According to the Stanford Children's Hospital report, nearly 110,000 children ages 5 to 14 were treated in hospital emergency rooms for baseball-related injuries in 2009. In addition, three to four children suffer fatal injuries while playing baseball each year, resulting in the highest fatality rate among sports for children ages 5 to 14. Despite this, baseball remains a widely popular sport among collegiate and youth athletes with over 2.4 million children worldwide participating in Little League Baseball alone.

During 2015, 1,673 schools offered varsity college baseball teams, with average athletic scholarships of $14,737 for Division I athletes. Of these 1,673 schools, 229 are NCAA Division I, 269 are NCAA Division II, and 384 are NCAA Division III programs. From 2010 to 2016, Division I NCAA championships were won by six different universities (South Carolina 2010, 2011; Arizona 2012; UCLA 2013; Vanderbilt 2014; Virginia 2015; Coastal Carolina 2016). Division II championships were earned by Southern Indiana (2010 and 2014), West Florida (2011), West Chester (2012), Tampa (2013 and 2015), and Nova Southeastern (2016). During this same time period, Division III championships were claimed by Illinois Wesleyan (2010), Marietta (2011 and 2012), Linfield (2013), Wisconsin-Whitewater (2014), SUNY Cortland (2015), and Trinity (2016).

Important associations and organizations involved in managing youth baseball include Little League Baseball (www.littleleague.org), American Amateur Baseball Congress (www.aabc.us), National Association of Intercollegiate Athletics (www.naia.org), and National Amateur Baseball Federation (www.nabf.com), among others.

Sources

College Baseball & Scholarship Opportunities, 2016. n.d. Accessed September 7, 2017, at http://www.scholarshipstats.com/baseball.html.

National Federation of State High School Associations. n.d. *Participation Data.* Accessed September 7, 2017, at http://www.nfhs.org/ParticipationStatics/ParticipationStatics.aspx.

Sports Injury Statistics. n.d. Stanford Children's Health. Accessed September 7, 2017, at http://www.stanfordchildrens.org/en/topic/default?id=sports-injury-statistics-90-P02787.

2014–15 High School Athletics Participation Survey. Accessed September 7, 2017, at http://www.nfhs.org/ParticipationStatistics/PDF/2014-15_Participation_Survey _Results.pdf.

Basketball

Basketball was born in a YMCA gymnasium in Springfield, Massachusetts, in 1891. Developed by Dr. James Naismith, the goal of the game was to shoot the ball into a peach basket—thus the name basketball. Eventually, after having halted game play to retrieve the ball from inside the basket, the bottoms of the baskets were cut out. Popularity of the game took off with the formation of the first U.S. college basketball team at Vanderbilt University in 1893. The first American local leagues originated in large East Coast cities such as New York City, Philadelphia, and Boston. In 1896, the first recorded professional basketball game was held in Trenton, New Jersey. In 1936, basketball became an official Olympic sport with the United States defeating Canada 19–8. The first televised games were aired in February of 1940. The National Basketball Association (NBA) was established in 1949. By the end of the 20th century, the NBA had grown into a multi-billion-dollar enterprise and a significant part of American sports culture.

Today, more than 300 million people play basketball worldwide, and it remains one of the most popular youth sports. According to a 2016 report issued by the National Physical Activity Plan Alliance, however, there has been a decrease in youth basketball participation in the United States.

- According to the 2014 National Physical Activity for Children and Youth Plan, basketball was the second most prominent school sport among U.S. high school females with over 430,000 organized programs.
- 541,479 high school male players participated in basketball programs in 2015.

In 2009, injuries within the sport included more than 170,000 children between the ages of 5 to 14 who visited the emergency room for basketball-related injuries. According to the National Athletic Trainers Association, sprains were the most common type of injury, accounting for 43 percent of total injuries.

In 2015, 2,029 colleges sponsored varsity level basketball programs. The average NCAA Division I basketball scholarship was $14,958 for male and $16,022 for female athletes. Approximately 5.7 percent of male and 6.2 percent of female high school basketball players continued to compete at any college level, with about 1 percent of both male and female high school basketball players competing at NCAA Division I schools. Women's basketball programs are maintained at 99 percent of NCAA schools, the highest of any female team sports.

Sources

College Basketball & Scholarship Opportunities, 2016. Accessed September 7, 2017, at http://www.scholarshipstats.com/basketball.htm.

National Physical Activity Plan Alliance. *2016 United States Report Card on Physical Activity for Children and Youth.* Accessed September 7, 2017, at http://physicalactivityplan .org/reportcard/2016FINAL_USReportCard.pdf.

Sports Injury Statistics. n.d. Stanford Children's Health. Accessed September 7, 2017, at http://www.stanfordchildrens.org/en/topic/default?id=sports-injury-statistics-90-P02787.

Bowling

Although games similar to modern bowling have been played as far back as 3200 BC, American bowling originally was played on outdoor lawn bowling greens. By the end of the 19th century, bowling had evolved from a ninepin into a tenpin game. In response to unstandardized variables of the game, such as ball type and weight, the American Bowling Congress was created in 1895. Two decades later, in 1917, the Women's International Bowling Congress (WIBC) formed to support female participation in bowling tournaments. The first collegiate bowling competition was held April 8, 1916, just previous to the formation of the WIBC. Currently, World Bowling is the governing body of both ninepin and tenpin bowling. The game is played in more than 90 countries with professional bowlers competing in the World Championships.

Bowling is not as popular in American culture as it once was. The number of bowling alleys in the United States fell from 5,400 in 1998 to 3,976 in 2013. However, with new options for bowling participation, including after-work happy hours and diverse bowling leagues, middle-aged bowling participation is on the rise. Meanwhile, youth bowling participation in the United States is a modest but nonetheless noteworthy subset of total sports participation:

- In 2015, 29,105 men and 26,110 women high school students participated in bowling programs.
- Each year, the top 80 men and 64 female U.S. college teams compete regionally to qualify for the Intercollegiate Team Championships, a nationally televised competition.
- The Northeast supports a higher number of bowling programs than any other geographic region of the United States.

Major youth bowling organizations include the United States Bowling Congress and the International Candlepin Youth Bowling Association, each of which holds youth bowling tournaments in girls' and boys' leagues. According to the Insurance Information Institute, Americans suffered about 17,000 bowling-related injuries in 2015. Of those, 1,500 were suffered by children between the ages of 5 and 14, and another 2,100 occurred to participants between the ages of 15 and 24. The most common bowling-related injuries include elbow, shoulder, and wrist tendonitis. Nearly 100 American colleges and universities offer bowling scholarships. In 2015, 141 colleges sponsored varsity-level bowling programs. The average NCAA Division I athletic scholarship for women was $15,969. In 2015, 2.7 percent of male and 4.7 percent of female high school bowlers continued on to compete at any college level. There are more than 3,500 college bowling athletes that compete annually in more than 80 BOWL-certified tournaments.

Sources

College Bowling & Scholarship Opportunities, 2016. Accessed September 7, 2017, at http://www.scholarshipstats.com/bowling.html.

Insurance Information Institute. *Sports Injuries.* 2015. Accessed September 7, 2017, at http://www.iii.org/fact-statistic/sports-injuries.

International Bowling Museum and Hall of Fame. *History of Bowling.* Accessed September 7, 2017, at http://www.bowlingmuseum.com/Visit/Education/History-of-Bowling.

Statista. *Number of Participants in Bowling in the United States, 2006–2015.* Accessed September 7, 2017, at http://www.statista.com/statistics/191898/participants-in-bowling-in-the-us-since-2006.

Witsil, Frank. 2015, May 10. "Is Bowling in Its Final Frames or Will It Roll On?" *USA Today.* Accessed September 7, 2017 at http://www.usatoday.com/story/money/business/2015/05/10/bowling-final-frames-roll/27070351.

Cheerleading

Cheerleading originated in the United States as an all-male sport as early as 1877. It wasn't until 1923, at the University of Minnesota, that women were incorporated into cheerleading. During this time the sport of cheerleading developed immensely with the introduction of tumbling and acrobatics. Female involvement in cheerleading received an additional boost during World War II, when many male college students joined the U.S. military. In 1948 Lawrence "Herkie" Herkimer helped form the National Cheerleaders Association (NCA). Herkie's contributions to cheerleading include the first cheerleading clinic held by the NCA, the cheerleading uniform supply company Cheerleading & Danz Team, the cheerleading jump that came to be known as the herkie, and the spirit stick. Professional cheerleading originated during the 1950s. The National Football League held the first recorded cheer squad who cheered for the Baltimore Colts. Modern-day cheerleading began during the 1980s with advancements in stunt sequences and gymnastics. Additionally, during the 1980s all-star teams originated with the formation of the United States All-Star Federation (USASF). Today, cheerleading is closely associated with American football and basketball.

Cheerleading remains predominantly an American sport with an estimated 1.5 million participants in all-star cheerleading. Most American schools have organized cheerleading programs. Cheerleading can range from cheering to advanced physical activity. Routines commonly range from one to three minutes and contain components of tumbling, jumping, dancing, cheers, and stunting. Major youth competitions include the International Cheer Union World Championships, National Cheerleading Championships, and Pan-American Cheerleading Championship. Organizations in the United States, such as the Universal Cheerleading Association, host year-round camps and competitions for cheerleaders from seventh grade through college. Pop Warner also offers opportunities for youth to become involved in the sport, offering cheer and dance programs for beginner, intermediate, and advanced participants.

Within the United States participation rates include:

- In 2014 approximately 3.46 million individuals (aged 6 years and older) participated in cheerleading programs.
- 40 percent of all cheerleaders participated within the sport 60+ days per year, making the sport one the highest rates of frequent participation.
- 94 percent of U.S. participation in cheerleading is female.

Although injury rates in cheerleading tend to be lower than in other school sports, the accidents that do occur may be more severe. Although concussions can result from cheerleading-related injuries, strains and sprains are more common, covering half of all cheerleading injuries.

Individuals searching for scholarships should look to associated organizations and associations such as the American Association of Cheerleading Coaches and Administrators (AACCA) and the National Council for Spirit Safety and Education (NCSSE). Cheerleading is not considered an NCAA athletic event, and there are no Olympic cheerleading events. However, many professional sports leagues feature cheerleading squads, including the NBA, NFL, MLB, and NHL.

In the United States, participating associations and organizations include the United States Cheerleading Association (www.uscheerleading.com), United States All Star Federation (www.usasf.net), and Varsity Spirit (www.varsity.com).

Sources

Being a Cheerleader: History of Cheerleading. n.d. Accessed September 7, 2017, at http://www.varsity.com/event/1261/being-a-cheerleader-history.

Children's Hospital Colorado. *Cheerleading.* Accessed September 7, 2017, at https://www.childrenscolorado.org/doctors-and-departments/departments/orthopedics/programs/sports-medicine-center/sports-injuries-we-treat/cheerleading.

Number of Participants in Cheerleading in the United States, 2006–2015. Accessed September 7, 2017, at http://www.statista.com/statistics/191651/participants-in-cheerleading-in-the-us-since-2006.

Cross-Country

Cross-country competitions, which originated in English schools in the 19th century, are unique from other running sports in that they take place on open-air courses that cover natural terrain such as forest areas and grass-covered fields. The first national championship was established in 1876. Harvard was the first college to introduce cross-country as a training event for track and field in 1880. In 1903 the first International Cross Country Championships were held. Cross-country was introduced into the Summer Olympic Games in 1912 with Sweden taking the gold medal. In 1962, the International Amateur Athletic Federation (IAAF) gained jurisdiction over the sport as the governing body of worldwide cross-country and track and field. IAAF set rules for both men's and women's cross-country events and established the World Cross Country Championships. Today, the World Cross Country Championship is the highest regarded international competition in cross-country running. In the sport, runners are judged both as individuals and as a team. Fall and winter are the most common seasons of participation. The Junior Olympic Cross Country program runs annually with more than 3,000 youth runners competing in the USA Track & Field National Junior Olympic Cross Country Championships.

Youth participation rates in the sport of cross-country have steadily grown since the early 2000s, especially for female athletes:

- During the 2014/2015 season, approximately 250,981 male and 221,616 female high school students participated in cross-country programs.
- During the same season, 18,310 men and 19,598 women ran cross-country in U.S. colleges.

In 2015, 1,538 schools sponsored varsity level cross-country programs. The average Division I athletic scholarship was $14,918 for men and $15,958 for women cross-country athletes. Approximately 1.8 percent of male and 2.5 percent of female high school cross-country runners continued to compete at a Division I school, while 7.0 percent of male and 8.6 percent of female high school cross-country runners continued to compete in college overall.

Leading associations and organizations for the sport include USA Track & Field (www.usatf.org), Cross Country for Youth (www.crosscountryforyouth.org), and the International Association of Athletics Federations (www.iaaf.org).

Sources

College Cross Country & Scholarship Opportunities. Accessed September 7, 2017, at http://www.scholarshipstats.com/crosscountry.htm.

Number of Participants in U.S. High School Cross Country. 2009–2016. Accessed September 7, 2017, at http://www.statista.com/statistics/267951/participation-in-us-high-school-cross-country.

Field Hockey

Field hockey is one of the oldest athletic events, as historians have documented the existence of early versions of the sport dating as far back as nearly 3,000 years to the Greek classical era. Modern-day field hockey was adopted into English public schools during the mid-19th century. In 1886, cricket players attempting to develop a sport to be enjoyed during the winter season created the rules for modern field hockey. Increased popularity of the new sport led to the formation of the sport's first organizing body, the Hockey Association in London. Field hockey first appeared in the Olympic Games in 1908 with only three participating teams: England, Ireland, and Scotland. The International Hockey Federation (FIH) formed in 1924 and remains the sport's international governing body. Women's field hockey made its debut as an Olympic event in 1980.

In most countries there is an even balance between male and female participation in field hockey. In the United States, however, field hockey is predominantly a female sport. Field hockey has historically been played on grass or turf fields, but it is increasingly common for games to be played indoors on artificial turf.

Participation in field hockey programs is as follows:

- During the 2014–2015 season, 60,687 high school students participated in field hockey programs.
- The overwhelming majority of high school field hockey athletes in the U.S. are female.

- Both collegiate and high school participation is highest on the East Coast of the United States.

During the 2008–2009 season, the overall injury rate in NCAA field hockey was 6.3 per 1,000 athlete exposures. The sport requires a significant amount of running and uses equipment made of rigid materials, making muscle strains and contusions the most common injuries in NCAA field hockey.

In 2015, 275 universities sponsored varsity level field hockey programs. Of the more than 60,000 high school field hockey athletes in the United States, 8.9 percent went on to compete at the collegiate level in 2015, with 2.6 percent competing at NCAA Division I programs. The average NCAA Division I field hockey scholarship in 2015 for females was $15,571, and $6,511 for Division II schools. From 2010 to 2016, NCAA Division I championships in women's field hockey were won by Syracuse (2016), Connecticut (2014, 2013), Princeton (2012), and Maryland (2011, 2010).

Within the United States, leading associations and organizations include USA Field Hockey (www.teamusa.org), National Field Hockey Coaches Association (www.nfhca.org), and Field Hockey USA (www.fieldhockeyusa.org).

Sources

Athnet. *History of Field Hockey.* n.d. Accessed September 7, 2017, at http://www.athletic scholarships.net/history-field-hockey.htm.

College Field Hockey & Scholarship Opportunities. Accessed May 3, 2018, at http://www .scholarshipstats.com/fieldhockey.html.

NCAA. *Field Hockey Injuries: Data from the 2004/05–2008/09 Seasons.* Accessed September 7, 2017, at https://www.ncaa.org/sites/default/files/NCAA_FieldHockey_Injuries_HiRes.pdf

Football

Though associated with the sport of rugby football, American football is set apart by rules developed by Walter Camp, considered by many to be the "father of American football." Included in these rules were the formation of the line of scrimmage, new down and distance rules, and the legalization of interference. Professional football originated in 1920 as the American Professional Football Association. However, the first recorded football player to receive pay-for-play was William "Pudge" Heffelfinger, who received a $500 contract to play for the Allegheny Athletic Association in 1892. The American Professional Football Association's name eventually changed to the National Football League (NFL), which became the professional league as it is today.

The first youth football league was founded in 1929 as a four-team league called the Junior Football Conference. The league eventually changed its name to Pop Warner in honor of the iconic coach from Temple University, Glen "Pop" Warner. Today, Pop Warner is the largest and oldest youth football program in the world with all 50 states holding associated programs.

Participation in American football is high throughout the United States:

- Eleven-player football remains the leading sport among young male athletes.
- In 2015, 1,114,253 male and 1,698 female high school athletes participated in football programs across the country.
- In 2015, 92,052 male athletes competed in U.S. college football programs.

Though very popular among youth athletes, football players are subject to various types of injuries. The most common type of injury for college football players is knee injuries, which account for 17.1 percent of all football injuries. Concussions are also fairly common among football players, and their long-term health impact has become a high-profile and controversial issue for football players of all ages, from elementary school players to NFL veterans.

During the 2015 season, 8.2 percent of high school football players went on to compete in college football at any level. There are 129 NCAA Division I FBS programs, 125 NCAA Division I FCS programs, 171 NCAA Division II programs, and 248 NCAA Division III programs. The average scholarship for NCAA Division I FBS players in 2015 was $19,557 (85 scholarships per team). The average scholarship for NCAA Division I FCS players was $11,631 (63 per team) and $5,315 for NCAA Division II athletes (36 per team). From 2010 to 2017, NCAA Division I FBS championships were won by Clemson University (2016), Alabama (2015, 2017), Ohio State (2014), Florida State (2013), Auburn (2010).

Leading associations and organizations that shape youth football in the United States include Pop Warner (http://www.popwarner.com), National Youth Football Organization (www.playnyfo.com), American Youth Football and Cheer (www.americanyouthfootball.com), and United Youth Football and Cheer (www.unitedyfl.com).

Sources

College Football & Scholarship Opportunities. Accessed September 7, 2017, at http://www.scholarshipstats.com/football.html.

Football Overview. Accessed September 7, 2017, at http://www.popwarner.com.

The Journey to Camp: The Origins of American Football to 1889. Professional Football
   Researchers Association.

NCAA. *Football Injuries: Data from the 2004/05-2008/09 Seasons.* Accessed September 7, 2017, at https://www.ncaa.org/sites/default/files/NCAA_Football_Injury_WEB .pdf.

Golf

The first game of golf recorded was played with a stick and leather ball in 1297. Although highly disputed in nations around the world, modern-day 18-hole golf is credited to be a Scottish invention. The oldest surviving account of golf rules, titled *Articles and Laws in Playing at Golf,* were written in 1744 and intended for the Company of Gentlemen Golfers. Although the sport was played in America as far back as the colonial era, it was not until the late 19th century that golf attained any level of popularity. In 1848 a new golf ball was developed called the "guttie." The guttie was a much more affordable option than the previous ball, which had been made of feathers and leather, and it allowed greater numbers of people to pursue and enjoy the sport. In 1894 delegates from competing national amateur championship tournaments met to form the United States Golf Association (USGA), which remains the main governing body of the sport's professional ranks.

- The National Golf Foundation estimates that nearly 25 million individuals participated in golf activities in 2014.
- Female participation in golf continues to grow in high school golf athletics.
- During the 2014/2015 season, approximately 148,823 male and 72,582 female high school students participated in golf programs.
- 7.2 percent of male and 7.8 percent of female high school golf athletes go on to compete in college.

Injuries in golf tend to be less severe than in other sports. Wrist injuries are one of the most common injuries for both amateurs and professionals, accounting for up to 27 percent of all golf-related injuries. Together, the lower back, elbow, and wrist account for approximately 80 percent of all injuries sustained by golfers.

In 2015, 1,320 NCAA schools sponsored varsity level golf programs. The average NCAA Division I scholarship is $15,060 for male and $16,062 for female golf athletes. Of high school golfers, 1.8 percent of male and 2.6 percent of female high school players later compete at Division I schools. From 2010 to 2016, NCAA Division I men's championships were won by five programs: Oregon (2016), LSU

(2015), Alabama (2014, 2013), Texas (2012), and Augusta State (2011, 2010). In the same years, NCAA Division I women's championships were won by seven programs: Washington (2016), Stanford (2015), Duke (2014), Southern California (2013), Alabama (2012), UCLA (2011), and Purdue (2010).

Important associations and organizations include the U.S. Kids Golf (www.uskidsgolf.com), United States Golf Association (www.usga.org), and American Junior Golf Association (www.ajga.com).

Sources

College Golf & Scholarship Opportunities. Accessed September 7, 2017, at http://www.scholarshipstats.com/golf.htm.

Number of Participants in U.S. High School Golf, 2009–2016. Accessed September 7, 2017, at http://www.statista.com/statistics/267958/participation-in-us-high-school-golf.

Stachura, Mike. 2015, April 30. "Number of Golfers Steady, More Beginners Coming from Millennials." *Golf Digest.* Accessed September, 7, 2017, at http://www.golfdigest.com/story/number-of-golfers-steady-more.

Gymnastics

Gymnastics originated in early Greek civilizations to assist in bodily development. Early forms of gymnastics included running, swimming, jumping, throwing, grappling, and even weight lifting. The sport was introduced into American schools in the 1830s. The International Gymnastics Federation (FIG) was formed in 1881, organizing international competition. Around this same time, the Amateur Athletic Union replaced small clubs and organizations as the governing body of American gymnastics. In 1970, the United States Gymnastics Federation, also known as USA Gymnastics, was established as the national governing body of gymnastics within the United States. Recent trends in the sport include young athletes, particularly girls, beginning gymnastics at an earlier age, performing more difficult skills and spending more time practicing. There are two forms of international gymnastics: artistic and rhythmic. Artistic gymnastics primarily focuses on strength, balance, and agility. Artistic gymnastics allows for both male and female competition. Men compete in vault, pommel horse, still rings, parallel bars, high bar, and floor. Women compete in vault, balance beam, uneven bars, and floor exercise. Rhythmic gymnastics primarily focuses on flexibility, grace, dance and hand-eye coordination.

- In 2014, approximately 4.62 million Americans (aged 6 years and older) participated in gymnastics programs.

- In 2015, 2,079 men and 18,557 women high school students participated in gymnastics programs.
- According to the University of Pittsburgh Medical Center Sports Medicine, gymnastics has one of the highest injury rates among girls' sports, with nearly 100,000 injuries each year.

In 2015, 86 colleges sponsored varsity level gymnastics programs. The average Division I athletic scholarship for gymnastics was $16,249 for men and $16,349 for women. That same year, 15.7 percent of males and 7.9 percent of female high school gymnasts continued to compete in college, with 14.1 percent of men and 5.6 percent of women pursuing the sport at the Division I level.

In the United States, participating associations and organizations include USA Gymnastics (https://usagym.org), United States Association of Independent Gymnastics Clubs (www.usaigc.com), and the National Association of Intercollegiate Gymnastics Clubs (www.naigc.net).

Sources

84 Schools Sponsored Varsity Level Gymnastics Teams during 2016. Accessed September 8, 2017, at http://www.scholarshipstats.com/gymnastics.html.

Number of Participants in Gymnastics in the United States, 2006–2015. Accessed September 8, 2017, at http://www.statista.com/statistics/191908/participants-in-gymnastics -in-the-us-since-2006.

Strauss, Michael. "A History of Gymnastics from Ancient Greece to Modern Times," Scholastic.com, n.d. Accessed September 8, 2017, at http://www.scholastic.com/teachers /article/history-gymnastics-ancient-greece-modern-times.

Ice Hockey

Ice hockey evolved from simple games played in the 18th and 19th centuries using a stick and a ball. The creation of modern-day ice hockey is credited to Canada with the first games taking place in the 1850s. In the 1870s, students at McGill University in Montreal, Canada, formed the original set of rules. The first organized indoor match was played at Montreal's Victoria Skating Rink in March 1875. A circular piece of wood replaced the use of a ball to keep it inside the rink and away from harming spectators. Ice hockey leagues began to form in the 1880s, and professional hockey began around the turn of the century. The Stanley Cup was first awarded in 1893 to recognize the Canadian amateur champion and later became the championship award for the NHL. Ice hockey was first played in the winter

Olympic games held in 1920. Today, USA Hockey sponsors youth programs for boys and girls across the country, including player development camps and regional and national tournaments, and it provides a wide array of developmental resources for players and coaches.

- During the 2014–2015 season, approximately 35,875 male and 9,418 female high school students participated in ice hockey programs.
- Amateur hockey participation in the United States is increasing.
- Female participation in ice hockey is increasing in the United States.
- During the 2013–2014 season, Minnesota held the highest hockey participation with 54,507 total players. Minnesota is known as the "State of Hockey."

As a contact sport, ice hockey players do suffer injuries. Common injuries within the sport include shoulder, elbow, and wrist injuries. Joint injuries and joint separations are also common and occur from checking into the boards around the rink as well as falling on the ice. Concussions also occur in rare instances at all levels of play.

Of the high school ice hockey players in the United States, 0.3 percent of male and 18.4 percent of female high school players continue to compete at the collegiate level, with 3.6 percent of male and 6.7 percent of female high school players going on to compete for NCAA Division I programs. In 2015, 168 colleges sponsored varsity level hockey programs: 61 NCAA Division I, 8 NCAA Division II, and 81 NCAA Division III. Foreign students make up 21 percent of male NCAA ice hockey athletes and 26.9 percent of female NCAA ice hockey athletes. The average NCAA Division I athletic scholarship was $14,945 for male and $14,456 for female hockey players in 2015. From 2010 to 2016, NCAA Division I men's championships were won by North Dakota (2016), Providence (2015), Union (2014), Yale (2013), Boston College (2012), Minnesota Duluth (2011), and Boston College (2010). During the same years, women's NCAA Division I championships were won by Minnesota (2016, 2015, 2013, 2012), Clarkson (2015), Wisconsin (2011), and Minnesota-Duluth (2010).

USA Hockey (www.usahockey.com) is the leading governing body for youth hockey in the United States.

Sources

Number of Participants in U.S. High School Ice Hockey, 2009/10 to 2015/16. Accessed September 8, 2017, at http://www.statista.com/statistics/282093/participation-in-us-high-school-ice-hockey.

168 Schools Sponsored Varsity Level Ice Hockey Teams during 2015. Accessed September 8, 2017, at http://www.scholarshipstats.com/hockey.html.

USA Hockey. *2013–2014 Season Final Registration Reports.* Accessed September 8, 2017, at http://assets.ngin.com/attachments/document/0039/9585/2013-14_Final_Report.pdf.

Lacrosse

Lacrosse originated as a stickball game played by American Indians as far back as the 17th century. The name came from the use of a curved stick, also known to French settlers as "crosse." Modern lacrosse was formed in 1856 with the creation of the Montreal Lacrosse Club (MLC) and the introduction of regulating rules. No protective equipment was worn in traditional lacrosse; however, modern-day lacrosse features a variety of equipment, including helmets and padding, to protect participating athletes. Lacrosse first became an Olympic sport in 1904. U.S. Lacrosse was founded in 1998 as the national governing body of lacrosse. John Hopkins University (NCAA Division III) holds the oldest lacrosse tradition, having formed a team in 1893.

- The sport experienced continuous growth in both male and female high school participation from 2009 to 2016.
- Lacrosse is the fastest-growing sport for high school athletes in the nation.
- Lacrosse has seen growth at the collegiate level as well, with an additional 39 schools developing lacrosse programs in 2014 alone.
- During the 2014–2015 season, approximately 108,450 male and 84,785 female high school students participated in lacrosse programs.

The most common injuries in youth lacrosse are contusions and lacerations. However, in men's lacrosse, concussions are observed more frequently due to the increased physical contact in the game. Lacrosse-related injury rates average to 6.3 injuries per 1,000 athlete-exposures.

Of the more than 180,000 high school lacrosse athletes in the United States, only 2.8 percent of male and 3.9 percent of female players compete at NCAA Division I schools, but many more compete at NCAA Division II and III schools. In 2015, 576 universities sponsored varsity lacrosse programs. The average lacrosse athletic scholarship during the 2015 collegiate season was $14,151 for male and $15,365 for female student athletes. The average team size at the collegiate level is 45 athletes for men's teams and 30 athletes for women's teams. The national governing body of youth lacrosse in the United States is U.S. Lacrosse (www.uslacrosse.org).

Sources

Lincoln, A. E., et al. (2014, July). "Rate of Injury among Youth Lacrosse Players." *Clinical Journal of Sport Medicine, 24*(4). Accessed September 8, 2017, at http://www.ncbi.nlm.nih.gov/pubmed/24157466.

Number of Participants in U.S. High School Lacrosse, 2009/10 to 2015/16. Accessed September 8, 2017, at http://www.statista.com/statistics/267959/participation-in-us-high-school-lacrosse.

U.S. Lacrosse. 2015, April 21. *National Lacrosse Participation Grows 3.5 Percent in 2014.* Accessed September 8, 2017, at https://www.uslacrosse.org/blog/national-lacrosse-participation-grows-35-percent-in-2014.

Soccer

Although known as soccer in the United States and a few other countries, the majority of the world refers to the sport as football, including all of Central and South America, the Middle East, and most of Europe, Africa, and Asia. The earliest findings of soccer originate from China during the 2nd and 3rd centuries BC. The basic structure of modern soccer can be traced back to England, where the sport's popularity at several colleges and schools in the early 1800s led to the development of the Cambridge Rules. The Cambridge Rules, which set soccer apart from the sport of rugby, opted not to allow conduct such as tripping or carrying the ball.

Today, soccer is one of the most popular sports in the Americas and Europe:

- In 2014, U.S. Youth Soccer had 3.06 million registered players.
- Soccer is the third most played team sport in the United States, behind basketball and softball.
- In 2015, 432,569 high school male athletes participated in soccer programs.
- Among the top 10 boys sports, in 2015 soccer registered the largest gain with an additional 15,150 participants.
- In 2013, the estimated number of soccer-related injuries among children ages 19 and younger were approximately 171,000.

There are more than 1,000 universities across Canada and the United States that support men's and women's soccer programs. In 2015, there were 335 NCAA Division I schools offering 205 men's and 332 women's soccer programs. The average scholarship amount received for a Division I student athlete in 2015 was $14,490 for men and $16,186 for women. The average NCAA Division I scholarship awarded in 2015 covered only about 34 percent of the average soccer athlete's college costs. About 7.9 percent of male and 9.6 percent of female high school soccer players continued on to play in college as of 2015. From 2010 to 2016, six different schools won the NCAA Division I Men's Championship including Stanford (2016, 2015), Virginia (2014), Notre Dame (2013), Indiana (2012), North Carolina (2011), and Akron (2010). For the NCAA Division I Women's Championship, titles from 2010 to 2016 have been won by Southern California (2016), Penn State (2015), Florida State (2014), UCLA (2013), North Carolina (2012), Stanford (2011), and Notre Dame (2010).

In the United States, participating organizations and associations include U.S. Youth Soccer (www.usyouthsoccer.org), United States Soccer Federation (www.USSsoccer.com), U.S. Club Soccer (www.usclubsoccer.org), American Youth Soccer Organization (www.ayso.org), and many more.

Sources

College Soccer and Scholarship Opportunities. Accessed September 8, 2017, at http://www.scholarshipstats.com/soccer.html.

Lincoln, A., et al. 2011. "Trends in Concussion Incidence in High School Sports: A Prospective 11-Year Study." *American Journal of Sports Medicine*, 30(10).

Trends in Youth Soccer. n.d. Accessed September 8, 2017, at http://travelingteams.com/trends-in-youth-soccer.

Softball

The game of softball originated in Chicago, Illinois, in 1887. It spread quickly throughout the Midwest, where it was known by a variety of names, such as *indoor baseball*, *diamond ball*, and *pumpkin ball*, among others. Walter Hakanson introduced the name *softball* at a National Recreation Congress meeting in 1926. In response to the game's increasing popularity, a set of standardized rules was established in 1934. The sport was appealing to baseball players looking for an indoor option during the off-season but gained so much popularity as its own outdoor sport that the International Softball Federation was formed in 1952. The Amateur Softball Association (ASA), founded in 1933, submitted its first team for competition in the first Women's World Championship in 1965 and its first national men's team to a World Championship in 1966. The ASA was named the national governing body by the United States Olympic Committee. In 1991, softball was added to the roster for the 1996 Summer Olympics. Softball was then removed from the Olympic program for the 2012 and 2016 games but is slated to return for the 2020 Summer Olympics.

- Softball held a 1.6 percent increase in participation in youth ages 6–17 in 2015.

- In 2015, 373,892 female and 1,453 male student athletes participated in high school softball.
- Today, the Amateur Softball Association (ASA) holds competitions in every U.S. state and holds a membership of over 230,000 teams.

In 2009, almost 110,000 children ages 5 to 14 were treated in emergency rooms for injuries related to softball or baseball. Many softball injuries occur from overuse of shoulders and elbows. In 2015, there were 289 Division I NCAA teams. Each team played an average of 51.2 games.

In 2015, 8.3 percent of high school softball players continued on to play at the collegiate level. There are many NCAA colleges that offer softball programs including 289 Division I schools, 264 Division II schools, and 392 Division III schools. The NCAA provides scholarships for softball athletes. NCAA Division I programs provide 12 scholarships per team, and Division II provides 7.2 scholarships per team. The average scholarship amount on 2015 was $15,296 for Division I programs and $7,335 for Division II programs. Though Division III softball student athletes do not receive scholarships, other forms of financial aid are available. From 2010 to 2016, Division I college softball championships were won by five different schools: Oklahoma (2016, 2013), Florida (2015, 2014), Alabama (2012), Arizona (2011), and UCLA (2010).

In the United States, participation organizations and associations include the Amateur Softball Association–America (www.teamusa.org/USA-Softball), USA Softball (www.teamusa.org/USA-Softball), and the National Softball Association (www.playnsa.com).

Sources

College Softball & Scholarship Opportunities. Accessed September 8, 2017, at http://www.scholarshipstats.com/softball.htm.

History of Softball. n.d. Accessed September 8, 2017, at http://www.athleticscholarships.net/history-of-softball.htm.

Stanford Children's Health. n.d. *Sports Injury Statistics.* Accessed September 8, 2017, at http://www.stanfordchildrens.org/en/topic/default?id=sports-injury-statistics-90-P02787.

Swimming

Competitive swimming emerged during the 1830s in England in response to the first indoor pool being constructed in 1828. The breaststroke was the first recognized competitive form of swimming. John Trudgen developed the freestyle stroke, also referred to as the hand over hand stroke, in 1873. The first national governing body, the Amateur Swimming Association, was formed in 1880 in response to the growing popularity of the sport. By the end of the 19th century many European countries had established swimming federations, including Germany, France, and Hungary. Women's competitive swimming gained attention quickly with the first swimming championship held in 1892. Men's swimming was included as an Olympic event during the first games held in 1896 in Athens. Female swimmers were first allowed to compete in the Olympic games in 1912. Approximately 137,087 male and 166,838 female high school students participated in swimming programs during the 2014/2015 season.

- Water sports, including swimming, have increased in U.S. participation rates from 2010 to the present.
- In the *2016 Participation Report* published by the Physical Activity Council, individuals who did not participate in swimming programs, in all age groups, indicated swimming for fitness as one of their top three activities of interest.

In 2015, the average NCAA Division I swimming scholarship was $15,725 for male and $16,224 for female athletes. Approximately 7.5 percent of male and 7.8 percent of female high school swimmers continued to compete at the collegiate level that year, with 2.7 percent of male and 3.1 percent of female high school swimmers competing at Division I schools. In 2012, NCAA male swimmers held an injury rate of 4.00 injuries per 1,000 hours of training. Female swimmers held 3.78 injuries per 1,000 hours of training. Shoulder pain is the most common injury with 91 percent of swimmers ages 13 to 25 having experienced forms of shoulder pain at least once.

USA Swimming (www.usaswimming.org) is the national governing body for competitive swimming in the United States.

Sources

College Swimming & Diving Scholarship Opportunities. Accessed September 8, 2017, at http://www.scholarshipstats.com/swimming.htm.

Number of Participants in U.S. High School Swimming and Diving, 2009/10 to 2015/16. Accessed September 8, 2017, at http://www.statista.com/statistics/267977/participation -in-us-high-school-swimming-and-diving.

Physical Activity Council. *2017 Participation Report.* Accessed September 8, 2017, at http:// www.physicalactivitycouncil.com/pdfs/current.pdf.

Tennis

The original form of tennis, known as royal tennis, is believed to have originated in northern France during the 12th century. Athletes would compete by striking the ball with the palm of their hand. It wasn't until the 16th century that rackets were incorporated into game use. Courtyards were first used as arenas for game play. Today, tennis is played on three different types of courts: clay, hard surface, and grass (though the latter is not as common due to maintenance demands and susceptibility to weather impacts). Tennis can be played as a singles match (one player per side) or a doubles match (two players per side). Tennis became part of the Summer Olympic Games in 1896.

- During the 2014/2015 season approximately 157,240 male and 182,876 female high school students participated in tennis programs.
- During the 2014/2015 season 10,183 male and 10,782 female tennis players competed at the college level.
- In the year 2014, the Tennis Industry Association held 2.14 million youth ages 6–12, and 2.23 million youth ages 13–17, participating in tennis programs within the United States. This is a 1 percent increase from the previous year.

In 2015, injury rates for tennis included five injuries per 1,000 participation hours. Lower limb injuries, including ankle, knee, and thigh, are the most common. The majority of tennis-related injuries do not require hospitalization.

In 2015, 1,194 colleges sponsored varsity level tennis programs providing opportunities for 10,183 male and 10,782 female athletes. The average scholarship amount for Division I tennis players was $15,115 for male and $16,166 for female athletes. About 4.4 percent of male and 4.1 percent of female high school tennis players continue on to compete at the collegiate level, with roughly 1 percent of players (both male and female) competing at Division I schools. The United States Tennis Association, USTA (www.usta.com) is the national governing body for the sport of tennis in the United States.

Sources

College Tennis & Scholarship Opportunities. Accessed September 8, 2017, at http://www.scholarshipstats.com/tennis.htm.

Number of Participants in U.S. High School Tennis, 2009/10 to 2015/16. Accessed September 8, 2017, at http://www.statista.com/statistics/267993/participation-in-us-high-school-tennis.

2015 State of the Industry: Tennis. Accessed September 18, 2017, at https://www.tennisindustry.org/PDFs/research/2015-SOI-SHORT-VERSION.pdf.

Track and Field

Track and field not only includes running events but events such as relays, hurdles, high and long jump, shot put, discus, and many others. In the United States, track and field competitions date back to the 1860s. With the development of the Intercollegiate Association of Amateur Athletes of America, the United States' original athletic group, the first collegiate race was held in 1873. The first NCAA national championships were held in 1921 and were for male athletes only. However, women's track and field was represented in the Olympic Games soon after in 1928. United States of America Track and Field's (USATF) largest youth program is the Junior Olympics, which features almost 70,000 youth athletes competing in track, field, and cross-country championships.

- 1,057,358 high school student athletes participated in track and field programs during the 2014–2015 season.
- Participation in high school track and field in 2015 included 578,632 male and 478,726 female athletes.

The *American Journal of Sports Medicine* has reported that up to 90 percent of track and field injuries are in direct relation to overuse. Runner's knee, Achilles tendinitis, and plantar fasciitis are the most common track and field–related injuries.

In 2015, 1,184 American colleges and universities sponsored varsity level track and field programs featuring 34,900 male and 34,309 female athletes. The average NCAA Division I track and field athletic scholarship in 2015 was $14,869 for male and $15,905 for female athletes. In 2015, 5.8 percent of male and 6.9 percent of female high school track and field athletes competed in college; of those former high school athletes, 1.8 percent of males and 2.6 percent of females competed at NCAA Division I schools.

In the United States, leading associations and organizations involved in track and field for youth include USA Track & Field (www.usatf.org/youth.aspx), U.S. Track & Field and Cross Country Coaches Association (www.ustfccca.org), and International Association of Athletics Federations (www.iaaf.org).

Sources

College Track & Field and Scholarship Opportunities. Accessed September 8, 2017, at http://www.scholarshipstats.com/track.htm.

National Federation of State High School Associations. *2014–15 High School Athletics Participation Survey.* Accessed September 8, 2017, at http://www.nfhs.org/Participation Statics/PDF/2014-15_Participation_Survey_Results.pdf.

Shaginaw, Justin. 2014, May 12. "Scholastic Sports Injuries: Track and Field." *Philadelphia Inquirer.* Accessed September 8, 2017, at http://www.philly.com/philly/blogs/sports doc/Scholastic-sports-injuries-track—field-.html.

Ultimate Frisbee

Although disk sports have been played throughout history, the origins of ultimate frisbee are credited to Joel Silver, in Maplewood New Jersey, in 1968. Silver had developed the game while at a summer camp in Mount Hermon, Massachusetts, during the summer of 1967 and returned to Maplewood to present a frisbee team to his school student council. Early versions of the game featured 20 to 30 players per team and included American football characteristics such as running with the disk, a line of scrimmage, and a series of downs. The game of "ultimate" has traditionally resisted rules-enforcing referees and has instead invoked the honor system. The professional leagues, however, have employed referees. There are two professional leagues in the United States, the American Ultimate Disc League (AUDL) and the Major League Ultimate (MLU). USA Ultimate is the governing organization over the sport of ultimate frisbee within the United States. The USA Ultimate Youth Division began in 1988 and currently includes more than 400 club- and school-based teams with approximately 14,000 student-athletes.

Participation rates include:

- In 2014, approximately 4.53 million individuals within the United States (aged 6 years and older) participated in ultimate frisbee programs.
- In 2015, USA Ultimate, the governing body for the sport of ultimate frisbee in the United States, held 53,362 members with 17,973 college-aged participants and 13,651 youth.

According to the *Journal of Athletic Training,* in 2014, 1,317 ultimate frisbee-related injuries were reported with a 12.64 incidents per 1,000 athlete-exposure rate. Running, overuse, and collisions were the top three reasons for injury for both men and women's ultimate disk-related injuries. Although the injury rates for men and women's ultimate were similar, men were three times more likely to separate or dislocate their shoulders while women were seven times more likely to injure their knee. Ankle sprains are the most common injury.

Scholarship opportunities are limited for ultimate athletes. There are more than 700 college teams within Northern America including both mixed and women's-only teams. A list of scholarship opportunities can be found on the USA Ultimate webpage (www.usaultimate.org). Currently, ultimate frisbee is not an NCAA-affiliated sport. The majority of games are played at an intermural level on college campuses. USA Ultimate does hold a college division that began in 1984 and has over 700 participating college teams. Formalized regular seasons began in 2010.

Participating associations and organizations include USA Ultimate (www .usaultimate.org) and the World Flying Disk Federation (www.wfdf.org).

Sources

Number of Participants in Ultimate Frisbee in the United States from 2006 to 2015. Accessed September 8, 2017, at http://www.statista.com/statistics/191967/participants -in-ultimate-frisbee-in-the-us-since-2006.

Swedler, D., et al. 2015, April. "Incidence and Descriptive Epidemiology of Injuries to College Ultimate Players." *Journal of Athletic Training, 50*(4).

Youth Division. Accessed September 18, 2017, at http://www.usaultimate.org/youth.

Volleyball

Volleyball, originally called Mintonette, was developed in 1895 in Holyoke, Massachusetts, by the Young Men's Christian Association's (YMCA) physical education director William G. Morgan. In 1920, rules were instituted that included the regulation of three hits per side of the net. The United States Volleyball Association (USVBA) was founded in 1928 to represent the sport both nationally and internationally. With the development of the USVBA also came the first annual national open championship. The first Volleyball World Championships were held in Prague, Czechoslovakia, in 1949. In 1996, two-player beach volleyball became recognized as an Olympic Games event. Today the game is popular in many countries including Brazil, Russia, Europe, China, and the United States.

- Approximately 59,591 female and 2,701 male high school athletes participated in volleyball programs during the 2014–2015 season and 2,512 male and 26,915 females competed in U.S. college volleyball programs.
- 2,575 high schools within the United States participated in volleyball programs during the 2014–2015 season.
- 76 percent of USA Volleyball members are junior females, ages 10–18.
- Amateur Athletic Union volleyball holds more participation among youth females than any other female team sport.

Including games and practices, the accumulative injury rate in NCAA volleyball is 4.3 injuries per 1,000 participants. The most common volleyball injuries include ligament sprains (28.2 percent) followed by muscle strains (21.7 percent), tendinosis (7.5 percent), and contusions (4.6 percent).

During the 2015 season, 1,787 colleges sponsored varsity volleyball programs. The average scholarship amount for NCAA Division I volleyball athletes during 2015 was $14,851 for males and $15,960 for females. NCAA college female beach volleyball held 60 varsity teams during the 2015–2016 season and is the fastest growing sport in Division I. Though popular with both high school and college athletes, only 0.7 percent of male and 1.2 percent of female high school volleyball players went on to compete for NCAA Division I programs in 2015. More than 95 percent of NCAA schools participate in women's volleyball. The top NCAA Division I programs for women's volleyball include Florida, Stanford, Nebraska, California, USC, Texas, Hawaii, Penn State, UCLA, UNI, Washington, Minnesota, Dayton, Illinois, LSU, Iowa State, Colorado State, San Diego, Arizona, Cincinnati, and Tulsa. The top NCAA Division I and Division II programs for men's volleyball include Stanford, BYU, Cal State Northridge, Hawaii, Penn State, Pepperdine, USC, UC Irvine, UCLA, Ohio State, UC Santa Barbara, Long Beach State, Loyola, Ball State, and UC San Diego.

In the United States the leading associations and organizations governing youth volleyball include Amateur Athletic Union (AAU) Volleyball (www.aauvolleyball .org), United States Youth Volleyball League (www.usyvl.org), and USA Volleyball (www.teamusa.org).

Sources

American Volleyball Coaches Association. 2015, December. *Volleyball Fast Facts.* Accessed September 8, 2017, at https://www.avca.org/res/uploads/media/VOLLEYBALL -FAST-FACTS-12-15-.pdf.

College Volleyball & Scholarship Opportunities. Accessed September 8, 2017, at http:// www.scholarshipstats.com/volleyball.htm.

National Federation of State High School Associations. *Participation Data.* Accessed September 8, 2017, at http://www.nfhs.org/ParticipationStatics/ParticipationStatics.aspx.

NCAA. *Women's Volleyball Injuries.* 2008–2009. Accessed September 8, 2017, at https:// www.ncaa.org/sites/default/files/NCAA_W_Volleyball_Injuries_WEB.pdf.

This Was How Volleyball Was Introduced. Athnet.com. Accessed September 8, 2017, at http://www.athleticscholarships.net/history-of-volleyball.htm.

Wrestling

Wrestling dates as far back as 5,000 years ago to one of the earliest urban societies, the Sumerians. Recognized as one of the oldest forms of combat, archaeologists have found historical traces of wrestling in Ancient Egypt. Wrestling was the determining event of the Pentathlon during the Ancient Olympic Games (708 BC). There is evidence of wrestling being practiced by both nobility and the common class during the European Medieval era. Professional wrestling originated as traveling teams during the 1830s in France. Modern-day freestyle wrestling was introduced first in 1904. In 1921 the International Federation of Associated Wrestling Styles (FILA) formed and regulated amateur wrestling. In 1927 the rules of collegiate wrestling were published and followed by the first NCAA Wrestling Team Championship the next year on the campus of Iowa State College. The point system, which decides matches in the absence of a fall, was developed in 1941. In 1983 USA Wrestling became the national governing body of amateur wrestling. Female wrestling was recognized as an Olympic discipline in 2014 during the Athens Games.

- Female high school participation in the sport of wrestling has grown from 804 in 1994 to 11,496 in 2015. Meanwhile, 258,208 male high school students participated in school wrestling programs during the same 2015 season.
- Wrestling ranked seventh of all boys' sports in participation in American high schools in 2008–2009, with California accounting for the highest number of high school wrestlers (26,374).

As of 2015 there were 28 colleges that sponsored a female varsity wrestling program. In 2015, 350 colleges sponsored varsity level wrestling programs for men. The average Division I athletic scholarship was $13,359 for male and $13,746 for female wrestlers. About 3.9 percent of male and 3.7 percent of female high school student wrestlers continue on to compete at the collegiate level. There are 73 NCAA Division I wrestling programs with an average of 9.9 scholarships offered per team. General requirements for a college wrestling scholarship include finishing within the top 25 in your weight class and state, participating in both high school and summer tournaments, qualifying as a state championship competitor, being an FILD Junior National participant, being a varsity starter, and holding multiple high school tournament wins. Some of the most recognizable NCAA Division I wrestling programs include Cornell, Iowa, Oklahoma State, Penn State, Minnesota, Virginia Tech, Oklahoma, Lehigh, Rutgers, Boise State, Michigan, Missouri, Nebraska, Northwestern, Wisconsin, Ohio State, Iowa State, Kent State, American, Illinois, Oregon State, Cal Poly, Pittsburgh, Purdue, Central Michigan, and Wyoming.

During the 2006/2007 season, high school wrestling held an injury rate of 2.33 injuries per 1,000 athlete-exposures. For college athletes, the injury rate was 7.25 per 1,000 athlete-exposures. Injury rates were higher in matches than practices in both categories.

In the United States, key associations and organizations involved with youth wrestling include the National United Wrestling Association for Youth (www .nuwaywrestling.com), USA Wrestling (www.teamusa.org), USA Wrestling Kids National Teams (http://www.teamusa.org/usa-wrestling/team-usa/kids-national-teams), and National Wrestling Coaches Association (www.nwcaonline.com).

Sources

College Wrestling & Scholarship Opportunities. Accessed September 8, 2017, at http://www.scholarshipstats.com/wrestling.html.

College Wrestling Scholarships and Recruiting. Athnet.com. Accessed September 8, 2017, at http://www.athleticscholarships.net/wrestlingscholarships.htm.

National Federation of State High School Associations. *2014–15 High School Athletics Participation Survey.* Accessed September 8, 2017, at http://www.nfhs.org/Participation-Statics/PDF/2014-15_Participation_Survey_Results.pdf.

National Wrestling Coaches Association. *Wrestling's Facts and Resources.* Accessed September 8, 2017, at http://www.nwcaonline.com/nwcawebsite/savingwrestlinghome/facts.aspx.

Shaginaw, Justin. 2014, February 5. "Statistics on Wrestling Injuries." *Philadelphia Inquirer.* Accessed September 8, 2017, at http://www.philly.com/philly/blogs/sportsdoc/Statistics-on-wrestling-injuries.html.

United World Wrestling. *History of Wrestling.* Accessed September 8, 2017, at https://unitedworldwrestling.org/organization/history.

Selected Bibliography

Books

Andrews, James. 2013. *Any Given Monday: Sports Injuries and How to Prevent Them, for Athletes, Parents, and Coaches.* New York: Simon and Schuster.

Barcelona, Robert, Mary Sara Wells, and Skye Gerald Arthur-Banning. 2015. *Recreational Sport Management: Program Design and Delivery.* Champaign, IL: Human Kinetics.

Bissinger, Buzz. 2015. *Friday Night Lights: A Town, a Team, and a Dream* (25th anniversary ed.). Boston: Da Capo Press.

Coakley, Jay. 2010. *Sports in Society: Issues and Controversies.* Colorado Springs, CO: McGraw-Hill.

De Lench, Brooke. 2006. *Home Team Advantage: The Critical Role of Mothers in Youth Sports.* New York: HarperCollins.

Dohrmann, George. 2010. *Play Their Hearts Out: A Coach, His Star Recruit, and the Youth Basketball Machine.* New York: Random House.

Eckstein, Rick. 2017. *How College Athletics Are Hurting Girls' Sports: The Pay-to-Play Pipeline.* Lanham, MD: Rowman and Littlefield.

Engh, Fred. 2002. *Why Johnny Hates Sports: Why Organized Youth Sports Are Failing Our Children and What We Can Do about It.* Garden City Park, NY: Square One.

Ewing, Martha, and Vern Seefeldt. 1990. *American Youth and Sports Participation.* Lansing, MI: Youth Sports Institute at Michigan State University.

Farrey, Tom. 2008. *Game On: How the Pressure to Win at All Costs Endangers Youth Sports, and What Parents Can Do About It.* New York: Random House.

Graham, Robert, Frederick P. Rivara, Morgan A. Ford, and Carol Mason Spicer (Eds.). 2014. *Sports-Related Concussions in Youth: Improving the Science, Changing the Culture.* Washington, D.C.: National Academies Press.

Green, Ken, and Andy Smith. 2016. *Routledge Handbook of Youth Sport.* New York: Routledge.

Hartill, Michael J. 2016. *Sexual Abuse in Youth Sport: A Sociocultural Analysis.* New York: Routledge.

Holt, Nicholas L. (Ed.). 2016. *Positive Youth Development through Sport* (2nd ed.). New York: Routledge.

Hyman, Mark. 2009. *Until It Hurts: America's Obsession with Youth Sports and How It Hurts Our Kids.* Boston: Beacon Press.

Hyman, Mark. 2012. *The Most Expensive Game in Town: The Rising Cost of Youth Sports and the Toll on Today's Families.* Boston: Beacon Press.

Lomax, Michael E. (Ed.). 2008. *Sports and the Racial Divide: African American and Latino Experience in an Era of Change.* Jackson: University of Mississippi Press.

McCarthy, John, Lou Bergholz, and Megan Bartlett. 2016. *Re-Designing Youth Sport: Change the Game.* New York: Routledge.

Messner, Michael A., and Michela Musto (Eds.). 2016. *Child's Play: Sport in Kids' Worlds.* New Brunswick, NJ: Rutgers University Press.

O'Sullivan, John. 2013. *Changing the Game: The Parents' Guide to Raising Happy, High Performing Athletes and Giving Youth Sports Back to Our Kids.* New York: Morgan James.

Overman, Steven J. 2014. *The Youth Sports Crisis: Out-of-Control Adults, Helpless Kids.* Santa Barbara, CA: Praeger.

Ryan, Joan. 1995. *Little Girls in Pretty Boxes: The Making and Breaking of Elite Gymnasts and Figure Skaters.* New York: Doubleday.

Sabo, Don, and Philip Veliz. 2008. *Go Out and Play: Youth Sports in America.* East Meadow, NY: Women's Sports Foundation.

Vealey, Robin, and Melissa Chase. 2016. *Best Practice for Youth Sport.* Champaign, IL: Human Kinetics.

Websites

Aspen Institute Project Play: Reimagining Youth Sports in America, https://www.aspenprojectplay.org

Center for the Study of Sport in Society, http://www.sportinsociety.org

Institute for the Study of Youth Sports, http://edwp.educ.msu.edu/isys

Maine Center for Sport and Coaching, http://www.sportsdonerightmaine.org

MomsTeam Institute of Youth Sports Safety, http://momsteaminstitute.org

National Alliance for Youth Sports, https://www.nays.org

National Association for Sport and Physical Education, http://www.aahperd.org/naspe

National Council of Youth Sports, http://www.ncys.org

National Institute for Sports Reform, http://www.nisr.org

Positive Coaching Alliance, https://positivecoach.org

About the Editors and Contributors

Editor

SKYE G. ARTHUR-BANNING, PhD, is an associate professor and emphases area coordinator of the community recreation sport and camp management area within PRTM at Clemson University, SC. His primary research interests are centered around amateur sport and, specifically, sport development. Lately he has focused his work mainly on adaptive sport and rehabilitation as well as sportsmanship and ethical behavior. Skye has coauthored a textbook, *Recreational Sport: Program Design, Delivery, and Management*; edited two other books, *Youth Sport in America: The Most Important Issues in Youth Sports Today* and *Sports Global Influence: A Survey of Society and Culture in the Context of Sport;* and has been published in many peer-reviewed journals and mainstream media publications. He currently serves as the head of officials for the International Federation of CP Football, a Paralympic sport that includes individuals with cerebral palsy, traumatic brain injury, stroke, and other neurological impairments.

Associate Editors

P. BRIAN GREENWOOD is an associate professor in the Experience Industry Management department at Cal Poly, San Luis Obispo. Dr. Greenwood's discipline-specific research centers on sports-based youth development includes a research grant with the San Francisco Giants Community Fund in conducting an annual comprehensive evaluation for their flagship program, the Junior Giants. In his career in higher education, he has presented at more than 75 local, regional, national, and international academic and professional conferences and workshops, including a speaking engagement at the White House in 2009 to highlight the state of youth sports during the economic recession.

MARY SARA WELLS is an associate professor in the Department of Health, Kinesiology, and Recreation at the University of Utah. Her research focus is on community recreation, youth development, and youth sport, and she has been working directly with youth sport organizations across the country to develop better programs for participants for more than 10 years.

Contributors

GREG BACH is the vice president of communications for the National Alliance for Youth Sports and is the author of eight books on coaching youth sports.

MEGAN BARTLETT is the chief program officer at Up2Us Sports, where she oversees Coach Across America, the nation's first sports-based national service program; a ground-breaking coach training and certification program; and all efforts to build the capacity of organizations using sport to promote youth health and academic achievement and decrease youth violence. She was formerly the national program director for America SCORES, a soccer, creative writing, and service-learning program. Megan has an MA in urban policy and planning from Tufts University and is the coauthor of an upcoming book on redesigning sports for positive outcomes.

PAUL CACCAMO is a 25-year veteran of the nonprofit sector. He has helped to establish numerous nonprofits that focus on youth development, sports and physical activity, and education. He lectures and writes on the impact of sports on youth and community development. He founded the America SCORES national office in 1999 and Up2Us in 2009. He received his master's degree in public policy from the John F. Kennedy School of Government at Harvard University and his bachelor's degree at Georgetown University's Edmund Walsh School of Foreign Service. Paul has received numerous academic awards and citations for leadership, including one of Harvard's most prestigious graduate awards for innovation in the design of social service programs.

TROY CARLTON, MBA, MS, is a doctoral candidate in the Department of Parks, Recreation and Tourism Management at North Carolina State University.

LAURENCE CHALIP is the Brightbill/Sapora professor and head of the Department of Recreation, Sport and Tourism at the University of Illinois. He has worked extensively on matters of youth sport development, including service on the

Scientific Advisory Board for Project Play. His work examines sport policies and the effects those have on the quality of sport programming.

ASHLEY M. COKER-CRANNEY is an adjunct instructor at West Virginia University. She received her PhD in sport and exercise psychology from West Virginia University, her master's in counseling from West Virginia University, and her master's in psychosocial aspects of sport from the University of Utah. Ashley uses a wide variety of quantitative and qualitative research methods to study sport deviance, including issues related to disordered eating/exercise behaviors, playing injured, excessive violence, criminal behavior, and substance abuse.

R. BRIAN CROW is a professor of sport management at Slippery Rock University and conducts research on hazing in sport, the fan experience, and marketing in numerous sectors of the sport industry. He is actively involved as a consultant and speaker throughout North America.

BRANDI M. CROWE, PhD, LRT/CTRS, is an assistant professor in the Department of Parks, Recreation and Tourism Management's Recreational Therapy program at Clemson University. Her research interests include the role of leisure within stress/coping processes, and the use of complementary and alternative medicine as treatment for individuals with disabling conditions.

JOHN ENGH is the chief operating officer of the National Alliance for Youth Sports. He has made hundreds of presentations around the world on the importance of training volunteer coaches involved in youth sports, and he also is interviewed frequently by national media on this topic, as well as on other youth sports issues.

BARRY A. GARST, PhD, is an associate professor of youth development leadership at Clemson University and the former director of program development and research application with the American Camp Association. His applied research focuses on factors that influence youth program outcomes, with an emphasis on the needs and concerns of parents.

STEPHANIE P. GARST is the executive director of the US PLAY Coalition, a nonprofit organization housed at Clemson University that promotes the value of play throughout life. She earned her bachelors of business administration from the University of Texas at Austin and her master's in counseling and human development from Radford University. She has over 20 years' experience in community programming and informal education in camp, museum, and higher education settings. At

Clemson University, Stephanie not only runs the US Play Coalition, but she also teaches for the travel and tourism concentration. Stephanie is married to Dr. Barry Garst. They have two young daughters, Savannah and Laurel. She loves good food and good music . . . and she is a huge 1980s pop culture fan!

B. CHRISTINE GREEN is a professor of sport management and director of the Sport+Development Lab at the University of Illinois. She has consulted with sport organizations throughout the world on matters of sport development. Her work examines the nature and quality of youth sport experiences with a particular focus on the means to enhance youth sport participation.

BRANDONN S. HARRIS is an associate professor and director of the graduate sport and exercise psychology program at Georgia Southern University. He is a certified consultant with the Association for Applied Sport Psychology (CC-AASP) and is also listed on the United States Olympic Committee (USOC) Sport Psychology Registry. He currently serves as the coordinator for the Youth Sport Special Interest Group for AASP, as well as the chair of the AASP Ethics Committee. As a researcher, he conducts, publishes, and presents his work in the areas of youth sport, coach and athlete burnout, and professional/ethical issues in sport psychology. As a practitioner, he has consulted with youth and collegiate athletes, teams, parents, and coaches on a variety of sport psychology–related topics. Dr. Harris holds two master's degrees in sport and exercise psychology and community counseling from West Virginia University. His PhD in sport and exercise psychology was also completed at West Virginia University.

W. HUNTER HOLLAND received his BA in recreation management from Appalachian State University and a master's degree in outdoor recreation from Ohio University. Currently, he is pursuing a PhD at Clemson University, studying the influence of wilderness-based continuing education programs for K–12 educators. Mr. Holland's research interests are primarily focused on outdoor-recreational activities and their link with personal and professional development in participants. Hunter has worked for professional outdoor recreational organizations for more than 11 years, including Alaska Mountain Guides Climbing School Inc., the International Wilderness Leadership School, and the North Carolina Outward Bound School.

J. BENJAMIN JACKSON III is an assistant professor of orthopaedic surgery at the University of South Carolina. There he serves as a head team physician and is concussion certified. He has an active research protocol that is studying novel tools for the measurement of concussions in soccer.

JEFF JAMES, PhD, is Mode L. Stone distinguished professor of sport management and department chair, Florida State University.

MICHAEL KANTERS, PhD, professor and coordinator, Masters of Parks, Recreation, Tourism & Sport Management, North Carolina State University.

ERIC LEGG is an assistant professor in the School of Community Resources & Development at Arizona State University. His research and teaching focus on community sports and youth development. Previously, he worked for seven years in sports programming for a municipal parks and recreation agency He is also the founder/president of a community-based nonprofit sports organization, national volunteer chair with the United States Tennis Association, and a certified professional tennis instructor.

ERIC W. MACINTOSH is an associate professor of sport management at the University of Ottawa, conducting research on organizational behavior and marketing topics such as culture, leadership, corporate image, and brand authenticity. He has worked with many national and international sport organizations and is the coeditor of *International Sport Management*.

REED MALTBIE is the chief content officer and lead presenter for Changing the Game project. He holds master's degrees in both education and sport performance. An accomplished soccer player, he was a member of Davidson College's 1992 NCAA Final 4 Team. When he isn't coaching on the fields, he is speaking to and training coaches, parents, students, and sports clubs. Coach Reed also serves as an expert writer for SoccerNation.com, SoccerParenting.com, *Amplified Soccer* magazine, and is finishing the edits on his forthcoming book *What's Your Echo?*

WILLIAM MELTON is a senior orthopaedic resident at the University of South Carolina. He helps care for their athletes as well as those from surrounding high schools and colleges.

ERIN L. MORRIS is an assistant professor in the Sport Management department at the State University of New York at Cortland. Her research focuses on women's sport development and women's participation in sport. She has experience working in youth sport as a hockey coach and soccer official, and working in community recreation.

AUBREY NEWLAND is a sport and exercise psychology professor in the Kinesiology Department at California State University, Chico. Her research interests include youth sports, coaching, and motivation. Specifically, Dr. Newland is interested in how to optimize sport experiences for participants by providing a caring motivational climate, fostering evidence-based coaching practices, and facilitating better coach education.

YOUNG SUK OH is a graduate research assistant (PhD) in the Parks, Recreation and Tourism Management department at Clemson University. His research focuses on sport development and management, youth development through sport, adaptive sport, and consumer behavior in sport. He has experience working in youth sport as a physical education teacher, and working in sport management and marketing agencies.

JOHN O'SULLIVAN started the Changing the Game project in 2012 after two decades as a soccer player and coach on the youth, high school, college, and professional level. He is the author of the best-selling book *Changing the Game: The Parent's Guide to Raising Happy, High-Performing Athletes, and Giving Youth Sports Back to Our Kids,* and also *Is It Wise to Specialize?* O'Sullivan is a regulator contributor to SoccerWire.com, and his writing has been featured in many publications, including the *Huffington Post* and *Soccer America.* O'Sullivan is an internationally known speaker for coaches, parents, and youth sports organizations, and has spoken before TEDx, the National Soccer Coaches Association of America, IMG Academy, and at numerous other events throughout the United States, Canada, and Europe.

JUSTINE J. REEL, PhD, LPC, CMPC, is an associate dean of research and innovation within the College of Health and Human Services at the University of North Carolina Wilmington. She also has a tenured position as full professor within the exercise science program at UNCW. She also is a licensed professional counselor and certified mental performance consultant. Her research interests include body image, eating disorders, and obesity prevention.

WILLIAM RUSSELL is a professor at Missouri Western State University in the Department of Health, Physical Education, and Recreation. Dr. Russell teaches sport and exercise psychology, sport sociology, and research methods courses. His primary area of research interest is psychological outcomes from youth sports and sport specialization.

JAMES SANDERSON (PhD, Arizona State University) is president of Sanderson Media Group. His research interests include the influence of social media and sport, and youth sport, particularly issues of health and safety and family communication.

NICHOLAS SCHLERETH is an assistant professor of recreation and sport management at Coastal Carolina University. Dr. Schlereth completed his PhD in sport administration and his MBA in strategic management and policy at the University of New Mexico. His research spans strategic management in sport organizations and small businesses, stakeholder management, and risk management.

RONALD E. SMITH is a professor of psychology and director of the clinical psychology training program at the University of Washington. His major research interests are in personality, stress and coping, and sport psychology intervention. Dr. Smith has published more than 200 scientific articles and book chapters, and he has authored or coauthored 34 books and manuals.

FRANK L. SMOLL is a professor of psychology at the University of Washington. His research focuses on coaching behaviors in youth sports and on the psychological effects of competition. Dr. Smoll has published more than 135 scientific articles and book chapters, and he is coauthor of 22 books and manuals on children's athletics.

ELLEN J. STAUROWSKY is a professor of sport management in the Center for Sport Management at Drexel University. Dr. Staurowsky is internationally recognized as an expert on social justice issues in sport including college athletes' rights, the exploitation of college athletes, gender equity and Title IX, and the misappropriation of American Indian imagery in sport. She is coauthor of *College Athletes for Hire: The Evolution and Legacy of the NCAA's Amateur Myth* and editor of *Women and Sport: Continuing a Journey of Liberation and Celebration.*

PRESTON J. TANNER is an online program coordinator, internship coordinator, and lecturer in parks, recreation, and tourism at the University of Utah. He holds a bachelor of science degree in exercise and sport science; a master of science degree in exercise and sport science (psychosocial aspects of sport emphasis); a master of business administration (marketing emphasis) from the David Eccles School of Business; and is a doctoral candidate in parks, recreation, and tourism at the University of Utah. His teaching interests include sport trends, sport business, leisure behavior, marketing strategy, financial management, professional preparation, coaching, entrepreneurial recreation, teaching in higher education, and online education. His research interests include sport spectator satisfaction, loyalty, and sense of community in sport.

PHILIP VELIZ is an assistant professor at the University of Michigan's Institute for Research on Women & Gender. Dr. Veliz has multiple publications that address the association between adolescent substance use and sport participation, which have appeared in the *American Journal of Public Health*, the *Journal of Adolescent Health*, and the *International Review for the Sociology of Sport*. His personal research interests include the sociology of sport, substance use, and the impact of sport within public education. His most recent research focuses on the provision of sports among girls and boys in public high schools. Moreover, he is currently engaged in several projects that examine how involvement in sport either encourages or deters substance use among adolescents.

JACK C. WATSON II is a professor and chair of the Department of Sport Sciences at West Virginia University. He is a certified consultant with the Association for Applied Sport Psychology (CC-AASP) and is also listed on the United States Olympic Committee (USOC) Sport Psychology Registry. He is a past president of the Association for Applied Sport Psychology. His research interests include professional development issues in applied sport psychology (e.g., ethics, supervision, and mentoring), youth sport, and anger and aggression issues in sport. As a licensed psychologist in West Virginia, he has experience working with athletes across multiple age levels, sports, and ability levels on a variety of sport psychology–related topics. Dr. Watson also has a great deal of experience coaching youth sport teams in baseball, softball, basketball, and soccer.

CAIT WILSON is a PhD candidate in the Department of Health, Kinesiology, and Recreation at University of Utah. She is also a research assistant for the American Camp Association. Her research is focused on youth development in summer camp and sport settings.

Index